Health at School
Caring for the Whole Child

Health at School

Caring for the Whole Child

Wanda Nash SRN MA(Ed)
Muriel Thruston SRN SCM HV

With an historical introduction by
Monica E. Baly SRN SCM HV BA PhD

Foreword by
Dr Kingsley Whitmore
Community Paediatric Research Unit
St Mary's Hospital Medical School, London

Illustrations by David Parkins

Heinemann Nursing
London

First published 1985
by William Heinemann Medical Books
London WC1B 3HH

ISBN 0–433–23051–7

Typeset by Wilmaset, Birkenhead, Merseyside
Printed in Great Britain by
The Bath Press, Avon

Contents

Acknowledgements

Acknowledgement

I would like to acknowledge all those—whether children, parents, or staff—who are learners and educators at the Cedars School, Southampton. From them I learnt more than can be put into one book.

My personal acknowledgement is to the patience and encouragement shown by so many people. Starting with the librarians of various medical and educational units, Mrs Catherine Dobson deserves special mention. The patience of Mrs Kathleen Sharpe, our typist, has been sorely tried. Perhaps most of all, I tested the patience of my husband and our daughters—Lois, Poppy, Phoebe and Jo—who through thick dust and thin meals have nonetheless stuck by the project. These are the people who have become the proving ground of many of the ideas in this book, and I thank them.

Wanda Nash

Personal Brief

Wanda Nash has spent much of her working life as Nursing Sister with children who have physical handicaps at an LEA school. As chairman of the Hants School Nurses Association she has shared the experiences of nurses working in every type of school in this country, as well as visiting the United States and building up many contacts and ideas there. As a mature student, Wanda Nash graduated from the University of Southampton with a Masters Degree in Education. She won the Heinz Education Ward for her research, and has since been a Research Fellow at Southampton. She is married (to a senior clergyman) and has four daughters (three of whom are on their way to becoming therapists—in psychiatry, speech, and art. The fourth hopes to enter Law).

Acknowledgement

My contribution to this book is written in salute to all the school nurses I have encountered during my nursing career; and in particular to two people whose humanity and professional skill are of the highest order, and whose sensitivity and caring for the whole child shine through everything that they do: Mrs Joyce Beckwith, lately Nursing Sister at St Giles School for the Physically Handicapped, Croydon, and my son-in-law, Mr Keith Pearson, Year Tutor, Wilsons School, Wallington.

Muriel Thruston

Personal Brief

Muriel Thruston is the mother of five children; she returned to nursing as a health visitor and school nurse. Her views on the importance of maintaining the highest professional standards of training and practice led her to accept the position of Community Nurse Training Officer for Croydon District Health Authority. She was the only nurse member of the Warnock Committee of enquiry into Special Educational Needs. Her current activities include examining, assessing, lecturing and writing on a variety of health-related topics.

Personal Brief

Monica Baly, a former Area Officer for the Royal College of Nursing, is the author and editor of several major nursing texts, including *Nursing and Social Change*, 2nd edn. (1980), *A New Approach to District Nursing* (1981) and *Professional Responsibility*, 2nd edn. (1984). Her doctoral thesis examined the history of the Nightingale Fund and its legacy for nursing.

Foreword

Times change and we must all try to move with the times. This book is important because it epitomises the quiet transformation that is taking place in educational nursing. Both the public image and the self-image of school nurses are beginning to change as they become aware of their particular forte and realise their potential in health promotion. The changing epidemiology of childhood has necessitated a change in the style of health services for children and educational nursing has been quick to respond and could even be said to be forcing the pace at which health services in schools adapt to modern times.

But there are also other reasons why this book is important. First, while it offers practical advice on the more mundane methods of nursing care in schools, its authors do not shrink from delving into the very nature of educational nursing. And, by adopting a philosophical and psychological approach, they venture into crucial but as yet unexplored aspects of the health care of school children. The book is a forceful exposition of the need for school nurses to be child-oriented rather than task-oriented in their work.

Second, the book stresses the opportunities for health education that exist in every situation in which the school nurse may find herself. And third, the central chapters of the book demonstrate the authors' conviction that the relationship between the pupil and the nurse is all important in modifying the child's attitude towards his or her own health care. For this reason, attention is paid to how this relationship can be objectively but unobtrusively fostered.

And finally, *Health at School* is important because it contains much that should be of interest to teachers and school doctors. The chapter on sessions especially is written as much for teachers as for nurses. For school doctors, the book will be a challenge to review *their* role and methods and to share in a new kind of partnership with school nurses in providing health services in schools.

Kingsley Whitmore
London

Introduction

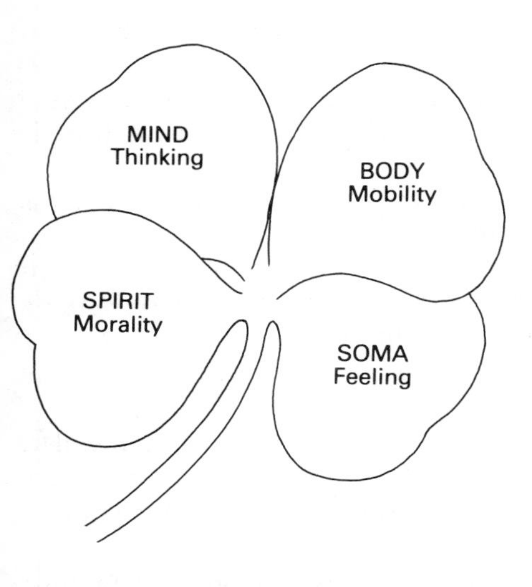

Living is a risky business. The theme of this book concerns the efforts of all staff who work in school to convince children that there is zest in living in spite of the risk. Anyone who is interested in the wholeness of a child's way of life is by definition interested in his health, and by balancing the different skills to be found within the school, each child can discover how to balance his own strengths and weaknesses. The adults who attend to him with a listening eye and an open ear will have a share in the work and in the reward—future citizens who recognise their own values and can live with a feeling of self-worth.

We open with a description of the wide scenario within which the health care of the school child has evolved—through historical, social and legal change. This is followed by a look at the models of health and disease that are current, and the position from which a worker in health can draw out a value-base. Our theme then focuses on the statutory responsibilities of the school nurse working with the school doctor, and her roles, skills, tools and opportunities. The chapter on general health education at school narrows down still further to concentrate on self-care, in particular that of the child with special needs. These are seen as wholeness deficits rather than as labels.

The overall content of the book has been influenced by the following beliefs:

- that relationships have an over-all significance in health behaviour.
- that authority and autonomy are being questioned, and fluidity is being introduced into attitudes that have been traditional.
- that child development is many-faceted and interdisciplinary and that cooperation is vital.
- that community care with all its untidy ends has goals that are

equally valid but different from the neat discipline of hospital care.

- that prevention is often preferable to cure, and that there is a certain disillusionment at present about medical care that is disease-oriented.
- that the concepts which under-gird the Education Act 1981 stress the needs of the whole child and not just his impairments.
- that parents and siblings should be encouraged to participate in the management of child problems and not just to be onlookers while professionals take the responsibility.
- that to enable a child to say 'I have discovered' is as important as enabling him to say 'I have been told'.
- that self-awareness may be the hallmark of what has been called the 'Me' generation, but that this must extend to an awareness that other people have their own experiences that are equally valid.
- that knowledge of myself and my needs includes an understanding of the environment in which I live and of the needs of others who share it. I should ensure that a balanced care of resources and people are all part of my world.

Throughout this book we are offering new goals. The old goals of education were success and achievement. But good pay, comfortable living and good health can no longer be expected as if they were rights. They are bonuses. In real life there are features of 'unsuccess' to be met—uncertainty, stress, dislocation and change. The new goals are to equip each child to cope with the inevitable risks that are in life, as well as with its zest, and thereby to suggest ways of significant living that do not rely on continuous paid work and hypothetical 'happy families'.

In tackling these far-reaching issues we have tried to avoid stereotypes. However there are at least two conventions we have kept to for the sake of brevity and clarity. The first involves pronouns: we have generally used she/her to refer to any adult worker and he/him to refer to any child. The second is that some issues which are fundamental to all human beings have been left implicit. These include an individual's allegiances—to community, friends, family, self and God—and his personal understanding of religion and sexuality. Such important subjects are general to all and not specific to this book.

Our chief aim is to advance a service which succours all children. For this, we have taken a holistic approach to health and school, which emphasises the interaction of mind, body, spirit and feeling in the building up of personality. It will have achieved its goal if it does something towards the realisation of the inter-relatedness of all people working at school, whatever their age, and whatever their occupation. We are all in it together.

1 The Setting

by Monica Baly

The Historical Background

Two hundred and fifty years ago most children were not educated. Education for the lower orders, the vast majority of the population, was considered unnecessary and inappropriate, and the children from these classes were made to work. On his travels around the British Isles in 1724–27, Daniel Defoe recorded in his book *Tour Through the Whole Island of Great Britain* that

> There was not a child in the town or the villages around it of above five years old, but, if it was not neglected by its parents and untaught, could earn its bread.

He also noted with approval that in the Dales 'hardly anything above the age of four years old but its hands were sufficient for its support'.

Attitudes to the labour and education of children were mixed, however. There was a desire to use their labour, but there was also a desire that they grow up as Christians and this meant teaching them to read. Several decades earlier, in 1698, the Society for Promoting Christian Knowledge (SPCK) had been founded. It provided many schools in the early part of the eighteenth century, but these schools soon had to compete with the Industrial Revolution which was claiming children for the mines, workshops and factories. Eventually SPCK's educational schemes foundered because of the shortage of teachers.

At the end of the century, Dr Andrew Bell and the Quaker Joseph Lancaster, each in their different and separate ways, demonstrated that the problem of lack of teachers could be overcome by the 'monitorial system' in which teachers taught the older children who in turn taught the younger—this was probably the system within which Jane Eyre taught at Lowood School. Two societies were founded to promote the system and both are still in existence, the British and Foreign Schools Society and the National Society for Promoting the Education of the Poor (now the Society for Promoting Religious Education). Within 20 years, these two societies had founded numerous schools. These schools existed within a patchy and haphazard system, however, and this led Samuel Whitbread in 1807 and Lord Brougham in 1820 to put forward 'national' schemes. Finally in 1833, the House of Commons voted £20 000 to assist the National and British Societies to build up their schools—the government having bowed to the pressure of the Church that education was essentially a religious matter.

In the same year, the government set up an Education Committee of the Privy Council with Dr James Kay (later Sir James Kay Shuttleworth) as the secretary.[1] Dr Kay held office for ten years during which he laid the foundations of the elementary education system which lasted until 1944. He also abolished the monitorial system and set up a teacher training college at Battersea (this is of interest to nurses because before Battersea College became the Polytechnic of the South Bank, it was the training college of many early health visitors). Her Majesty's Inspectorate of Schools also dates from this time. In spite of these advances, however, progress was slow throughout the nineteenth century because strong sectarian resistance by both the Church of England and the non-conformists undermined all efforts at central reform.

The war between labour and education continued, with industrialists relying on cheap child labour and parents relying on the children's wages, until 1870. In that year, W. E. Forster, Vice President of Education in the Gladstone administration, piloted through the Elementary Education Act in the face of fierce opposition. This Act was a compromise but it gave the government the power to set up School Boards which could provide schools out of public funds if there was no voluntary Church school—hence the term 'Board School'. One effect of the Act was an accelerated school building programme, many in the distinctive late Victorian Gothic style which makes looking for the date over the door almost unnecessary. However, the Act did not make school attendance compulsory; it merely gave the Boards the power to make it compulsory if they wished, and many did not.

From the point of view of the development of nursing, these schools were important in that they provided elementary education for girls. This was followed by an upsurge of secondary education—especially in the endowed schools—some of the products of which were to find their way into nursing. This rise in educated women was one of the reasons for the increase in recruitment to nurse training in the 1880s.[2]

With the Elementary Education Act came a concern about the health of school children. In 1892 The Metropolitan and National Nursing Association, which had been founded by William

Rathbone with the help of the Nightingale Fund, sent a Nightingale nurse, Amy Hughes, to look after the health of the children in the school in Chancery Lane. Miss Hughes was shocked by the poor health of the children, but it was the Boer War and the national shock at the state of health of many of the army recruits that caused the real concern about child health. In 1904 the Interdepartment Committee on Physical Deterioration made forceful recommendations on how to improve child health. These included the training of mothers by organisations such as the Salford Lady Health Missioners (one of the forerunners of health visitors); the need for Health Societies; feeding arrangements for school children; physical training and games; and, striking a modern note, combating juvenile smoking.

Meanwhile, in 1899 a Board of Education was set up and in 1902 the Balfour Education Act enacted the new authorities which had been created by the Local Government Act of 1888—the Local Education Authorities (LEAs). Their statutory duty was to provide elementary education for all children until 14 years of age. LEAs were also given powers to grant aid for the provision of education beyond the elementary level. Some education authorities were diligent in the provision of secondary education, but some were laggard and the situation was complicated by the fact that minor authorities provided elementary education only.

The greatest cause of controversy about the LEAs arose, however, from the fact that they could make grants to religious and endowed schools; these institutions would then reserve a quarter of their places for 'scholarship' children with the LEAs paying the fees. This situation continued until 1944 and is historically important because it explains why 'good' schools are unevenly distributed. Even today parents will move to an area where there is more choice of schools, especially of the formerly endowed schools.

The 1904 report on physical deterioration formed the basis for much of the social legislation which the Liberals brought in after their landslide victory in 1906, although steps to improve school health had already been taken in some areas; in 1905, for example, the London County Council had set up its own School Medical Service and even before this 85 other authorities had employed doctors and nurses to advise.[3,4]

In 1907 a School Medical Service was established by the Education (Administrative Provisions) Act. The arrangements for this service were conducted by the Board of Education with Dr George Newman (later Sir George) as its first and distinguished head. Unfortunately the general practitioners, who were already aggrieved about the inroads that the outpatient departments of hospitals made into their income, resisted the Act.[5] In order to placate their lobby, school doctors and nurses were allowed to provide only limited treatment and, in theory at least, children were to be referred to a general practitioner. As most parents could not afford a doctor, much of the disease and dysfunction discovered went untreated.

Almost coinciding with this Act was the Education (Provision of Meals) Act 1906. This Act faced stiffer opposition than the 1907 Act providing medical services in schools. Its Bill caused a storm of protest and a leader in *The Times* condemned it as making 'serious inroads into the personal responsibilities of parents'.[6] It was this attitude—that parents must be paupers before children could have free meals—combined with the limitations of the school health service, that caused the health of army recruits at the outbreak of World War I to be little improved.

As part of the Reconstruction Plan for a 'land fit for heroes', the Education Act of 1918 (the Fisher Act) extended the duties of the LEAs:

- to provide medical treatment and inspection for all children in elementary schools and for medical examinations of children in secondary schools.
- to provide treatment for minor ailments, defective vision, dental disease and enlarged tonsils and adenoids (although such treatment was to be paid for by the parents except in needy cases).

Sadly, the more ambitious parts of the Act foundered in the post-war depression. The compulsory leaving age was raised to 14 years, however, and in 1924 the Labour Government requested that the Board of Education enquire into the organisation, objective and curriculum of courses of study, other than in grammar schools, for children up to the age of 15 years. This led to the Haddow Committee whose report was to be the cornerstone of English education for the next quarter of a century.[7] The main recommendation was that there should be primary education for all until the age of 11 years, after which there should be secondary education in a 'Senior' or 'Modern' school lasting until 15 years. By 1939 about two-thirds of the elementary schools were reorganised along these lines. A further development occurred at the outbreak of World War II: the Spens Committee recognised that these schools were giving a 'general education' and that the time was ripe for secondary education to develop along three broad lines—Grammar, Modern and Technical.[8] The stage was set for the post-war Education Act.

The School Health Service expanded throughout the inter-war period but the services were complicated and uneven. In 1919 the new Ministry of Health took overall control, however, and Sir George Newman was the Chief Medical Officer of Health at the Board of Education. Each authority was a law unto itself: the large cities tended to run a full-time service with a specially recruited corps of doctors and nurses, and progressive authorities like the

London County Council ran their own training schemes. The scale of pay and conditions of service varied from authority to authority. Other LEAs included the School Health Service as part of the duties of the health visitor, by arrangement with the medical officer. In the days when the health visitor had a distinct geographical area, this arrangement was advantageous, since the health visitor could follow through children she had known as toddlers and she was a valuable point of reference about home and housing difficulties. This advantage has been largely lost with 'group attachment' schemes, the increased mobility of the population and the heavy demands made of health visitors by the ageing population.

Whether the improved standard of health for army recruits in 1939 was due in any measure to the School Health Service and to school meals is difficult to say, but wartime evacuation revealed that many children were still ill fed—some did not know what it was to sit down to a meal—many were verminous, and poor health and behavioural problems often formed a vicious circle, each exacerbating the other. The horror stories of evacuation probably account for the reason why the Education Act of 1944 piloted through by Mr R. A. Butler went through without the religious or sectarian controversy or the reactionary sentiments that had bedevilled previous Acts.

The Butler Act made sweeping changes in public education which was divided into three stages: primary, secondary and further education—the latter accounting for all education for individuals past school age. All fees were abolished in schools maintained by the LEAs but voluntary schools were given the choice of being aided or controlled; grant-aided schools retained their right to denominational religious worship and to appoint their own teachers. Furthermore, for the first time, authorities were required to consider the need to provide nursery schools for children under the age of five years.

Since 1944 there have been a number of developments. The Education Act of 1964 gave LEAs the power to establish primary and secondary schools with different age limits. Amending Acts progressively reduced the level of contributions towards school building due from managers of voluntary aided schools and, most importantly, the Education Act of 1976 gave the Secretary of State the power to compel LEAs to organise secondary schools on comprehensive lines.

The School Health Service since 1944

Section 48 of the 1944 Act required all LEAs to provide medical inspection at appropriate intervals for pupils attending schools or county colleges maintained by them. It also required LEAs to make arrangements to provide free medical treatment for pupils attending any school or county college that the LEAs maintained. Moreover, Section 78(c) empowered authorities to make arrangements with independent schools to participate in the school health and in the school meals service.

Perhaps most important from the point of view of the school nurse was the clause that required authorities to have regard for the needs of children suffering from any disability of body and/or mind and to seek out and ascertain these needs. The categories were at that time defined as blind pupils, partially sighted pupils, deaf pupils, partially hearing pupils, educationally subnormal pupils, epileptic pupils, physically handicapped pupils, pupils suffering from speech defects and delicate pupils. It was national policy that handicapped pupils should, as far as possible, be educated in normal schools. By 1973, however, the idea of fixed categories had fallen into disrepute and it was subsequently abolished.[9] Nevertheless special treatment is still provided when necessary in ordinary schools, special schools, special schools in hospitals, and in hospital for individual children.

'Delicate' children still form the largest group of handicapped pupils with the chief ailments of the 1970s being asthma, bronchitis, diabetes, obesity and emotional disturbances.

The other large category—from 5 to 10% of the school population—is the educationally subnormal group who under the Education (Handicapped Children) Act of 1970 have been transferred from the jurisdiction of the Department of Health and Social Security to the Department of Education and Science. All subnormal children are now entitled to education in schools.[10]

Among the many problems facing the School Health Service since 1944 has been the fact that, in common with other welfare services, the main and most enthusiastic users of the service have been the higher socioeconomic groups. Often parents with the least need are the most ready to talk to the school nurse and the doctor as they tend to speak the same language.

Allied to the problem of the take-up of the services has been the whole question of cost. Because of rising costs, in 1959 the School Health Service Regulations stopped requiring a specific number of health checks and instead it was suggested that doctors and nurses should spend more time on selective inspection. One result of this was that, by the time of the Court Report in 1976, school medical inspections had fallen by 25%.

Under the National Health Service Reorganisation Act of 1973, the School Health Service was integrated into the NHS and came under the direct control of the DHSS. Locally the services were administered by the Area Health Authority with each authority having a Child Health Nursing Officer who was responsible for coordinating all the health services for children. Since the Patients First Reorganisation of 1982, this duty has fallen to the District Health Authorities. One disadvantage of the recent reorganisation is that the District areas are not coterminous with the boundaries of the LEAs; the LEAs have retained responsibility for the ascertainment of children in need of special education treatment and for the provision of special schools.

However, there have been new positive developments; for example, District Handicap Teams for the assessment and care of handicapped children have been set up. They consist of the community paediatrician, the nursing officer, the social worker, the principal psychologist and the teacher, with other specialists as required depending on the handicap.[11] Another important development is the awareness of school nurses themselves of the need for a group identity and they have been meeting both nationally and internationally to discuss and share common problems—not least of which is the need for a definite post basic training.

The Sociological Setting

Early Educationalists

When Defoe suggested that a child of five should earn its keep, he was referring to agricultural England, but the child as a miniature adult was not confined to the rural poor; for example, paintings by Reynolds or Gainsborough show stiffly dressed children of aristocrats. However, at the time that Reynolds was painting in the late eighteenth century, philosophers like John Locke of the Enlightenment were preaching a new gospel. Locke held that children were born with a blank mind—a *tabula rasa*—on which experience would write. Thus he challenged the idea of original sin which people at that time believed had to be beaten out of children. The most important influence on child education in the eighteenth century, however, was undoubtedly Jean Jacques Rousseau who saw children as unique individuals and who attributed evil, not to sin, but to society and to the departure from the natural state in which people were both good and happy. 'Man is born free but everywhere he is in chains', wrote Rousseau in *Du Contract Social*. In his novel *Emile*, published in 1762, Rousseau developed the theory that instruction should proceed by an appeal to the child's curiosity and by stimulating his intelligence rather than by imposing knowledge upon it. In his emphasis on the importance of the senses, Rousseau owed much to Locke and from this emphasis stemmed his ideas on maternal feeding, bodily freedom and physical training, and the exercise of judgement through sensory perception. Although Rousseau's three stages have no psychological basis, his ideas prepared the way for further critical appraisal. The idea of the innocence of childhood runs through the work of poets like Wordsworth and Blake, and Rousseau was a profound influence on such nineteenth century figures as Pestalozzi, Froebel and in our own day, Maria Montessori.

Changes in the Nineteenth Century

The nineteenth century is often thought of as a period of Dickensian childhood misery ruled by a 'spare the rod and spoil the child' philosophy. But it is a mistake to take history from fiction especially when the novelist is using polemic to make a point. Nineteenth century attitudes to children were much more complicated than those depicted by reformers like Dickens and Kingsley; the literate classes were bombarded with articles and magazines on how to be better wives and mothers, and on how to bring up children according to the ideas of Rousseau, Froebel and the more advanced in the medical profession.[12] The growing Victorian middle class was very conscious that the infant mortality was unacceptably high and magazines and journals blamed mothers for improper care.

> The omnipotent God never intended that nearly half the babies born in this country should die before they are five years old ... general ignorance of simple and safe remedies have been fatal causes.[13]

Mothers were urged to breast feed and middle class mothers became anxious as the evils of quack medicine and soothing syrups were hammered home. The anxiety over how to discipline children grew intense in the 1860s and it became an accepted principle of child care that the mother should direct the child positively through love, kindness and a soft manner. A popular book published in 1848, *Family Friend*, claimed that:

> In some families the children are continually addressed as tiresome plagues, mischievous brats and such like terms. In some families children are considered to be very good if they do not jump, sing, shout or make a noise and are as grave as penguins. But all this is in the direct opposition to nature! Such very good children are to be pitied.[14]

Admittedly such articles were mainly read by the middle classes, but it was a growing class and attitudes percolated downward, although there was a gap of about a generation between the classes. One important result was a reduction in family size for if the mother was to heed the advice of *Family Friend*, the size of the family could not remain the same. It was in this context that the Victorian family began to reduce the birth rate. Accordingly, the practice of birth control became increasingly acceptable and literature on the subject became more readily available.

The importance of the reduction of the birth rate after 1870 cannot be overemphasised. The reasons for a fall in the birth rate from 38 per 1000 population to 14 per 1000 in two generations are complicated, but they include a rise in large scale industry, the loss of security, the decline of religion, popular education, the growth and prestige of science, new attitudes to children, the emancipation of women and birth control.[15] One cause reacted with another and cause and effect were sometimes circular. Smaller families meant that there was more opportunity for the woman to develop as a person and for the children to be treated individually. Eventually this became accepted and expected—in other words, it became fashionable. Furthermore, the advent of smaller families was connected with the demand for longer schooling; children cost more due to schooling, so families *had* to be smaller. It was one thing to have ten children all earning in the fields or factories before the age of 12, it was quite another to have ten dependent until the age of 15 or older.

The limitation of family size was an important factor in the fall of the infant mortality rate; more care was given to fewer babies and there was less infection. But the fall in the infant mortality rate altered the ratio of the sexes because frail boy babies now survived to adulthood. In the late Victorian period, there were about 1060 females to every 1000 males[16] and that imbalance continued until World War II with the consequence that marriage was late. Men could afford to wait and for economic reasons often had to do so. After the 1950s, there was an equality in the numbers of the sexes and even an excess of males in the lower age groups. However, smaller families, partly brought about by two world wars, did not bring the millenium for children; although competing for attention in a large family had disadvantages, the world we have lost did have some advantages.

New Pressures on Families in the Twentieth Century

Earlier marriage in a sophisticated society led to innumerable problems. First, the bride and groom were likely to be only children or members of a small nuclear family and they tended to have no experience of bringing up younger brothers and sisters or of handling small babies. Second, the earlier the marriage occurred, the more likely was breakdown and divorce. Third, occupational change and mobility often meant that married children were no longer near the parental base for support. In essence what has happened is that, in the last 30 years or so, families have become more isolated with fewer people to bear one another's burdens. Responsibilities that were once borne by the wider family now are often shouldered by two very inexperienced young people and sometimes it is more than they can bear. Children need surrogate parents and spinster aunts had their uses.

One of the reasons for the limitation of family size was the emancipation of women and their desire to develop as individuals. With early marriage and childbearing over comparatively early, the mother had to face the boredom of the house or find work outside the home. Of course, working class wives have worked outside the home since the industrial revolution, the difference is that it is now a life-style that has spread to all classes and that is desired rather than viewed as a mere economic necessity.

The fact that nearly half of all married women are in some paid employment has had a number of consequences. The consumer market has cashed in on labour-saving devices of all kinds, not only with washing machines and dishwashers but with other streamlining devices as well so that houses are easier to run. The Victorian wife, even if she had a maid, often had her day fully occupied because the business of cooking, washing and cleaning and its organisation took so long. Now many things once made in the home like preserves, soft drinks, bread, cakes and cleaning materials are bought in the supermarket and few mothers do much in the way of dressmaking—with jeans and jump suits replacing frilly petticoats, there is little need. But there can be losses as well as gains. Conflict can be severe if the children are ill and need to stay at home, or if there is an income drop, for example, with the father's redundancy. When trouble such as a behavioural problem arises working wives are harder to help and visits by health visitors have to be made at night along with every other competing caller and to the background of the television.

If wives work, it is clear that some of the traditional roles of men and women must be reversed. There is no reason why household tasks should be allocated by gender, and there is no reason why the father should not change the baby, but it can be a situation that needs delicate handling, especially in times of crisis. Role reversal may jar if a father becomes unemployed and this may affect the children.

New Pressures on Children

Most parents strive to do their best for their children and to give them a stable and loving home, but there is no doubt that there are many more pressures on children than there were fifty years ago. First, most children are better nourished and they mature earlier; the 14 year old girl is no longer a 'slip of a thing', but rather she is wearing adult clothes. Second, as society becomes more technical and sophisticated, it demands longer education and a longer period of dependence on the parental home. Thus the period of adjustment from childhood to adolescence becomes longer and the period of conflict greater. Third, the criteria society uses for adulthood bears little relationship to physiological development. The age at which adolescents may marry, drive a car, sign consent to their own operation, be served in a public house are all arbitrary, and recently a new debate has been added about the right of the doctor to follow the rules of professional secrecy if a girl under 16 insists that her parents should not be told that she has been prescribed the contraceptive pill. Why should it be contemplated that the rule of secrecy be broken for a 15 year old but not a 16 year old?

The ambivalence towards the criteria for adulthood creates confusion in many areas, not least of which is the attitude to money. Children are often given more pocket money than previously. But children must learn to handle money and it depends on what they are expected to do with it whether this is a bad thing or not. Some adolescents are students struggling on a grant, others of the same age have a high percentage of disposable income for expenditure on leisure, clothes and social activities. It must be remembered, however, that 'constant, visible indulgence in such apparent non-essentials acts as a further irritant to parents who are themselves at this time economically most deprived and so envy and resentment form part of the changing relationship between the parent and the child'.[17] It must also not be forgotten that the life-style of the immediate school leaver is often longed for by the boy and girl still at school who do not yet have their own money.

In spite of the switch to comprehensive schools and the greater attention to the needs of the non-academic, school remains a competitive place from which those who either have no ability or no wish to compete long to escape. Physically mature and intellectually uninterested, they are bored and tend to seek excitement with their peer group outside. This may be harmless, like visits to discotheques or it may involve the wrecking of property simply because property symbolises adult values. Vandalism must be seen as a kicking against authority; often it is stimulated by the demands of school discipline which seem to conflict with the demands of the world elsewhere. Frequently, this group sees the demands of school life not as a preparation for a job, but for long-term unemployment and even more boredom. In this depressing outlook, any excitement for excitement's sake may be sought.

Another result of the limitation of family size has been the building of smaller houses and since World War II, more families have been housed in box-like houses or high rise flats where there is no separate accommodation for children and few safe play areas. Children cannot be banished to the nursery or to play in the back yard and even if they have a room of their own, children are now partakers of the adult world. This includes watching adult television with its violent films and often horrifying news. The cartoon in which a child, asked if he has seen a 'video nasty', replies 'yes, but the Falklands war was worse' rings a warning bell. Children who have been brought up with the nuclear debate think that the holocaust is at hand. The nineteenth century had its underworld of children who had to fend for themselves at an early age, but neither their activities nor the horrors of the Boer War were thrust at them *visually* every night of the year. On the other hand, there is the argument that children should be brought up to know the world as it really is rather than the happy make-believe land of childhood fiction. Striking a balance is not easy.

One of the most difficult problems the school nurse is likely to face is that of schoolgirl pregnancies. So far health education has failed on this subject, largely because not enough attention has been paid to the education of boys. According to Scholfield, sexual activity is taking place earlier than before and there is a 5 year gap between the first experience of sexual intercourse and the commitment to the use of contraception.[18] In 1982, 14% of the total births in England and Wales were illegitimate; and for the first time among teenage mothers, the number of illegitimate births outstripped legitimate births—29 000 to 27 000. Two years earlier, it was reported that there were some 4600 known pregnancies in girls under 16 of which 3000 ended in abortion.[19] Whether to put a schoolgirl on the pill and whether the parents should be told may be a medical matter, but school nurses cannot stand aside from the debate. When there are no supporting parents—for example, mother maybe unmarried with troubles of her own or, as has been known, the father maybe on a charge of incest—it is often Hobson's choice.

Morality based on chastity because of the fear of pregnancy is difficult to preach with oral contraceptives available. The trouble is that society is not sure to whom they should be available, and the network of communication in the teenage peer group is often confused and unreliable. Perhaps a shocked society is asking the wrong questions and perhaps the questions should be aimed at society itself and not the girls or the medical profession. One question might be why do children place such a premium on sexuality? If the child's mind is a *tabula rasa*, society—primarily the mass media—has much to answer for what it has written on those blank slates. A second question might be why can some children confide in doctors and nurses but not their parents?

Another way the young often find of dealing with conflict is to take alcohol or other drugs. Fortunately hallucinogens and amphetamines are now difficult to obtain due to restriction on their manufacture, but teenagers with initiative will find a way. Cannabis has probably excited more comment than it warrants except if it leads to the use of hard drugs like cocaine, heroin and morphine, but these are usually problems for the older age groups. Another reason for alarm is inhalant or glue sniffing which is becoming an increasingly serious problem, resulting in a number of deaths.

The legal drug of the young adult is, of course, alcohol; some young adults spend 40% of their disposable income on alcohol. However, in spite of the increase in pocket money, alcohol abuse is not likely to present the school nurse with a serious problem except in Colleges of Further Education. Nevertheless, the high incidence of serious drinking problems among adolescents—120 000 cases of convicted drunkenness a year—indicates the need for health education on the subject. The same applies to smoking. The latest report of the Royal College of Physicians suggests that 100 000 people will die prematurely because of disease caused by cigarette smoking, so children must be actively discouraged from smoking.

Most of the problems outlined stem from the 'You have never had it so good' society which arose out of full employment in the 1960s and the increasing expectation of increasing material benefits. This problem has been compounded by the reversal of economic trends with the current recession and the prospect of unemployment for so many adolescents. We have the values of the 1960s without the income to pay for them.

Western civilisation may never see full employment again, so the question has to be asked: for what are we educating children? In 1975 Professor R. Dahrendorf suggested in the Reith lectures that there was an urgent need to get away from the Protestant work ethic that has been the basis of a capitalist society where work is something a person is paid to do for so many hours a day. He argued in favour of a more flexible approach to paid work, leisure, voluntary work and retirement.[20] Education should, therefore, equip children at the basic level for all these experiences and it should reveal the many different doors through which they can pass later and not merely the one marked 'Paid Work'. Above all, education should equip children to adapt to change, and to understand and appreciate their own ability to make choices.

The Legal Setting

The Rights of Children

In the eighteenth century Locke said:

> All that a child has the right to claim from his father is nourishment and education and the things that nature furnishes for the support of life.[21]

He went on to emphasise that parental power is vested in both parents and that the government of children is not intended to be severe or arbitrary. Today, the United Nations General Assembly has elaborated on this theme, stating that a child has the right to adequate feeding, shelter and education within the laws of the country and to protection from exploitation, discrimination and mental and physical harm.[22] In England, if parents or guardians fail dramatically in these respects, they may be prosecuted and the child taken into care. Since 1946 the care of children has been vested in a Children's Department, and since 1972 at local level this has come within the ambit of the Social Services Departments of County Councils and Metropolitan authorities.

Children may legally come into care through a court order or because the authority is fulfilling its duty under the Children Act 1975. Court cases usually arise from matrimonial, wardship or criminal proceedings; in matrimonial cases, where it seems that neither parent should be given custody, the child may be committed to the care of the local authority. Court cases may also arise because of offences committed by children; children under the age of ten cannot be charged, but they may be taken into care. Other reasons for taking children into care are because the parents or guardians have been shown to be incapable of providing for the child or because the child has been abandoned. However, it must be stressed that the local authority has no power to keep a child against the wishes of the parents, although it does have a duty to ensure that as far as possible the child will have proper care. On rare occasions, and only after stringent conditions have been fulfilled, will an authority override the wishes of the parents.

Non-accidental Injury to Children

It follows that a child has the right not to be injured. To paraphrase Miss Nightingale, the first duty of the parents is to do the child no harm. It comes as a shock, therefore, to read the annual reports of the National Society for the Prevention of Cruelty to Children and to learn that hundreds of parents lose control and batter their children to death. The actual numbers involved and the reasons for this apparent growth in violence are difficult to assess, but the school nurse should be familiar with the literature on the subject.

Surveys show that the families at the greatest risk tend to be those where the parents are young, immature and unable to respond to the needs of demanding children. The analysis of recorded cases may be misleading because cases among the higher income groups may not be reported. It does seem, however, that the lower income groups—especially when associated with marital discord and unemployment—are heavily represented.

Confidentiality

In his oath, Hippocrates swore never to divulge what he had seen or heard in his practice and it has been a longstanding article of faith among doctors and nurses that the knowlege they have about patients should be regarded as confidential. No doctor or nurse breaks the principle of confidentiality lightly; indeed doctors have faced contempt of court proceedings rather than do so. But when a life may be in danger, confidentiality does raise enormous ethical problems. In the last analysis, the person with the information must make the decision and, indeed, the ability and willingness to make such decisions is the nub of professional responsibility. However, there are guidelines that the school nurse can follow if she is in the position of suspecting non-accidental injury to a child. (See Chapter 11.)

Information about Criminal Activities

In the course of her work, the school nurse may come across evidence that worries her and she may be uncertain as to where her first duty lies—to the child, to the parents or to society. It is unlikely that the school nurse will uncover overt criminal activities, although she may in the case of a home visit in the inner cities or among sixth formers. While she may decide to apply the Hippocratic principle to what she suspects is cannabis growing in the front garden, she will have different feelings about incest or the exploitation of children for prostitution. School nurses are not policemen and they must weigh the validity of their suspicions carefully; again they should consult a colleague who would be in the eyes of the law privileged to receive such information. But they should only initiate action if the priority of need is such that there is a danger to the child if action is not taken. In legal and ethical matters there is one overriding maxim: 'Act always so as to increase trust.'

References

1. James Kay was one of the first Health Commissioners. He was also known for his work with cotton operatives. See Baly, M. (1980). *Nursing and Social Change*, 2nd edn. p. 101. London: Heinemann Medical.
2. Maggs, C. (1983). *The Origins of General Nursing*. London: Croom Helm.
3. Fraser, D. (1973). *The Evolution of the Welfare State*, p. 144. London: Macmillan.
4. Dent, H. C. (1977). *Education in England and Wales*, p. 101. London: Hodder and Stoughton.
5. Abel-Smith, B. (1964). *The Hospitals*, pp. 173–219. London: Heinemann Educational.
6. *The Times* (1905). (Leading article) 5 Jan.
7. *Report on the Education of the Adolescent* (1926). London: HMSO.
8. *Report on Secondary Education with Special Reference to Grammar and Technical High Schools* (1938). London: HMSO.
9. *Report on the Committee on Handicapped Children and Young People* (1978). London: HMSO.
10. *Report on the Committee on Residential Care for the Mentally Handicapped* (1978). London: HMSO.
11. Slack, P. (1983). 'The healthy school child'. In *Community Health*

(Clark, J., Henderson, J., eds.), p. 161. Edinburgh: Churchill Livingstone.
12. Branca, P. (1975). *The Silent Sisterhood*, p. 110. London: Croom Helm.
13. Branca, P. (1975). *The Silent Sisterhood*, title page quote, from *Every Mother's Book*. London: Croom Helm.
14. Branca P. (1975). *The Silent Sisterhood*, p. 157. London: Croom Helm.
15. *The Royal Commission on Population* (1949). London: HMSO.
16. Maggs, C. (1983). *The Origins of General Nursing*, p. 41. London: Croom Helm.
17. Gunn, A. (1983). 'Becoming an adult'. In *Community Health* (Clark, J., Henderson, J., eds.), p. 164. Edinburgh: Churchill Livingstone.
18. Scholfield, M. (1973). *Sexual Behaviour of Young Adults*. London: Allen Lane.
19. Davies, S. (1980). 'What every child should know'. *The Times*, 21 Feb.
20. Dahrendorf, R. (1976). *The New Liberty*. London: BBC Publications.
21. Locke, J. (1946). *The Second Treatise* (Gough, J. W., ed.) Oxford: Basil Blackwell.
22. *Report of the UN General Assembly* (1959). Geneva: UN.

2 The Structures

> The connection between health and education is one of the most important aspects of paediatrics. In general, our understanding of disorders of learning is still rudimentary, and the problems of intellectual limitation, defective speech, inadequate reading ability, excessive clumsiness, disturbed behaviour, truancy, school phobia and delinquency create a formidable array of disability. These problems will yield only to the combined efforts of doctors, teachers, psychologists, social workers and others. Yet we have found a good deal of evidence that as yet services were not disposed to cooperate in the interests of the child.
>
> The Court Report, 1976

Interdependent services rely upon planning, communication and cooperation for the achievement of maximum efficiency, but since 1970 services involved with the well-being of children have been subject to frequent and drastic change. No matter how valid the reasons were for the change in the administrative structures, there is no denying that these reorganisations have had far-reaching consequences. Furthermore, health, education and social services still do not react well enough or quickly enough, either individually or collectively, to the signs of need; and children already suffering disadvantage for environmental, social or health reasons often suffer double disadvantage on account of poor services. It is, therefore, important for individual workers to have an understanding not only of the organisational arrangements of services other than their own, but also to have a sound knowledge of the procedures and working relationships which exist between them. It may be dependent upon the discrimination and persistence of health workers in school that appropriate contacts are made and constructive change takes place.

This section covers the basic structures of the Central Government Education Department, Local Education Authority (LEA) and services, the National Health Service (NHS), and District Community Services.

Central Government

The activities that the Government carries out for its citizens are involved with three main functions:

1. Making laws .... Legislative function
2. Ruling according to law .... Executive function
3. Judging violations of the law .... Judicial function

The system of government in this country works by the combined efforts of many individuals and bodies, each acting as a check on the other, and the rights and freedoms of the individual are derived largely from this system.

The Government Executive

This consists of the Prime Minister acting together with other members of the Government, who form a Cabinet which agree upon government policy. Cabinet Ministers have a collective responsibility to Parliament, and included among them are the Heads of Departments of State. These Ministers of State are individually responsible to Parliament for the actions of the Civil Servants in their Departments. The Department of Education and Science is the main executive arm of the central government for education.

In addition to its general executive responsibilities, the Department deals with university grants; Her Majesty's Inspectorate is responsible for the maintenance of national standards of education and acts as an information and advisory body (Fig. 2.1).

Local Government

Local authorities are given their powers by central government; they administer many services in their own areas, but the responsibility for some services is shared. In addition to their own sources of income, local authorities receive grants and borrow money from central government funds.

The structure of local authorities is governed by various Acts of Parliament or Local Government Acts and their administration is based on the local election of councillors. Each council must annually elect a mayor or chairman to preside over council meetings and undertake ceremonial functions.

The work of the council is carried out by an arrangement of committees and subcommittees. Some committees must, by Act of Parliament, be established and they are called Statutory Committees. The Local Council Education Committee is one of these (Table 2.1).

Local Government Services

The administrative structure of education services at local level is based on Local Education Authorities (LEAs) who are responsible for implementing the plans and policies of the Local Council Education Committee. Although the pattern of organisation within the Local Authority may vary, the functions and responsibilities remain broadly the same. (The Greater London Council and the six Metropolitan Counties are currently facing change and must be regarded as possible exceptions.)

Table 2.1 shows the structure of Local Council Education Committees.

Schools

The vast majority of children are educated in schools maintained by local authorities; only a small minority of parents are able to

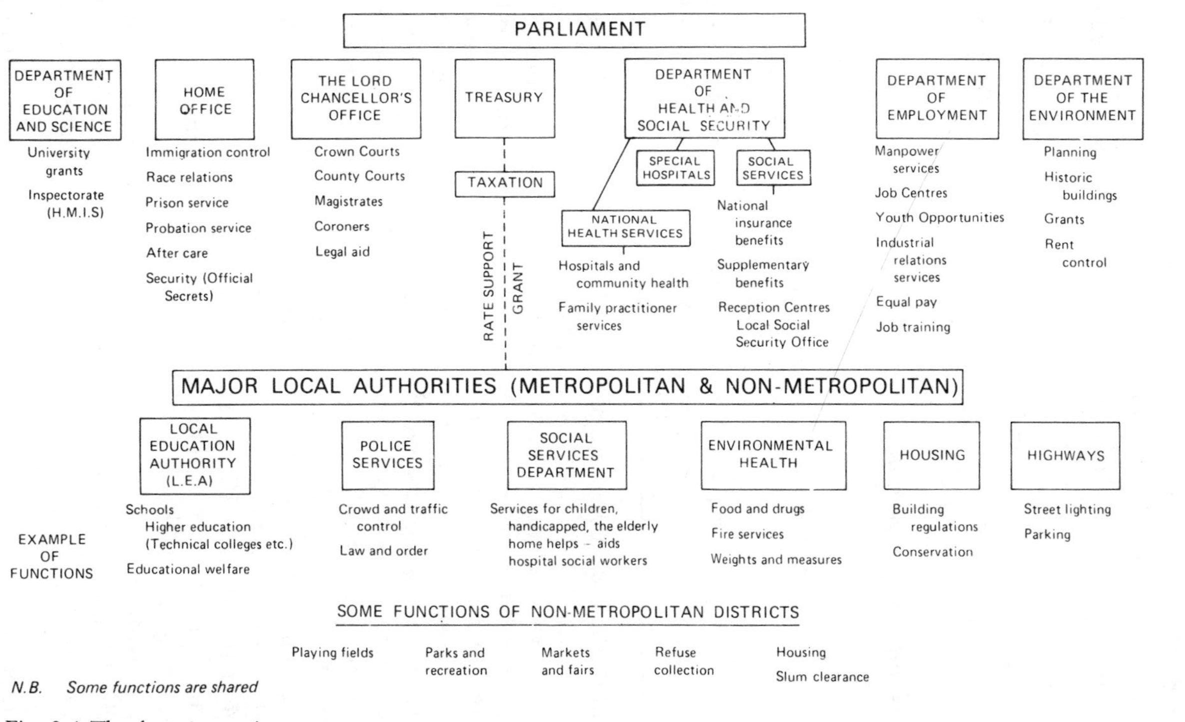

N.B. Some functions are shared

Fig. 2.1 The functions of government.

Table 2.1
The Local Council Education Committee

The Education Committee of a local authority provides for the planning and local representation of educational interests.

Model example of structure

Committee Constitution:	The mayor and 26 members of the elected local council. Five teachers serving in maintained schools and colleges. One representative from the local branch of the Association for the Advancement of State Education.
Subcommittee Structure:	1. Schools. 2. Further and Community Education. 3. Education Development and Finance.
plus *Special Committees.*	1. Education Joint Consultative Group (teachers and members). 2. Education Advisory Committee (members and representatives of various organisations with an interest in education).

opt out of the local educational system by sending their children to independent schools, a category which includes the great public schools as well as small establishments run for private profit.

The 1944 Butler Education Act established Primary, Secondary and Further Education, but the way in which the LEA organises its provision is subject to other important considerations. Since 1976 the Secretary of State has had the power to compel reorganisation of secondary schools on comprehensive lines, and most local authorities have abandoned selective schools in favour of this system. Within it, however, local authorities have the power to vary age limits within schools, and provision may include schools covering 11–18 years, 11–16 years with 6th form colleges, and 11–14 years plus 14–18 years; or a mixture of all three.

In addition to their rights under the 1981 Education Act, parents may insist that their children are educated in schools which provide for a specific religious education. In many areas, Church of England, Roman Catholic, Nonconformist, Jewish and other denominational schools are financially supported and approved as local authority provision.

In addition, there are a number of schools which, although outside the state system, may in certain circumstances be used by the LEA to meet the special educational needs of some children.

Non-maintained Special Schools

These are schools which have been set up by voluntary bodies. They are non-profitmaking concerns which receive financial support from charities or trusts; but the running costs of the majority are met almost entirely out of the fees paid by LEAs for pupils placed at the schools. They have to meet a number of conditions for approval as special schools and they receive visits from Her Majesty's Inspectorate. In return for compliance with conditions for approval, they may also receive grants towards capital projects.

Independent Schools

These are schools which prefer to remain independent of the state system. They have to be registered with the Department of Education and Science. Some are run by voluntary bodies, and some are profitmaking ventures. Among them are schools which cater wholly or mainly for handicapped children and under the Education Act (Miscellaneous Provisions) 1953, these schools may be used by the LEAs as special provision if they are deemed appropriate and subject to the Minister of State's veto. The Warnock Committee (1978) urged the need for closer supervision and inspection of these schools to ensure that they continued to maintain satisfactory standards of education and that the provision for individual children was appropriate to their needs. The Committee also recommended that the responsibility for following up the placement of a child in an independent school catering for pupils with special educational needs should rest with the person designated by the multiprofessional team which assessed the child's needs, and that part of the conditions of acceptance for the use of such a school should be that the school offer access to officers from the placing authority and the authority in whose area the school is situated. It further recommended that authorities should satisfy themselves that adequate health care is available before placing children in either non-maintained or independent schools catering mainly or wholly for children with special needs. Social Service Departments act *in loco parentis* in relation to any child who is placed in care, and the Committee recommended that no child with special educational needs should be placed in an independent school without agreement between the LEA and the Social Services Department.

Other Roles within the Education Service

Education Welfare Officers

In addition to checking on and enforcing school attendance, the Education Welfare Officer may be called upon to carry out many other non-teaching duties such as arranging school transport, providing information to individual families about entitlement to free meals, educational maintenance allowances and grants for school uniforms, and providing escorts for children to and from schools. In the course of these duties, they provide extra support to families and may keep schools informed of the particular home problems relating to some children. To some extent their services may overlap with other agencies and they provide a useful link between health, education and social workers.

Nursery Nurses

Nursery nurses work in a variety of settings including nursery schools, special units, hospitals, infant classes and residential homes for young children. Their skills in child care and knowledge of child development have been increasingly recognised. The syllabus for the Advanced Certificate of the National Nursery Examination Board includes a unit on children with special needs. In day nurseries and homes where the Portage System of developmental programmes have been used, nursery nurses have shown their ability to work with parents as well as with children with special needs.

Ancillary Workers

These are non-teaching assistants employed by the LEA, whose work involves care for children with special difficulties or disabilities; the help of an ancillary worker is often crucial to the effective placement of an individual child in an ordinary class. They are chosen for their sympathetic attitude to children and their experience as parents. They receive no specific training, although some schools provide short in-service courses for them. They may be employed as full-time or part-time helpers.

Residential Child Care Staff

Workers who undertake residential care in many ways act as parents and their contribution is vital to the effectiveness of boarding special schools. They provide a personal contact for children and create patterns of living which reduce the institutional effects of boarding schools. Child care staff may hold the Certificate of Social Service, but many have received no specific training, although this situation is changing. Nurses may also be employed in these schools to carry out nursing duties.

School Counsellors

The need for personal counselling for adolescents and young adults has received increasing recognition. Some schools may make provision for this by appointing a school counsellor who is available at specific times to listen in confidence to pupils' worries and concerns. The Warnock Committee pointed to the need for the development of courses offering the basic principles and skills required in counselling and organised preferably on an interprofessional basis. Children—like the rest of us—will choose their own counsellors, especially in the absence of a recognised service, and school counselling is as yet in its infancy.

Social Workers

Since the implementation of the Seebohm Report, Social Service Departments have had responsibilities for the care and welfare of handicapped children and their families. In some areas social workers may be linked to individual schools and in addition to their casework with families, they may provide some of the services which are associated with the Education Welfare Officer. In many authorities there are close links between the two services to ensure the best use of available resources.

Preschool Play Workers

Environmental problems, particularly in inner city areas, have led to schemes initiated by LEAs, whereby the families of children needing extra support and home stimulus are put in touch with a preschool play worker. She will visit the family on a regular basis to encourage and participate in play as a means of growth and development for the child. Often she also works to relieve the isolation and to extend the understanding of the parents, who may themselves have been deprived of warm parenting in their own childhood. There is a great need for appropriate modelling which can be offered—indirectly—by the play worker.

Hospital Play Therapists

The importance of play has been recognised as a valuable means by which children in hospital can express their anxieties and feelings of isolation and insecurity in what is for many of them a very threatening situation. Some hospitals use play therapists on the wards and also in outpatient departments. For children whose education has been punctuated by visits to hospital, there is a great need for the school staff and the play therapist to exchange visits and be familiar with both settings in order to provide a sense of continuity and security for the child.

School Nurses

School nurses may be found working in every different type of school, and the content of their work may vary to suit the needs of their employers. They may be employed as full-time, part-time or school term workers, they may be resident or non-resident and their work may range over several schools or be confined to one. Their titles may also vary according to their employment.

Within the Education Authority

Some LEAs employ their own school nurses who may work full-time or part-time within schools; they may also work with visiting school nurses from the school health service.

Independent and Non-maintained Schools

Independent and non-maintained schools may employ school nurses to undertake specific nursing duties. They may work alongside resident or non-resident care staff, and some are required to undertake non-nursing work as part of the school team. These schools may also have arrangements with the local school health service for the provision of immunisation and screening programmes which involve visits from health service school nurses.

School Matrons

Independent and non-maintained schools may employ persons as School Matrons to undertake a variety of duties which may include a nursing content. 'Some nursing experience' rather than specific nursing qualifications may be the prerequisite for appointment to the post, but in many cases school matrons will possess recognised nursing qualifications. It is to be hoped that increasing availability of approved school nurse courses will lead these schools to require school matrons to undertake an approved course before appointment or as soon as possible after appointment.

Because of the diversity of school nursing, its role and identity is taking time to develop and mature. Nevertheless, wherever and in whatever capacity the school nurse is employed, her overall objectives in relation to the children in her care remain the same. It is by building upon this principle that a strengthened body of service will continue to emerge.

The Health Service

> We travelled hard, but it seemed that every time we were beginning to form up in teams we would be reorganised, and later I was to learn in life that we tend to meet every situation by reorganising, and a wonderful method it can be for creating the illusion of progress while producing confusion, inefficiency and demoralisation.
>
> Petronius, Governor of Bithynia, 65 B.C.

In making a survey of the recent NHS reorganisations, one might be forgiven for thinking that some lessons are hardly learnt even after 2000 years; nevertheless progress in the treatment and prevention of disease and the recognition of positive health values has been achieved by community awareness and responsibility, goaded by individual skill and struggle.

The National Health Service Act 1946

This Act was designed to provide a comprehensive health service which consisted of three elements (Fig. 2.2):

1. Hospital Services
2. Separately contracted General Medical Practitioner and Dental Services.
3. Local Authority Community Health Services—embracing a separate administration for the School Health Service and the Maternity and Child Welfare Services.

The Act imposed a duty on every Local Health Authority to provide a health visiting and home nursing service, and Health Visitors/School Nurses were required to hold the Health Visitors Certificate. By 1974, however, because of the general shortage of Health Visitors, almost half the nurse-time in schools was provided by State Registered or State Enrolled Nurses who were not qualified Health Visitors and in many cases had received little or no specific training in school health work. Short courses in school nursing were set up from 1976 in an effort to make up some of the formal training deficiency.

Local Authority Social Services Act 1970

Between 1946 and 1971 local authority services were grouped with the personal social services under the direction of a Medical

Officer of Health. The general thrust of these services was supportive and preventive and because ill health is inextricably linked with poor social environment, health and social services were frequently involved with the same users. There was no single recognised pattern of administration, and social workers felt a need to improve their training and career structure. These factors led to a committee of enquiry being set up under Sir Frederic Seebohm, and eventually to the establishment of separate Social Service Departments in each local authority under the control of a Director of Social Services. This meant, in effect, that the community health services were now administratively isolated from both hospital and social services, and family doctors were isolated from all three.

Primary Health Care Teams

It was inevitable that, in the absence of proper machinery for cooperation, misunderstandings and conflicts of interest would arise, and community health surveys indicated that improvements were needed in the coordination and delivery of services. In some areas experimental schemes were set up whereby district nurses

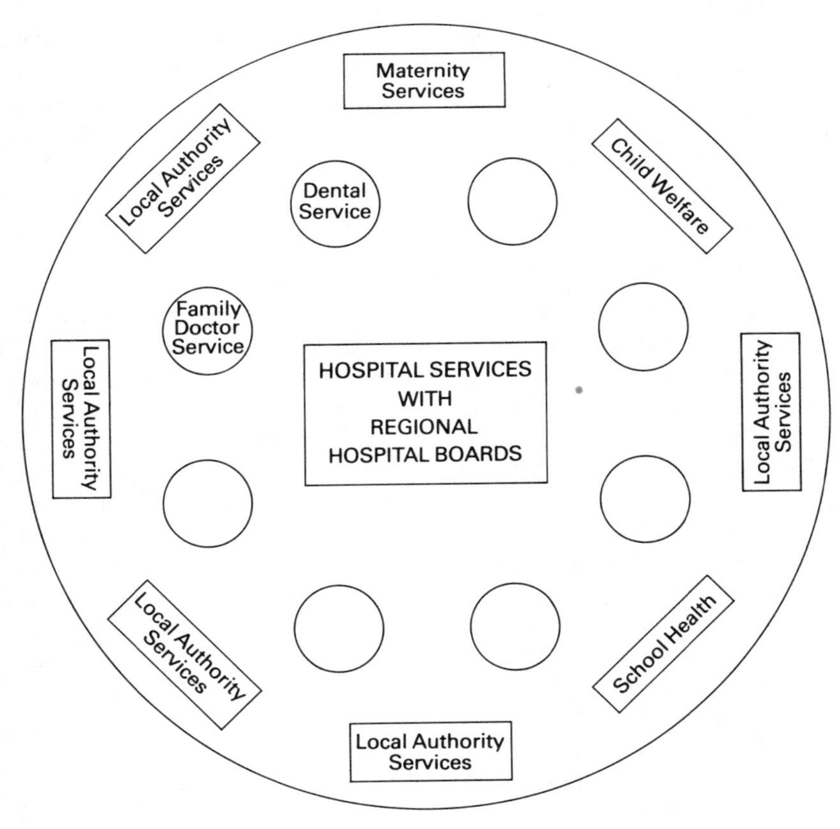

Fig. 2.2 The National Health Service organisation 1946–1973.

and health visitors were attached to groups of general practitioners, and in 1963 the Annis Gillie Committee on the Future Scope of General Practice recommended that district nurses, health visitors, midwives and social workers should be attached to medical practices to form *Primary Health Care Teams*.

Despite the practical and administrative difficulties, the team concept was generally welcomed, but in some instances the establishment of specific teams proved impracticable; these were:

1. some inner city areas where doctors worked from rented lock-up surgeries.
2. areas where there was a highly mobile population; the Health Visitor who was geographically based was often able to provide a better service.

Nevertheless, the importance of a team approach was established and gradually communication between groups of workers improved. Each group became more aware of the contribution the others make to the health care service as a whole.

Health Centres

Under the 1946 National Health Service Act, health authorities were empowered to build health centres which would provide facilities for general practitioner, dental and pharmaceutical services, hospital outpatient sessions and community health and welfare sessions. The establishment of such centres has been slow to develop for a variety of reasons, and in the present economic situation some authorities have been forced to put their plans into cold storage.

The National Health Service Reorganisation Act 1973

This Act sought to sweep away the traditional preoccupation of medical and nursing education with disease and the care of the sick and to provide a single comprehensive system of primary and supporting health care (Fig. 2.3). Increased understanding of the causation of disease and its links with environmental, social and emotional problems had opened the way for greater emphasis on the preventive health service and on the need to overcome the separation which existed between hospital, local health authority and general practitioner services.

The Secretary of State for Social Services was to preside over the Department of Health and Social Security and be responsible for central planning, advice and monitoring of the service as a whole.

Fourteen *Regional Health Authorities* were established, each with one or more university medical schools within its boundaries. Each Region comprised between three and eleven Area Health Authorities and there were 90 Areas in all. For the day to day running of the services, 75% of the Areas were again subdivided into Districts based on a population of up to 400 000, and each

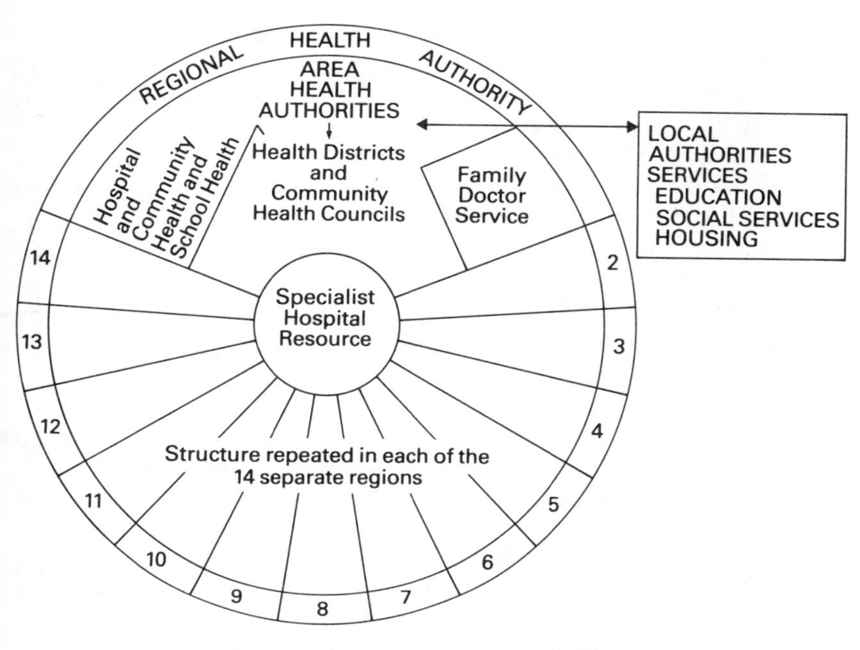

Fig. 2.3 The National Health Service reorganisation 1974.

contained a district general hospital. The remaining 25% of Areas were one district area authorities.

Each *Area Health Authority* was served by an Area Team of Officers responsible for planning and monitoring the performance of the health districts. Health services in Wales and Scotland were established on broadly similar lines.

The *Family Doctor Services* remained subcontracted to the NHS; the terms of their contracts with the newly established Family Practitioner Committees were laid down in specific regulations covering the provision of a 24 hour service.

A reorganisation of this magnitude, however carefully planned, invariably throws up unforeseen difficulties. The removal of community and school health services from the local authorities to the new Area Health Authorities in order to group them with hospital services created particular difficulties in communication and planning.

In the London area only four of the sixteen health authority boundaries corresponded with those of the individual London boroughs, and therefore some authorities had to serve on several separate planning and consultation committees where previously they had served on one. Services had to adapt to different patterns of work within different overlapping boundaries, and the proliferation of committees often led to confusion, frustration and aggravation and slowed down the process of decision-making and the efficient implementation of policy at local level.

In 1979 a Royal Commission on the working of the National Health Service was appointed. What emerged from the overall monitoring of services was a recommendation to streamline the management structure by cutting out one layer in the chain of responsibility. The Department of Health and Social Security then issued a document entitled *Patients First* in which, although it accepted the criticisms of the existing management structure, stressed the need to avoid another major upheaval in reorganisation. After widespread consultation and in keeping with government guidelines, each Regional Health Authority drew up a plan to define the geographical boundaries of the proposed new health authorities.

1981–1982 Management Restructure

Under this plan the old multidistrict Area Health Authorities were abolished and new District Health Authorities were set up, each based on a population of roughly half a million people (Fig. 2.4). They derive their authority from the Region and are directly accountable to it. This simplified structure is designed to provide a less cumbersome method of management and to facilitate and speed the flow of information and the process of decision-making—but many problems still remain. The promotion of health depends on many factors and services outside the scope of the NHS; local authority provision and environmental control create conditions which are also vital to the health of the community. There are still district health authorities whose boundaries are not coterminous with those of local government

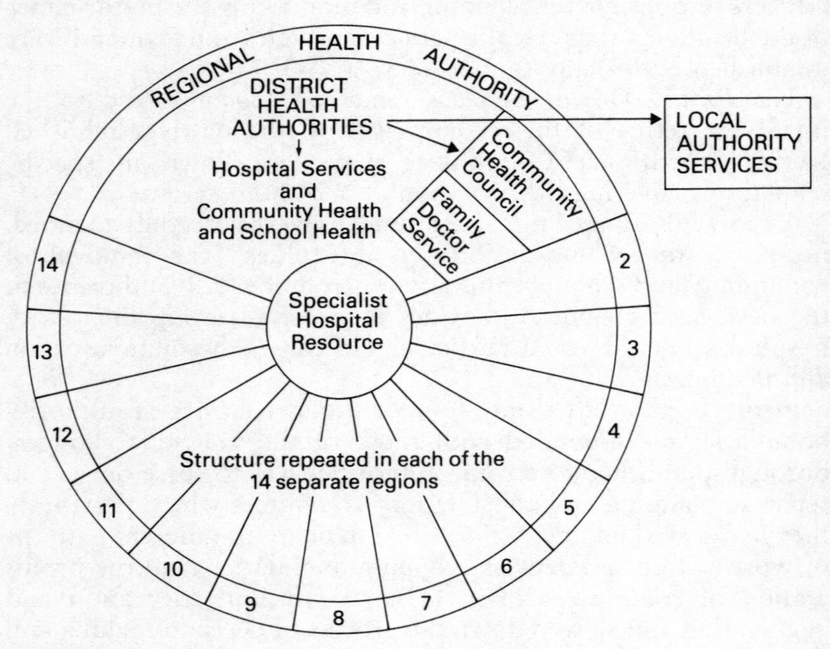

Fig. 2.4 The restructuring of the National Health Service 1981–1982.

areas, and efficient correlation of their services is essential if the health needs of the community are to be met.

The management of the NHS involves various professional and functional groups. The reorganisation was based upon the concept of self-management within each group and upon consensus or team management at Area level with group representation. On the positive side, it is argued that of necessity professional relationships are fostered and the interests and values of each group are involved and reflected in team decisions; on the other hand, this method of management may on occasion throw up situations where decisive action is made difficult and the compromise which results may provide a less effective service. Detractors of the system would argue that all health workers are accountable primarily to the community for the service they provide and that more heed should be paid to the voice of the consumer.

Community Health Councils

The Community Health Councils (CHCs) set up in 1972 were given the two-way task of representing the health needs of the local people to the health authority and of providing information to the public concerning the health services available in their area. Their work has been hampered and is in some ways ineffective due to lack of resources; although they can collect information, monitor and advise, no way has yet been found to compel health authorities and medical services to take sufficient note of their representations and to actively involve CHCs in decision-making and the process of change.

The Griffiths Report 1983

Even before the 1982 reorganisation was complete, another inquiry into management methods was set up under the chairmanship of Mr Roy Griffiths; its recommendations called for further change. In order to strengthen personnel management and provide more accountability for services, the report suggested a change in the management model involving the appointment of a general manager for each district health authority, coupled with radical changes in the system of budgeting. It pointed out the need to establish a system of financial control which would allow for comparison between individual levels of unit expenditure and the quality and quantity of services provided, in order to maintain cost-effectiveness overall; it also recommended that doctors should be more involved in management and the general oversight of services (Fig. 2.5).

It would be idle to speculate upon the outcome of these proposals; suffice it to say that they have been made in an attempt to rectify acknowledged deficiencies in the present system. As far as the proposed Unit Management Budgets are concerned, four demonstration districts have been chosen to operate the system from April 1984.

The debate about management continues; there are those who

maintain that consensus management has provided a democratic and flexible system, and that the benefits which have accrued from improved working relationships provide the best foundation for the growth and development of a caring and committed service. Others would argue that consensus management was part of an evolutionary process and that the time is ripe for a system which, while it recognises the contribution of the respective caring professions, will make its decisions with the needs of the consumer primarily in mind.

Organisations within the District Health Authorities

At the time of reorganisation, the administrative arrangements for each District Health Authority were made in consultation with their regional advisers; different patterns of organisation arose to suit different patterns of practice and different local health needs.

The provision of a *School Health Service* forms part of the statutory duty of the district health authority. In addition to the service provided for LEA schools, any independent or non-maintained school may make a request for some of these services

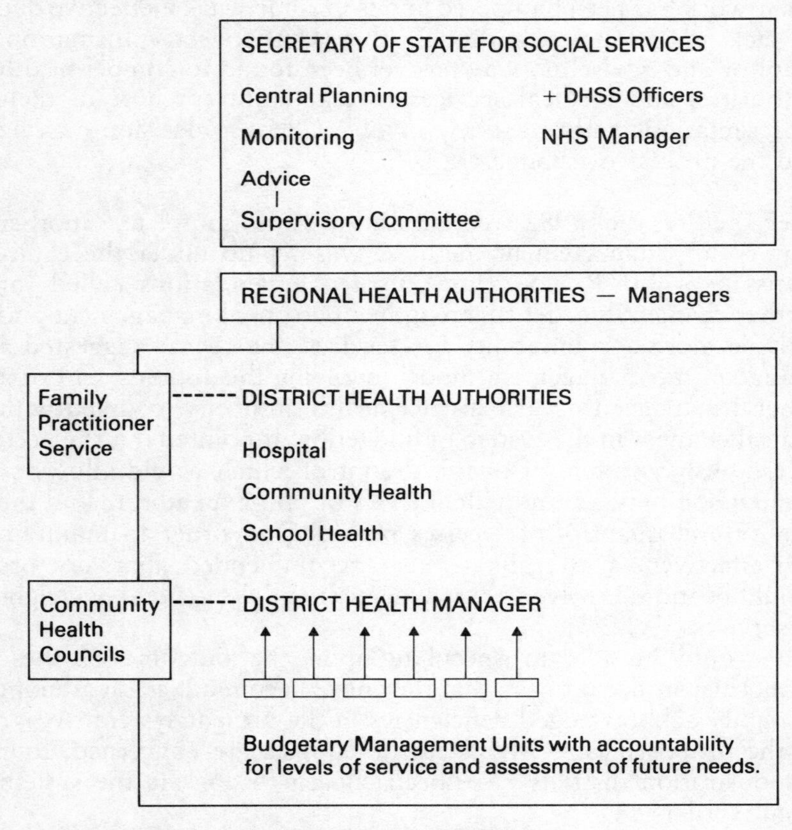

Fig. 2.5 Simplified Griffiths Management Model 1984.

to be made available to them and may come to an arrangement with the district health authority regarding their provision. The Warnock Committee recommended adequate health care as an essential prerequisite to the placement of children in these schools when it is proposed to use them as special educational provision.

The District Medical Officer carries overall responsibility for coordinating child health services, including school health services; and the Specialist in Community Medicine (Child Health) is directly accountable to the LEA for NHS functions in relation to the education service. This includes providing advice and having executive responsibility for the school health service provision and ensuring that the medical and other health service staff are available for these functions. The Specialist in Community Medicine (Child Health) will work closely and consult with the appropriate District Nursing Officer who has overall management control of nurse managers and nurses in the field of school health.

School Nurses Employed by the School Health Service

Peripatetic School Nurse

These nurses work with school doctors and are responsible with them for the health surveillance and health screening of a number of schools. Many district health authorities now follow the Court Committee recommendations and provide specifically named doctors and nurses for schools.

Comprehensive School Nurse

Large comprehensive schools may have one full or part-time school nurse or a nurse who works also with the infant and junior schools which feed into it. This system provides a greater continuity and availability of information and expertise and encourages the growth of teamwork and health education activities between education and health staff.

Special Schools

School nurses in special schools work mainly for one school; in addition to health surveillance, they undertake clinical nursing duties according to the needs of their pupils. They may be responsible for a nursing team which includes nursing auxiliaries, for whom they provide short in-service training programmes. They work closely with teachers, speech therapists, occupational therapists, physiotherapists and classroom ancillary workers.

Within their role, they develop a particular expertise which is indispensable to the care and education of many children. They develop and take part in programmes of independence training for children and they may also undertake home visiting and advise parents on the management and care of their child. They provide a link with hospital resources and may be required to run clinics in the school for a variety of hospital consultants.

As the process of educational integration evolves, these nurses should provide an invaluable advisory and support service for their colleagues in ordinary schools.

School/Clinic Nurses

In some health districts school nurses may be employed in a dual capacity. In addition to their work in schools, they may work in a wide variety of clinic settings; for example, Child Health, Enuresis, Ophthalmic, Audiology, Family Planning and Youth Advisory clinics.

School Nurse Administration

There are three main patterns of administration and accountability within the school nursing service:

1. School nurses work alongside their health visiting colleagues and are accountable to them.
2. School nurses work alongside their health visiting colleagues, and both are accountable to a nurse administrator who holds the Health Visiting Certificate.
3. School nurses may work alongside their health visiting colleagues, but be accountable to a school nurse administrator whose experience in school health work provides a valuable source of specialist information and support; because of the statutory requirement under the 1946 National Health Service Act for Health Visitors/School Nurses to hold the Health Visiting Certificate, this school nurse administrator will herself be accountable to a nursing officer who is so qualified.

Under the present system of training the career structure is virtually halted for the school nurse who does not hold the Health Visiting or District Nursing Certificate. Experience, performance, training and qualifications are all ingredients which are essential to the development of a career structure and in the case of the school nurse, the break in the training and qualification pattern is a stumbling block to progress. The key to its removal may well be found in the hands of the United Kingdom Central Council for Nursing, Midwifery and Health Visiting (UKCC), which carries overall responsibility for training policy and the development of nurse education.

Nurse Education, Registration and Professional Conduct

The Nurses, Midwives and Health Visitors Act 1979

In June 1969 a committee on nursing, chaired by Lord Briggs, was set up to review the role of the nurse and midwife in the hospital and community, and the education and training required for that role. The Briggs Report was presented to Parliament in October 1972. It recommended that there should be a single central body responsible for professional standards, education and discipline in nursing and midwifery; it proposed an initial foundation training course consisting of five modules which would lead to the Certificate of Nursing, and further modules which would lead to the Certificate of Higher Education and would take the place of the various post-basic nursing certificates. Although the recommendations were accepted in principle, resulting legislation did not appear until 1979 with the passing of the Nurses, Midwives and Health Visitors Act.

The UKCC

The Act provided for a United Kingdom structure of statutory bodies consisting of a Central Council (UKCC) and four National Boards of Nursing, Midwifery and Health Visiting (England, Northern Ireland, Scotland and Wales). They replaced the nine bodies which had been previously responsible for registration, education and training and professional conduct of all nurses, midwives and health visitors in the United Kingdom. The five bodies are independent, but work closely with each other. The UKCC's responsibilities include:

1. Policy and drafting of the rules to govern training, education, registration and professional conduct.
2. Maintenance of a single, up-to-date professional register, which is computer based and is designed to include all the qualifications approved by the UKCC.
3. The UKCC is also required to establish and improve standards of training and education in order to maintain professional competence.
4. The UKCC's Health Committee will enquire into all cases of alleged unfitness to practice due to ill-health, and the Professional Conduct Committee will adjudicate on cases of alleged misconduct referred to it by the National Boards. These two committees have the power to remove names from the register and to reinstate them.
5. Under EEC Regulations, the UKCC will assume responsibility for implementing its directives.

The UKCC has produced a Code of Professional Conduct which seeks to set guidelines for nurses, midwives and health visitors. (This can be obtained from the UKCC, 23 Portland Place, London W1N 3AF.)

The National Boards

The Boards are responsible for ensuring that the policies of the UKCC with respect to education and training are carried out. They provide or give approval to institutions to provide training and education courses for nurses, midwives and health visitors. The Boards also control examinations. They investigate cases of alleged misconduct and may refer such conduct to the UKCC Professional Conduct Committee.

Each National Board is required to establish Standing Committees for Midwifery and Finance; there is also a Joint Committee of the UKCC and the National Boards which is called the Health Visiting Joint Committee. The Act provides for persons who are not members of the Board to be appointed as members of a standing committee, and provides for a majority on the committee to be persons who have worked in the professional field with which it is primarily concerned. In this way it is hoped to safeguard the interests of special groups. The interests of school nurses are represented on the Health Visiting Joint Committee.

The Briggs Committee plan for an integrated system of nurse training and education has to some extent been overtaken by events. The European Community Regulations will now have to be taken into account. These require the mutual recognition of diplomas and qualifying certificates and the coordination of conditions of practice. The European Commission issues directives which have been negotiated by the Permanent Committee of Nurses; it will be the responsibility of the UKCC to implement these directives.

Under the original training plan, the learner would remain a health services employee with *apprentice status* and both employer and employee would be subject to existing Labour Laws. These include the Contract of Employment Act 1971, the Health and Safety at Work Act 1975 and the Employment Protection Act 1975. However, at the time of its proposal, the Royal College of Nursing—along with other professional bodies—was in favour of *student status* for learners, as this would allow for greater flexibility and freedom in the planning and implementation of training courses.

Given that a basic course leading to the Certificate of Nursing is established, modules leading to the Higher Certificate of Education could well include a compulsory basic community module, followed by further modules in health visiting, district nursing or school nursing. In this way a position of equal qualification would become available to school nurses.

The Social Services

> Personal Social Services, education, housing and the environmental services are, in some respects, as important for the health of children as the health services themselves.
>
> The Court Report, 1976

Social services may be statutory or voluntary. Like the health and education services, they grew and developed in a largely *ad hoc* manner and in response to the special needs thrown up by a changing society.

The present administrative structure of the personal social services was established under the Local Authority Social Services Act 1970. The Act aimed to provide a family-orientated pattern of social service by bringing together various functions of local authorities into a single Social Services Department. The responsibilities of these departments include the provision of a home help service and services for children and disabled, mentally ill and mentally handicapped and elderly people. The Departments are under the control of a Director of Social Services and their administration falls broadly into three main divisions.

Resource, Management and Development Services

In addition to Finance and Personnel Divisions, central resources will normally include departments of Information, Records and Statistics; developmental services may include research, planning and training facilities. The liaison, coordination and development of voluntary services may also be part of the central resource. Furthermore, authorities maintain separate specialist departments for the assessment of handicapping needs and the provision of aids, equipment and adaptations.

Field Work Services

The training of social workers is basically generic, and because of this, a teamwork plan has evolved which allows for specialisation within each group of social workers. Each Area Team aims to provide the knowledge and expertise required to meet the wide range of community need. It should also be a source of growth and support for the individual social worker.

The Central Council for Education and Training in Social Work was set up in 1971 as the body responsible for the promotion of training for all personal social services staff (CCETSW).

Social workers may be involved with children, their families and their schools in a number of different settings:

1. Day nurseries, special units, playgroups and opportunity groups, family welfare centres and nurture groups.
2. Child-minding and foster home services.
3. Children with hearing impairment, visual impairment or severe physical or mental handicapping conditions.
4. Children in Special Schools.
5. Family and Child Guidance Services.
6. School Psychological Services.
7. Children or parents in hospital.
8. Children at risk of non-accidental injury.
9. Children involved with court proceedings.
10. Liaison with residential child care workers and children's homes.

Residential and Child Care Services

Children may come into the care of the local authority on a temporary or long-term basis, and the arrangement may be voluntary or by court order. Court cases usually arise from matrimonial, wardship or criminal proceedings. Children may come into care because they have been abandoned or because, for reasons of illness or family breakdown, the children cannot be suitably provided for at home or with relatives.

Children may be committed to the care of the Local Authority in matrimonial or wardship proceedings where it seems that neither parent should be given custody. Court cases may also arise from offences committed by children; children under ten cannot be charged, but they may be taken into care.

Educational provision for these children will vary according to individual circumstances. Many will attend local schools in the normal way, some may attend day or boarding special schools with social work support and a very small number, because of the nature of their offences, may be educated in closed units. Within any of the institutional settings, whether children's homes, boarding schools or closed units, there exists a need to promote and develop positive health values and in this respect, the role of the locally based health visitor or school nurse has yet to be developed. Children in a relatively isolated or closed situation will often respond in a more creative way to those who do not appear to be directly involved with their destiny; and health-based discussions may well provide opportunities for children to air and review their opinions in an objective setting. Skilled and sensitive handling of the subject matter can provide the conditions of relaxation and eagerness to learn which may not be present on the more formal occasions.

Voluntary Organisations

The future of voluntary organisations was the subject of an enquiry by the Wolfenden Committee in 1978. The Committee described 'The Voluntary Movement' as a living thing:

> New organisations are formed to meet newly discerned needs. Others die. Yet others change their emphasis or venture into fresh fields. Relations with statutory authorities constantly change with new legislation or changes in administration, there is nothing static about the scene.

While many older organisations have become national institutions working for those in need, more recent years have seen the growth of national and self-help groups that are often increasingly specialised—for example, the Downs Children's Association and the National Deaf Children's Association. Some groups concentrate upon a particular aspect of help for a particular disability such as the production of talking books for the blind. Others concentrate on research or on social work and are instrumental in pioneering the provision of new and improved services to meet the changing needs.

Most voluntary bodies aim to secure a better public understanding of the special needs of certain groups within our society; in many cases they exert pressure upon central and local government for better public provision.

Work with the professionals in health, education and social services is a vital function of voluntary organisations. Care is not the prerogative of the caring professions—although they should be an exemplification of it. 'Living care' must constantly remain in touch with the reality of need, and it is this reality which voluntary organisations strive to present. Community care involves the community itself and therefore enhances the importance of health education and of the link between enlightened health attitudes and a thriving society.

The school health worker who sees herself not only as a professional, but also as a part of the total community dynamic, has much to gain, much to learn and much to give in partnership with the living voluntary movement.

Health Education

Health is a human value. CHILDREN LEARN WHAT THEY LIVE.

> If a child lives with criticism, she learns to condemn.
> If a child lives with hostility, he learns to fight.
> If a child lives with ridicule, she learns to be shy.
> If a child lives with shame, he learns to feel guilt.
> If a child lives with tolerance, she learns to be patient.
> If a child lives with encouragement, he learns confidence.
> If a child lives with praise, she learns to appreciate.
> If a child lives with fairness, he learns justice.
> If a child lives with security, she learns to have faith.
> If a child lives with approval, he learns to like himself.
> If a child lives with acceptance and friendship, he or she learns to find love in the world.
>
> (Poster issued by the Scottish Health Education Unit)

Modern health education has its focus in the Health Education Council. The Council was set up in 1968 as a limited company with funding from central government. Its stated objectives are:

1. To promote and encourage education and research in the science and art of healthy living and to promote the principles of hygiene and encourage the teaching thereof.
2. To assist and coordinate the work of all statutory bodies in carrying out their powers and duties under the Public Health Acts and other statutes, relating to the promotion or safeguarding of Public Health or the prevention or cure of disease in so far as such work comprises health education and propaganda.

Regional Health Authorities may choose to establish District Health Education Departments and LEAs may choose to appoint health advisors or health coordinators of health education. There is as yet no accepted pattern of provision.

An established Health Education Department can assist in the planning and promotion of health education programmes in schools and may provide the necessary resources. It may also act as a bridgehead between health and education authorities and assist in the planning of joint health teaching ventures.

3 Special Education

> If it can somehow be demonstrated that to educate is to care, and often to cure, then whatever the details of the future system, the battle will have been won.
>
> Mary Warnock, 1978

Whereas the development of mainstream education had its origins in religious motivation and charitable enterprise, special educational facilities grew primarily out of a recognition of social need. The prosperity and survival of the individual in society is linked with his ability to produce goods or provide services. In the 18th century, when child labour was the rule and the Poor Law provision offered only the barest means of subsistence, concern for the plight of the deaf and the blind, and later the physically handicapped, led to the establishment of protective institutions by charitable and individual enterprise. Their early objectives were to provide industrial and vocational training in order that certain categories of people might earn a living rather than be a charge on the State. The training was generally limited to these ends and provided on an all-age basis. Many of these institutions relied upon the profits of their workshops.

By 1870 when statutory provision of education for children between 5 and 10 years was enacted, these charitable institutions had begun to recognise and provide for the separate needs of children—although some handicapped children were educated in ordinary schools, often with no special assistance. Many of these charitable institutions offered a genuine educational element in addition to training. Because of their existence as a special educational resource, the right to special education became linked with separate categories of handicap; and as the quality and availability of education improved, state special schools were set up as additional or alternative provision.

By 1945, 11 separate categories were recognised. Children were perforce educated either in ordinary schools with no special rights to special educational treatment, or they were assigned to one of the categories. This meant that children with more than one handicap had to be arbitrarily separated out according to one of their disabilities. The deaf and blind child had to be educated as either deaf or blind, and the low IQ child with spina bifida had to be treated as either physically or mentally handicapped. Both professionals and parents became increasingly aware of the inadequacies of this system.

Parents themselves were better educated and they pressed for equality of educational opportunity for all their children. The wheel had turned a full circle. Special schools had set out to provide opportunities where previously none had existed, but in post-war Britain they were often regarded as second-best and outdated alternatives to the ordinary schools. In particular, their isolation and separation from mainstream education was increasingly questioned. The educational system which had developed was analogous with that of two children engaged in parallel play, but with increasing awareness of the advantages and difficulties confronting them as they were inexorably drawn towards imaginative and cooperative integration of their activities; successive acts of Parliament describe this progress.

1760–1870 Separate Categories of Special Philanthropic Interest

The Blind

The first school for the blind in Great Britain was established by Henry Dannett in Liverpool in 1791. It gave training in music and manual crafts to pupils of both sexes and all ages; other ventures followed, but it was not until 1835 that the Yorkshire School for the Blind offered a genuine educational element combined with industrial training, and set out to teach reading, writing and arithmetic. The first senior school for the blind was founded in 1866 at Worcester, and was named 'College for the Blind Sons of Gentlemen'.

The Deaf

The first schools for the deaf followed a similar pattern. In the early 1760s, Mr Thomas Braidwood opened an 'Academy for the Deaf and Dumb' in Edinburgh; it selected paying pupils to be taught to speak and read, and in 1792 the 'Asylum for the Support and Education of the Deaf and Dumb Children of the Poor' was opened in London under the direction of Mr Braidwood's nephew. As support for the venture grew, other Braidwood schools were opened, notably the branch at Margate. The education provided was extremely limited and subordinated to training for commercial ends. By 1870, schools had been founded in many places, including Donaldson's Hospital in Edinburgh (now Donaldson's School).

Physically Handicapped Children

The first separate provision was made in 1851 when the 'Cripples Home and Industrial School for Girls' was founded at Marylebone, and a similar 'Training Home for Crippled Boys' was set up in 1865 at Kensington. The children contributed to their own support by making goods for sale.

Mentally Handicapped Children

Before the middle of the 19th century, mentally handicapped children who required custodial care were committed to all-age workhouses and infirmaries. The first specific provision was the 'Asylum for Idiots' established at Highgate in 1847, and by 1870 there were five similar institutions, three of which offered some form of training and education. The children were later separated from the adults and followed a programme of simple teaching and manual work. By 1870 four separate categories of handicap were clearly discernible.

1870–1921 Centralisation of Responsibility

The Forster Education Act of 1870 established School Boards to provide elementary education for children from 5 to 10 years in areas where there were insufficient places in voluntary schools, and although school attendance was not compulsory, and the Act did not specifically include disabled children, the building of extra schools and increased availability of education led some authorities to provide special classes.

In 1874 the London School Board established a class for the deaf at a public elementary school and subsequently arranged for the teaching of blind children in its schools; but many boards made no such provision, and the physically and mentally handicapped children who attended elementary schools had to derive what benefit they could from ordinary classes.

As each successive Education Act conferred more statutory powers and duties upon education authorities, they also brought into focus the special educational needs of children unable to benefit from existing provision. The establishment of voluntary and independent schools continued alongside statutory provision and in some ways acted as a spur to further legislation.

As a result of a Royal Commission set up in 1886, the Elementary Education Blind and Deaf Children's Act 1893 was passed. It introduced the compulsory provision of education for the blind from 5 to 16 years and for the deaf from 7 to 16 years, and school boards were given the power to pay grants beyond the age of 16 years in order to establish pupils in a trade.

The Commission also considered the needs of mentally defective children and defined three categories: the Feebleminded, Imbeciles and Idiots. A further committee of enquiry envisaged that a medical officer appointed by the school board would decide whether a particular child would be educated in an ordinary school, in a special school or not at all. Sadly, these categories gave rise to considerable difficulties over the years. Many children were not presented for examination and assessment, as anxious parents lived in fear that their child might be certified as ineducable or might have to suffer the stigma attached to placement in a special school.

The Commission recommended that epileptic children should attend ordinary schools wherever possible, and that otherwise school authorities should provide for them in special residential schools or pay for their maintenance in a voluntary institution. The Education Act 1899, which followed as a result of this report, gave only permissive power in respect of mentally handicapped and epileptic children, and it was not until 1914 that these powers became a duty to provide special educational facilities for them.

1921–1944 Consolidation and Expansion of Categories

The Post-war Education Act 1921

This Act set out the statutory framework for special education and identified the compulsory provision which now extended to four categories of handicapped children. New stimulus continued to be provided by voluntary effort; trade schools, hospital and open air schools, and schools for physically handicapped children added to the available provision, although there were still many areas of deficiency.

Blind Children

The first nursery education for blind children was provided by the Royal National Institute for the Blind, who set up residential Sunshine Homes for Blind Babies; and in 1921 the Institute established Chorley Wood College as the first secondary school for blind girls.

Partially Sighted Children

Although the first provision for partially sighted children was made by London County Council in 1907, when myopic children in the Authority's blind schools were taught reading from large print rather than Braille, many authorities did not make adequate or suitable provision. As recently as 1934, the Committee of Enquiry into Problems relating to Partially Sighted Children found that many were being educated as though they were blind and recommended that as far as possible these children should be educated in classes within ordinary schools.

Deaf Children

The question of nursery education for deaf children could hardly arise at a time when formal education was not considered appropriate until the age of seven years. It was not until the Education Act (Deaf Children) 1937 that the statutory age of formal education was lowered to five years. The only school provision was in private schools, and the first grammar school provision was not made until 1946, when the Mary Hare Grammar School for the Deaf was founded for boys and girls.

Partially Deaf Children

The first special school for partially deaf children was set up by

Bristol Local Education Authority in 1906, and another was established in London shortly after; but as with the partially sighted, many children were either placed in ordinary schools where they were at a disadvantage, or in schools for the deaf where their residual hearing was insufficiently exploited. In 1938, the Committee of Enquiry into Problems relating to Children with Defective Hearing recommended additional help and support from visiting teachers for those attending ordinary schools, or attendance at special schools for the partially hearing. As a result of this report, some authorities set up special schools, but provision was less than adequate, and many children who would have benefited from local provision were sent to residential schools a long way from home and familiar surroundings.

Mentally Handicapped Children

In 1929 the Wood Committee on Mental Deficiency drew attention to the inadequacies in the assessment and provision for feebleminded children. It recommended that the system of certification should be abolished as the stigma attached to it led to many children not being ascertained as in need of special education. The Committee urged the development of more special schools and classes to cater for children who were retarded and failing to make progress in ordinary schools. The report also suggested that special provision should be regarded as a helpful variation of the ordinary school rather than something separate and humiliating.

Maladjusted Children

Maladjustment was not officially recognised as a form of handicap until the 1944 Education Act. At the end of the 19th century, University College (London) set up a psychological laboratory to study the behaviour of difficult children, and in 1893 the British Child Study Association was formed. London County Council appointed the first school psychologist (Cyril Burt) in 1913, and individual children could be referred to him by teachers, parents, doctors, magistrates and care workers. The treatment of children showing behavioural disturbances began to develop along multi-professional lines, and in 1927 the Child Guidance Council was formed. Hospitals and voluntary bodies set up clinics, and later some medical services established clinics which were, in part, maintained by education authorities. Until the 1944 Education Act, however, provision for these children was minimal, although some authorities paid for children to attend voluntary homes. In 1941 a Government Green Paper called 'Education after the War' recommended that maladjustment be recognised as a category of handicap, and that special schools should be set up on a regional basis.

Speech Defective, Delicate and Diabetic Children

By 1941 these children were recognised as requiring separate treatment; the Board of Education issued a Green Paper which recommended that legislation relating to the education of handicapped children be revised and updated. Support grew for the concept of a single framework of educational provision to include the special needs of handicapped children, and this found expression in the 1944 Education Act.

1944–1974 A Single Framework of Provision

The Butler Education Act 1944

The 1944 Act required LEAs, as part of their general duties, to ascertain special educational needs and make appropriate educational provision for all children from 5 years of age.

School Medical Service

Under the Act the service was renamed the School Health Service, and in 1945 the Regulations which followed the Act recognised 11 categories of educational provision. Maladjustment and Speech Defect were entirely new categories; Partial Blindness and Partial Deafness were extensions of existing categories; Delicate and Diabetic Children were now separated from the Physically Handicapped children.

The New Overall Structure

The Act established an overall structure of Primary, Secondary and Further Education for all children. In Scotland, the Education Act (Scotland) 1945 contained many similar provisions, but one important difference was the additional power to provide Child Guidance Services, to study backward and difficult children and to provide advice for parents and teachers. The Act recognised the importance of early discovery and treatment of educational disability, and the provision of educational psychologists in Scotland continued to grow at a greater rate than in England and Wales. Largely as a result of these initiatives, assessment by educational psychologists as an essential part of the multiprofessional team became established.

Ascertainment

Authorities were empowered to require parents to submit their children for medical examination subject to a lower age limit of 2 years, and the authorities were given discretionary powers to make educational provision from 2 to 5 years. Children who were ascertained as handicapped could now be educated in ordinary schools if this was considered appropriate to their needs; but there was little provision for parents' appeal against the authority's decision that a child required special educational treatment.

Mentally Handicapped Children

Certification of Defective Children was abolished, and children not considered capable of being educated in school were to be reported to the local authority for the purposes of the Mental Deficiency Act of 1913. The lower age of compulsory school attendance was reduced to 5 years and the right to remain beyond the age of 16 was established.

Developments after the 1944 Education Act

Deaf and Partially Hearing Children

Provision expanded from 1938, when the statutory age of school entry was lowered to 5 years. Following the report of the Lewis Committee of Enquiry in 1968, the need for early diagnosis of impaired hearing and for preschool advice and education was at last receiving recognition. Peripatetic teaching services were developed by many authorities, but not all. The report was mainly concerned with effective methods of deaf education, and urged the need for more research into the teaching of language. Units in ordinary schools were set up for partially hearing children. Not all of them were successful, however, in terms of the individual child, who had to grapple with problems of communication with teachers and classmates in order to participate fully in the life of the school.

In 1978 the Warnock Committee of Enquiry into Special Educational Needs recommended a single educational service for all hearing impaired children, to be organised on a regional basis and to include peripatetic teaching, special schools and units. It emphasised the importance of parents as partners in the education of their children and pointed to the continuing need for well planned evaluative research into methodology and the teaching of language. It also pointed out that there were many children in ordinary schools who suffer from temporary and episodic impairments of hearing which may lead to educational difficulties. Teachers need to be informed about children for whom this is a likely occurrence, and there should be a two way system of exchange of information between the teacher and the school nurse.

Blind and Partially Sighted Children

By 1955 blind and partially sighted children had been placed in separate schools, and some less seriously handicapped in these ways were being educated in ordinary schools. In 1972, the Vernon Committee of Enquiry into the Education of the Visually Handicapped made teacher training recommendations and urged greater flexibility of provision and placement. Although some education authorities appointed peripatetic teachers, many had little experience of working with very young children and parents.

The Royal National Institute for the Blind set up its own education advisory service for the parents of visually handicapped children, the advisors being trained teachers of the blind. The service works on a regional basis because the numbers of blind children are relatively small.

Mentally Handicapped Children

Concern regarding the exclusion of mentally handicapped children from school continued to grow, and in 1959 the Mental Health Act gave parents extra time in which to appeal against exclusion and the right to call for a review of placement after one year.

Parents were also given more information regarding the treatment, care and training of their child. This Act compelled more cooperation between local health and education authorities, but parents were still unhappy about the segregation and labelling of their children as ineducable. Finally in 1970 the Education (Handicapped Child) Act removed the power of the health authorities to provide training for these children, and the staff and buildings of Junior Training Centres were transferred to the education service.

Educationally Subnormal Children (Severe)—ESN(S)

Under the 1970 Education Act, *all* mentally handicapped children were now entitled to special education, and the new category of Educationally Subnormal (Severe) was formed. Many of the children had additional handicaps and required a wide variety of treatments and care.

Educationally Subnormal Children (Moderate)—ESN(M)

These children were seen as children of limited ability, and as children retarded by other conditions such as ill health, irregular attendance or lack of continuity in their education. Despite the continued increase in provision, large numbers of children remained in ordinary schools and were not being satisfactorily helped.

Although some education authorities appointed peripatetic teachers, many initiatives have come from parents and voluntary organisations, who have established self-help and support groups and have enlisted professional help and advice in playgroups, opportunity groups and parent workshops. Projects undertaken by the Hester Adrian Research Centre at Manchester University underlined the importance of early educational help and support for the families with handicapped children.

Physical Handicap and Epilepsy

The poor condition of many post-war schools, together with regulations which governed new school building, compelled the establishment of separate residential special schools to meet the need for increased provision. The purchase of large country mansions provided sufficient educational places, but at the expense of isolation for both children and staff. The need for special educational treatment became associated with placement in special schools. As the post-war difficulties were overcome, support grew for the principle of educating handicapped and non-handicapped children together by making more special provision in ordinary schools.

Delicate Children

Improvements in the standards of living and the provision of milk and school meals reduced the need for this provision. The majority of diabetic children were able to attend ordinary schools, but there was a continuing need to cater for children for whom life in an ordinary school was too strenuous. Asthmatic children, nervous children or those debilitated by poor environmental conditions benefited from this special provision.

The Education (Miscellaneous Provisions) Act 1953 permitted education authorities to use independent schools subject to the Minister's power of veto. Insufficiency of state provision compelled the use of independent schools, and in 1978 the Warnock Committee commented upon the difference between a school being regarded as efficient and one being regarded as suitable and made recommendations concerning appropriate access to these schools by the education authorities.

Maladjusted Children

Before the war, little provision was made for these children, but the post-war period saw an expansion in the quality and quantity of services. In 1955 the Underwood Committee of Enquiry on Maladjusted Children reported on the medical, social and educational problems relating to maladjusted children. It recommended that the maladjusted child should live at home wherever possible and attend an ordinary school or special class. It also recommended that there should be a comprehensive Child Guidance Service available to every local education authority and that this should involve the school psychological service, the school health service and child guidance clinics working in cooperation. Most local authorities accepted this pattern of provision and, in addition, hospitals were asked by the Minister of Health to cooperate with this service.

These recommendations highlighted the need for an increase of professional staff, and in 1968 the Summerfield Working Party urged the need for improved training for educational psychologists and a doubling of their numbers.

In Scotland the child guidance service developed much more rapidly, and valuable work was carried out in the field of assessment. In 1969 the Education (Scotland) Act made it a duty for Scottish authorities to provide a child guidance service, and the recommended ratio of educational psychologists to children was 1:3000. In England, on the other hand, the Summerfield Report recommended a ratio of 1:10 000.

In 1974 responsibility for the school health service passed from the local authorities to the newly created Area Health Authority: the Departments of Health and Social Security joined with the Department of Education and Science to produce a circular which recommended that the child guidance service should be based on a multiprofessional team in order to provide assessment, diagnosis, consultation and treatment, and to marshal other help and advice for the child and his family.

The Court Committee on Child Health Services, which reported in 1976, recommended that child guidance clinics and psychiatric hospitals be recognised as part of an integrated child and adolescent psychiatry service. Other far-reaching restructuring proposals were made which have not, as yet, been adopted. The Government did accept, however, the need for further progress and coordinated planning.

Children with Speech Defects

Provision for the needs of children who have severe communication difficulties is still in the process of development. Although Manchester Education Authority first employed a speech therapist in 1906, there was no recognised qualification for speech therapy until the College of Speech Therapists was formed in 1945 and became the recognised examining body. From then on, the treatment of children with speech defects increased, and in 1969 the Quirk Committee Report on Speech Therapy Services recommended expansion and unification of the service. Some authorities set up special units within ordinary schools, where speech therapists work alongside teachers. Development of provision has been hampered, however, by lack of qualified staff.

Children in Hospital

The National Health Service Act 1946 empowered regional hospital boards and teaching hospitals to use parts of hospital premises as special schools, by arrangement with local education authorities and voluntary bodies. Education in hospital presents the problem of combining continuity of teaching with the need for flexible programmes in a limited environment and subject to a wide variety of individual needs. The dictates of medical conditions and the treatments involved, the length of stay in hospital, and the wide age range of children create a particular challenge to teachers and caring staff. Many teachers of children in hospital lacked professional support and advice and easy access to educational resources. It was recognised that successful education of these children would depend on imaginative caring and close cooperation between hospital and teaching staff. The Warnock Committee proposed that education in hospital should be regarded as special educational provision, and that support for teaching staff should be provided by a Special Education Advisory and Support Service.

Community Homes and List D Schools

Under the Children and Young Persons Act of 1969, institutions for the maintenance and accommodation of children in the care of the local authority were designated Community Homes. They can be of three types: homes from which the majority of children attend local schools; homes with observation and assessment facilities; and homes with education on the premises.

The Warnock Report observed that the circumstances which may lead to children being taken into the care of the local authority are also likely to give rise to learning and behavioural difficulties. It recommended that teachers in these establishments should be in the service of the LEAs, and that regular support should be provided for them. The Committee observed that 'without good relations between community homes and schools there is a very real danger that the social and educational needs of the children concerned will be considered in isolation from each other and inadequately met'. As with hospital teachers, those based in community homes may also suffer the same professional isolation and lack of educational resource and support.

In Scotland broadly similar provisions are in force. Responsibility for the former remand and approved schools was transferred to social work departments in 1971 and this included responsibility for educational provision. These schools are known as List D Schools.

Nursery Education

The growth of home teaching and nursery provision has been slow. The 1944 Education Act gave permissive powers to provide nursery education from 2 years, but financial constraints and the post-war pressures to provide the ordinary and special education services limited the growth of nursery education, although the need was generally recognised.

The Warnock Committee recommended a substantial increase of nursery provision; this would correspondingly increase the educational opportunities for children with special needs. The Committee welcomed the involvement of parents and supported the need for a flexible range of provision which would include playgroups, opportunity groups and day nurseries in addition to nursery schools, classes and special units, and it suggested experimentation with mobile caravans to meet the needs of rural areas. It drew attention to the fact that many children suffer from more than one handicap and urged the development of multi-professional teams to work with members of the proposed new Special Education Advisory and Support Service. It also recommended the establishment of a comprehensive peripatetic teaching service which would cater, wherever possible, exclusively for children with disabilities or significant difficulties below school age and which would cover every type of disability or disorder. Within it there would be scope for specialisation, and children with sensory disabilities would be visited by teachers with related expertise. Teachers would need to have insight into the needs of parents and to cooperate closely with other professionals.

Progress Towards an Integrated Educational System

The 1944 Education Act went some way towards ensuring that within the statutory age limits there would be a sufficiency of provision for handicapped children with special needs—needs being defined in terms of specific categories of handicap.

It was envisaged that many handicapped children would be retained in ordinary schools, but the Act lacked the machinery to make this a practical possibility. Not only was there a dearth of adequately trained teachers and other professional staff, but there was a lack of suitable school buildings. Furthermore, ascertainment of special need was based on compulsory medical examination, which inevitably assigned a child to one of the 11 defined categories of handicap for which the law required education in special schools. This perpetuated and encouraged the growth of separate provision for separate groups of children, and set them apart from mainstream education. While this system provided opportunities for learning experience from which the child might otherwise have been debarred, it ignored his need to interact with all manner of other children and to find his own identity among his peers.

There was also a great increase in the knowledge and understanding of the developmental progress of children and its relevance to their education. It was recognised that learning handicap for the individual child could arise from a wide variety of social or emotional difficulties and could be of a permanent or temporary nature. Moreover there was not necessarily any direct relationship between medical disability and special educational need. Within ordinary schools there were many children who needed special help, and education authorities developed various forms of 'remedial education'.

Isle of Wight Study

The needs of individual children began to receive increasing attention. In 1964–65 a study of the incidence of intellectual and educational retardation, psychiatric disorder and physical handicap was carried out on the Isle of Wight. It covered children between 9 and 11 years, and from it came the prediction that at any one time approximately one child in six is likely to require special educational provision for varying periods of time.

Assessment

Support for integration grew and was given extra momentum in 1970 when the Education Department assumed responsibility for the education of all mentally handicapped children of school age.

Formal assessment procedures came under review as it was increasingly appreciated that handicaps overlap and are interrelated and that the needs of children with similar handicaps may be different. The success of education for the individual child could depend upon the accuracy of those who assess his needs. In 1975 the Department of Education issued a circular which emphasised the multiprofessional character of the procedures and urged the value of informality and parental participation. At the same time it introduced an improved set of forms for recording the educational, medical, psychological and other data needed to decide upon the special educational needs of the child. It also provided a summary sheet for use during assessment, placement and review.

The Court Committee

In 1974 responsibility for the school health service was transferred from the LEAs to the new Area Health Authorities, and at this time a Committee of Enquiry had been set up under the chairmanship of Professor Donald Court to review the child health services. It subsequently produced the report which was called *Fit for the Future*.

The Warnock Committee 1974–78

It was in this climate of opinion that the Committee of Enquiry into Special Educational Needs was set up under the chairmanship of Mrs Mary Warnock. Before the Committee reported in 1978, the Education Act of 1976 provided the Secretary of State with powers to compel reorganisation of secondary schools on comprehensive lines. Section 10 of the Act required LEAs to arrange for special education of all handicapped pupils to be given in county or voluntary schools, except where this was impractical, incompatible with efficient instruction, or unreasonably expensive. This part of the Act was not implemented, however, as the Secretary of State decided to await the findings of the Warnock Committee.

Special Educational Needs—The Warnock Report

The remit of the Warnock Committee was:

> To review educational provision in England, Scotland and Wales for children and young people handicapped by disabilities of body or mind, taking into account the medical aspects of their needs, together with arrangements to prepare them for entry into employment, to consider the most effective resources for these purposes, and to make recommendations.
>
> The Warnock Report, 1978

This was the first Government committee to review the educational provision for all handicapped children, whatever their handicap. It was clear from the Isle of Wight and other studies that the whole spectrum of educational need could not be met by the prevailing system of categorisation, because such a system was based more on medical diagnosis than on an adequate assessment of a child's educational needs.

The Committee maintained that education was concerned with the quality of living, and that, as such, education is a good to which we all have a right, regardless of our environment, status or handicap. The long term goals of education were defined as twofold:

> First, to enlarge a child's knowledge, experience and imaginative understanding and thus his awareness of moral values and capacity for enjoyment; and second, to enable him to enter the world after formal education is over as an active participant in society and a responsible contributor to it, capable of achieving as much independence as possible.

> The educational needs of every child are determined in relation to these goals. We are fully aware that for some children these goals can be approached only by minute, though for them, highly significant steps, while the second may never be achieved. But this does not entail that for these children the goals are different. The purpose of education for all children is the same; the goals are the same; but the help that individual children need in progressing towards them will be different.

The Committee was therefore concerned with the quality of educational provision and sought to establish a statutory framework which would include effective assessment of educational need, a flexible range of provision and appropriate training facilities for teachers and other professional staff.

It proposed that statutory categorisation of handicapped pupils be abolished, and that provision of special educational treatment be related to a child's individual needs as distinct from his disability. In order to safeguard the interests of children with severe, complex and long-term difficulties and disabilities, there should be a system of recording the special needs of those children who were judged to require provision not generally available in ordinary schools. This record would provide a detailed profile of their needs and be based on consultation with their parents and the findings of a multiprofessional team.

Out of its proposals the Committee identified three areas of priority:

1. the needs of children under five years.
2. basic and post-basic training.
3. education from 16 years.

With respect to children under 5 years of age, the report stated that:

> For some children ... education must start early and continue at home and at school and into adult life. Parents as much as teachers must see themselves as active educators, and both parents and teachers may need the help of other professionals in their endeavours. At every stage of our discussion the contribution of parents and non-teacher professionals to the education of the child has been at the front of our minds.

This is perhaps one of the most significant statements of the report; not only does it recognise the vital importance of good parenting and its effect upon the education of the child, but it acknowledges the need for support, advice and practical help for the parents themselves. When we consider that until 1970 some severely handicapped children were not thought capable of benefiting from educational services, this constitutes a crucial shift of emphasis which has far-reaching implications for all the professional services involved with the wellbeing of children and their families. It concerns itself not only with care, education and treatment outside the home, but with the quality of the environment into which a child is born, and with the need to provide the necessary support and help from birth as part of the child's special educational provision. For many five year old children, education in this sense is already five years too late. The better the provision we make for children under five, the better will these children be able to benefit from formal education in ordinary schools; more will be able to accept and be happy with this environment, and the gaps in development and experience will not be too great for teachers to respond to, and make provision for, in the ordinary school setting.

Parental Support: the *Named Person*

The special needs of the young handicapped child and his family are wide-ranging, and while many agencies are involved with helping these families, health visitors are the only automatic contact with all families. From the moment of diagnosis or discovery, almost all parents of handicapped children will need support, counselling, practical advice and information—and a single point of contact through which these can be obtained. A research project on services for these parents revealed a number of weaknesses and lack of resources in some areas (Laing, 1979). It also revealed that even where the levels of provision were satisfactory, parents were often unable to make the best use of them because there was no single source of information and communication between the different agencies was poor.

The Committee recommended that there should be a *Named Person* to whom the parent could turn for advice; this person would act as a general resource or a sort of 'Alpine Guide'. Because of her automatic contact with all families, the health visitor would fulfil this role in the first instance, although she might properly relinquish the responsibility to another worker if this proved to be more appropriate or more helpful.

Interprofessional Training

Both the Court and Warnock Reports urged the need for interprofessional training at local and national levels in order to improve the quality of advice and expertise available to parents, particularly in their own homes. Counselling skills needed to be linked with a greater knowledge of child development and the problems of management which are likely to arise in families with handicapped children.

Coordination and Planning of Services

Joint Consultative Committees were established in 1972 to advise health, education and social services in the planning, provision and coordination of arrangements to meet the needs of, among others, children and young people with disabilities and significant disabilities. The Warnock Committee regarded their work as vital for the development of services and supported the view that the establishment of District Handicap Teams could provide a professional link for both the *Named Person* and the family.

It would be impossible to over-emphasise the importance of early discovery and assessment of any difficulties and handicapping conditions which might be likely to affect the child's educational progress. Because of their early contact with families and their training in appreciating the educational significance of their observations, health visitors are particularly well placed not only to help and advise parents, but also to marshal additional resources. Their records should be designed to facilitate maximum use of their observations, and they need to maintain close contact with the education service and to foster their working relationships with other professionals, so that early educational opportunities are not wasted.

In the past some parents have complained of delay in diagnosis and assessment of needs. It is essential that effective systems of communication are established between hospitals, community health and local authority services to minimise delays and provide information for parents.

Within the Schools

The Committee envisaged a single framework of educational provision, within which there would be a system of assessment which aimed to identify children who needed additional or supplementary help in order to overcome their educational difficulties whatever they might be. Special needs could require:

1. the provision of special means of access to the curriculum through special equipment, facilities or resources, modification of the physical environment, or specialist teaching techniques.
2. the provision of a special or modified curriculum.
3. particular attention to the emotional climate or social structure in which education takes place.

Special education would encompass this whole range of need wherever it was provided and whether it was long-term or short-term or on a full time or part time basis. It was estimated that at any one time as many as one in six children might require some form of special educational provision. Within this group there would be many children whose needs could be met with appropriate support in the ordinary school. For children with severe or complex difficulties, however, a multiprofessional team would prepare a profile of the child's needs and the type of special education required. This would be embodied in a statement which would be available to parents and would oblige the local education authority to make suitable provision.

Although suitable provision could be made in non-maintained or independent schools as an alternative to local authority provision, these schools should be subject to regulations for approval laid down by the Secretary of State.

Transition from School to Adult Life

The needs of young people over the age of 16 were of great concern. Careers officers should be involved in assessment of future prospects at least two years before school leaving. Furthermore, there should be access to sixth forms and colleges, where appropriate support should be made available to enable handicapped students to attend ordinary courses of further education. For some, the prospect of life without employment raised the problem of how to achieve significant living without work: schools should give more help in developing vocational interests and social competence and suitable courses and special units should be developed in colleges of further education.

Teacher Training

The Committee envisaged that increasing numbers of children with special needs would profit from education in ordinary schools. Its main thrust, however, was to ensure the quality of provision wherever education took place. It therefore regarded advances in teacher training as essential to the progressive integration into ordinary schools of more children with disabilities. It recommended that a special educational element should be included in all initial teacher training courses, and that the teaching of child development should take account of different patterns and rates of development, the effects of common disabilities, and other factors whch might affect or hamper learning. Short in-service courses covering the same ground should be provided for the great majority of serving teachers. There should also be a range of special education qualifications in order to ensure adequate advice and support for all people involved with the special needs of children. Similar training should be provided for teachers in colleges of further education.

This was the overall plan. It was as though the concept of education had progressed from magic lantern shows, silent movies and talkies, to three dimension with wide-screen presentation. Because of its all-embracing view of the child and his needs, there were recommendations concerning the role and provision of health and personal social services, and the important contributions which could be made by other workers, independent schools and voluntary bodies.

Court, Warnock and Health Service

Both the Court and Warnock Committees recognised the need for a strong, effective and well-managed health service with adequate resources and well-trained personnel. The Court Report identified a body of knowledge and practice, both therapeutic and practical, which could be defined as educational medicine.

> The extent to which a child is able to benefit from education is directly related to how far his health and normal development have been promoted. The child health and education services must see themselves as engaged to a large extent upon different aspects of a

> common task and our proposals require the closest cooperation between them.
>
> The Court Report, 1976

Members of both committees were able to meet and discuss their common interests before the Court Committee reported in December 1976.

Fit for the Future—the Court Report on Child Health Services

The report proposed a reorganised structure of child health services based on comprehensive primary care linked with consultant support and hospital care. It envisaged family doctors and health visitors with special training in preventive and curative paediatrics. Health visitors would combine preventive and curative responsibility for children and be assisted by specially trained child health nurses and school nurses. In each health district, there would be at least one consultant community paediatrician, and a multiprofessional District Handicap Team to provide a special diagnostic, assessment and treatment service for handicapped children.

In the event the main proposal for a reorganised structure of paediatric services was not implemented, but the very thorough survey of child health services identified needs which were not being met. Many of the proposals to extend or improve existing practice have since been adopted by health authorities.

Court and Education

The primary objectives of the school health service in relation to the education of children and support of the schools and the local education authority were as follows:

1. To promote the understanding and practice of child health and paediatrics in relation to the process of learning.
2. To provide a continuing service of health surveillance and medical protection throughout the years of childhood and adolescence.
3. To recognise and ensure the proper management of what may broadly be described as medical, surgical and neurodevelopmental disorders in so far as they may influence, directly or indirectly, the child's learning and social development, particularly at school but also at home.
4. To ensure that parents and teachers are aware of the presence of such disorders and of their significance for the child's education and care.
5. To give advice and services to the local education authority, as required in the Education Act and the National Health Service Reorganisation Act.

It is interesting to compare the recommendations of these two committees to see what is common to both and what additions each thought necessary to their overall plans. Together they form a very comprehensive body of advice for further development.

Common Themes from the Reports

Parents: The need to provide professional advice, support and information concerning their children, their health and education, and to treat parents as partners and participants in the process of assessment and decision-making. Parents should have a known and readily available point of contact to facilitate advice and access to appropriate services.

Under Fives: A basic programme of health surveillance should be offered for all children, and an educational contribution should be available from birth should it be appropriate to the needs of the child and his family.

Coordination: Services should be planned and coordinated by Joint Consultative Committees, to facilitate adequate and efficient provision; and District Handicap Teams should be established to provide a coordinated service with multiprofessional input.

Training: There should be appropriate basic and post-basic training courses for teachers, doctors and nurses, and additional interprofessional courses should be established.

Information and Records: Health records should be kept for all children, and relevant information made available to education services; 10(B)M forms which provide teachers with advice and basic health information should be accessible and properly maintained. Personal and sensitive information should be under the control of the head teacher.

Practice and Provision: There should be a named school nurse and a named school doctor for every school, and health authorities should make adequate resources available to promote effective child health services in ordinary and special schools.

Research Centre: There should be regional interprofessional centres for research and information.

Many of these recommendations have the valuable purpose of encouraging the spread of existing good practice and improved cooperation and do not require significant additional resources.

Although the economic situation precluded large-scale expenditure, the impetus for improved provision had now been set in motion. This is reflected in the provisions of the 1981 Education Act.

The 1981 Education Act

The Act came into force from September 1982, and was passed as a direct response to the Warnock Report. Government money was not available to implement all its recommendations; however, the legislation is designed to provide the machinery for change.

It required local education authorities to review their educational provision and placed a duty upon them to identify educational need and to provide assessment on a multiprofessional basis. It strengthened the rights of parents and reaffirmed the Education Act 1976 which stated that wherever possible children should be educated in ordinary schools, subject to certain conditions.

The Act defines special educational need as a learning difficulty which calls for special educational provision, either:

1. because the child suffers from a disability which prevents or hinders him from making use of the educational facilities provided.
2. because he has greater difficulty in learning than the majority of children.
3. because in the case of a child under five, he has special educational needs if it is thought likely that he will fall into either of these two categories after he reaches the age of five.

Special Provision in Ordinary Schools

When a local education authority arranges special provision for a child, the 1981 Act reaffirms the conditions laid down in the 1976 Act—that taking into account the views of his parents, the child should be educated in an ordinary school provided:

1. he can receive the special education he requires without detriment to other children with whom he is being educated.
2. that this is compatible with an efficient use of educational resources.

It is the duty of the authority to enable the child to engage in as many of the school activities as is reasonably possible.

This definition of special educational need, and the way in which provision shall be made, highlights a series of important aspects which directly affect the responsibilities of health authorities, and their delivery of services to parents, and to education departments.

Identification of Needs

Because of the services that they provide, the health authorities have a clear responsibility to initiate the identification of special educational need and to inform parents of their intention to do so. In the case of a child under two years of age, the LEA may, with the consent of the parent, make an assessment of the child's educational needs and may record the needs of such children and make arrangements for their education.

Assessments

In their assessments, the LEA must seek appropriate advice (medical, social, psychological and other) and take into account any representations and evidence submitted to them, in order to ensure that educational provision is made in the light of all the available information, including the wishes of the parents.

All the nursing reports concerning the child will be coordinated by the health authority's designated nurse, who will provide liaison and a point of contact for the LEA. The designated nurse could be the Director of Community Nursing Services, or a nurse with special responsibilities for children with handicapping conditions.

Because of the multiprofessional nature of the assessment, some authorities have reviewed their Joint Consultative machinery and have established a children's coordinating committee. This committee would be responsible for the nomination of a key worker to marshal and coordinate the resources that are required and to provide support and information for parents.

The LEA has a duty to arrange assessments: parents themselves may request that an assessment of their child's needs be made.

In school, identification and requests for assessments will come mainly from teachers, but they may also be initiated by medical or nursing staff, child guidance clinics, psychologists, therapists and others.

Assessment Procedure

When a LEA proposes to make an assessment of educational need, it must inform the parents in writing of its intention, giving the name of an officer from whom more information can be obtained, outlining the procedure to be followed and informing the parents of their right to make representations and submit evidence. The parents also have a right to be present at the examination of their child.

If, as a result of the assessment, the authority decides against special educational provision, the parent may appeal to the Secretary of State, who may advise the authority to reconsider its decision.

Statement of Educational Needs

If, as a result of assessment, special educational provision is recommended, again parents have the right of appeal, and the educational authority must provide a Statement of Educational Needs. The parents have a right to see this statement, in order to assure themselves that the right decisions are being made in the interests of their child.

For those who submit reports to the assessment team, this raises the importance of careful and accurate recording of information, which may be used when decisions are made regarding the educational provision for children.

Statements must be reviewed on at least an annual basis and must be maintained and amended appropriately, in order to ensure that the provision continues to be that which is most suited to the needs of the child.

In addition to these safeguards, the Secretary of State may make regulations concerning assessments, particularly the way in which they are conducted and their review. He could, for instance, call for more frequent reviews in the case of particular children.

These are the main provisions of the Act as they affect the nursing services. It is one thing to pass an Act, but it is another to see that it is efficiently implemented. The Act is designed in a way which will allow LEAs maximum flexibility in their arrangements. Furthermore, each authority, having reviewed its provision and resources, is required to formulate a long-term plan which accords with the spirit of the Act.

Obviously the preparation of the plan, the quality of multidisciplinary cooperation and the availability of resources are of paramount importance, because the care of children will always be a multidisciplinary responsibility. The framework provides the setting within which people work together in the interests of children; the quality of education depends essentially upon their skill and insight, backed by adequate resources, efficiently deployed.

For the disabled child, learning to live on his own terms and to cope with his disability is a vital part of his education, without which he cannot prosper or make his full contribution to society. The more nearly he approaches his own potential for independence, the more effective will his education have become.

4 The Stance

Health workers in schools do not share a common role; they have job descriptions that differ from district to district, varied equipment and a wide range of expectations from their job. The role of the school health worker is still largely unmapped and ill defined; nevertheless, her stance can be given a more specific description.

What is meant by 'stance'? This is an ancient term which stems from Old French and Italian. It is defined in the *Oxford English Dictionary* as the position taken in preparation for action. It is the standpoint from which you work, at which you are seen and by which you are understood. It derives from 'stanza', a station or abode, and so it includes the attitudes, values and tastes of the occupier. It is that by which a person is identified, on which others will base their judgements, and through which they will take their lead towards yourself and, on occasion, towards the children you care for. So it is worth looking at closely.

It is particularly important that the person working in an educational establishment as the representative of health, should be seen by those trained in other disciplines to have sound attitudes towards child-care; the non-trained aides (NTA) and other ancillaries in the classroom, as well as the dinner ladies and the other staff concerned with upkeep and cooking, will look to the health worker for an example of how to respond to the children. An attitude is defined as the atmosphere created by a person's outlook or in the case of the *Concise Oxford Dictionary*, as 'settled behaviour, including opinion; settled mode of thinking'. If an attitude is to be settled and to influence others in settling theirs, it must grow out of positive thinking, to avoid giving the impression of inconsistency or confusion. Often those staff who are concerned with children's health are in an isolated position. Therefore, it is as necessary for them to be as sure of their value base as they are of their knowledge base. In the maze of ideas that are being explored today, especially those that concern health, education and morality, she will need to recognise and establish her own personal and professional stance.

This chapter will present the flavour of the living kernels of ideas, rather than a series of dried nutshells. It will concentrate on those ingredients of stance that are applicable to the working life of people who care for children's health in school (Fig. 4.1).

The personal foundation of beliefs about

Health
Illness and impairment
Dependence, independence and interdependence
Help
Risk-taking and control

are the bricks which constitute the framework
for the life and the work of the health worker

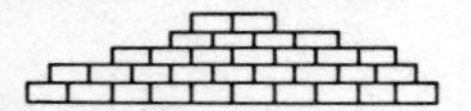

There are several models in health care. The model
she chooses will form the foundation from which she works

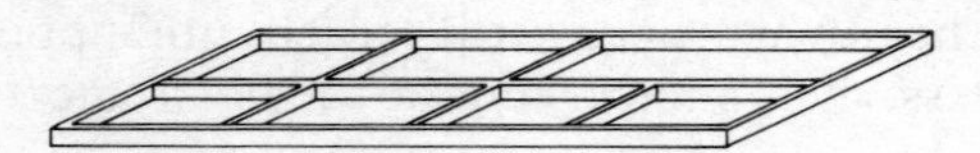

This foundation will determine how she

Interprets models of care
Translates issues of authority, autonomy and accountability
Values continuing education for herself
Values health education in school
Searches for health needs

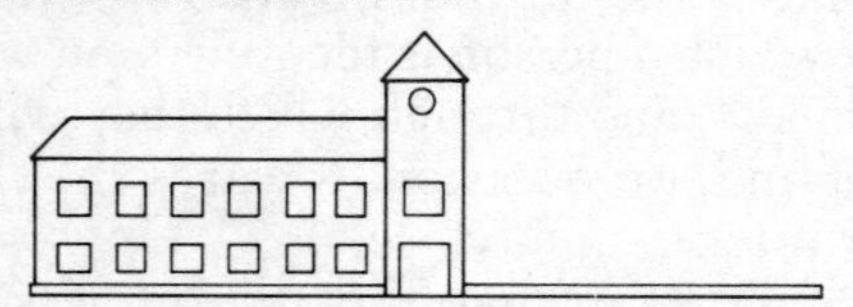

The stance will also determine how she
mobilises resources outside the school

Interdisciplinary opportunities
Tools provided by the state
Wellness facilities within the community

These will determine how she creates the whole structure
within which the child is to grow

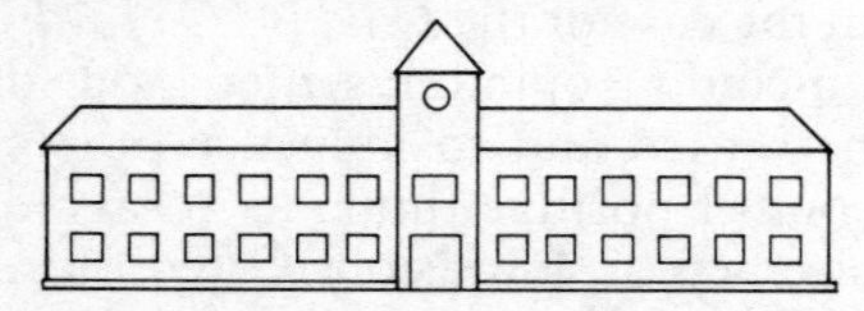

All of which are part of a holistic concept of life

Fig. 4.1 The stance of the health care worker in school.

The Value Base

Each health care worker has personal convictions about health, disease, impairment, dependence, help, coping with risk and the need for control.

Concepts of Health

Health might seem like a simple concept to those who accept their own idea as being universal, but in fact over the years and across cultures, there have been many different definitions of health. In earlier days, the idea of health was inextricably bound up with fears of the unknown—with fate, the stars and with forces beyond human control. In medieval times, good health was related to righteousness and bad health was seen as a just punishment for evil-doing.

In China health is seen as a balancing act between positive and negative forces—the yin and the yang. Chinese folk physicians are paid to keep their patients well; when their patients fall ill, their payments cease. By contrast, people who believe in voodoo can become fatally ill if they think that a spell has been cast upon them. Recently the power of expectation has been reversed—instead of expecting bad things to happen to the sick, in the West people who are ill expect benefits.

There are at least three distinct models of health found in our culture today: curative (the removal of disease) preventive (the prevention of illness), and educative and supportive (the promotion of wholeness).

The relationship between the attitude held by the carer and the expectation of the person who is cared for is such that the one seeks out the other and thereby their beliefs are confirmed. The health worker can similarly perpetuate desirable or undesirable health concepts in the impressionable children around her, depending upon her stance.

The notion of health as a static, achievable state is unrealistic. It is more helpful to think of health as a continuous developing process. It is a matter of adapting to the changing demands of being alive and of finding meanings which grow out of different challenges. It is an unravelling of the capabilities of the individual as he develops his optimum well-being. Life never stands still and it is in this developing process that the skills and values of the health worker can be an essential contribution.

The word 'health' itself derives from a stem common to several early European languages, including Anglo-Saxon. This same stem grew into many associated ideas, such as:

health — wholeness
heal — make whole
hale — sound in body and mind
hail — welcome, glad to see you
holy — belonging to God
holiday — relaxation

It is increasingly realised today that all these ideas play a part in the making of a truly well person. This interrelatedness can also be seen from the likely responses to the question—'are you feeling better?'—a question that can validly be interpreted in several ways.

- Yes I feel better, my headache has gone away (physical relief).
- Yes, I feel better, now the problem has been explained I can finish my homework (intellectual relief).
- Yes, I feel better because I understand why my mother was angry (reflection).
- Yes, I feel better since I kicked a goal myself (emotional relief).
- Yes, I feel better now I've given back the book I stole from my friend (moral relief).
- Yes, I feel better after that break away from it all (social relief).
- Yes, I feel better—I did it all by myself (expression of self-worth).

Concepts of Disease

Conversely, the many conditions in which a person is not at ease with his mind or body can be termed Dis–ease. The prefix 'dis–' or 'dys–' implies lack of or 'difficulty with', for example, discomfort, dishonesty, disability, dystrophy and dysfunction. Seen in this light, there are again several models of differing concepts of disease. In hospital, which is the primary base of all medical training, the diagnosis and treatment of organs and systems that are disordered is reasonably straightforward. Often measures can be taken to restore the diseased part to its fullest potential. Disease is thought of as a temporary affliction, in a particular area, which can generally be remedied or at least alleviated by the application of scientific methods. In hospitals, disease is thought to be caused by verifiable pathogens, and the principles of treatment that are appropriate to such conditions can also be applied to other presenting symptoms of disease. These principles involve the separating out of a specific cause by scientific enquiry and the mobilisation of the needed remedies (Table 4.1). There is not necessarily a link progressing between these tiers, and they are neither divisible nor distinct. The common cold may derive from all three aspects, whereas a severe case of meningitis may be confined to one. This model demonstrates the many factors which can be part of the aetiology of disease and the consequent variation in attitudes which are held by different people in the health services. Similarly, they place differing emphasis into the tiers, according to their degree of recognition of the process of disease.

Concepts of Illness and Impairment

Between these extremes of total wholeness and disease, there lies a range of conditions covered by the terms 'illness' and 'impairment'. Academic attempts to define these four states have proved

Table 4.1
Concepts of Disease

Separated scientific concept of disorder: biological dysfunction caused by pathogens, congenital malformation, endocrine disturbance, misuse of intake, accidental or intended violence *aggravated by* *Whole person concept of disorder:* disharmony of biopsychosocial balance breakdown in the interdependence of body/mind/spirit/soma failure of usual coping ability/behaviour dissatisfaction in personal relationships *aggravated by* *Environmental concept of disorder:* factors in the environment which predispose to imbalance, e.g. water or air pollution, bad housing or work conditions, private or public ignorance of hygiene; misuse of resources; political inappropriateness; purpose/direction in life felt to be lacking.

unsatisfactory. For our purpose here, illness and impairment apply to conditions that are less severe than disease and disability and have less effect—at least objectively—on the life-style of the individual.

Each person wants to be as far from death and as near to the goal of perfect health as his life-style permits. However, there is the grey area between these two polarities in which some discomfort is tolerated. How well it is tolerated, and for how long it is tolerated, depends upon each individual's expectancy of health and illness, and the expectations of those around him.

$$\text{Physical Death} \rightarrow \left\{ \begin{array}{c} \text{Desired direction} \\ \rightarrow \rightarrow \rightarrow \rightarrow \rightarrow \rightarrow \rightarrow \\ \text{Tolerated grey area} \end{array} \right\} \rightarrow \text{Perfect Health}$$

Where a person sees himself on this continuum, and where those nearest to him see him, may be different from where the health professional sees him. There is no exact spot to place him. The child, lacking experience with which to compare his condition, will lean heavily on the reaction of others to judge where his discomfort lies and how he should deal with it.

The point at which a person decides that his discomfort is more than he wants to put up with, or more than those near him want to manage, also varies. It is normal illness behaviour for most of the people not to go to the doctor for most of their complaints most of the time, and up to 90% of episodes that are self-identified as illness are entirely self-managed. This, in part, indicates the complex interactions between the physical and mental states of the individual and the social and working conditions in which he lives. Another factor may be a feeling that transferring authority over his body to others undermines his power to look after himself. Some, no doubt, welcome this transfer of responsibility. In either case, when a person becomes a patient, it is an event of considerable significance. The trigger which accelerates the action of going to the doctor is usually advice from an outside source. It may be a relative or a neighbour, but frequently it is the words of a nurse or health worker which starts the train of events. It must, therefore, be remembered that professional diagnosis itself can turn a situation that has been one of diffuse social and mental dissatisfaction into the full sickness process.

The Significance of the Stance of the Health Worker

Health personnel usually become involved with the grey area of bodily discomfort or emotional unease. They have the considerable responsibility of guiding the child's response to health and impairment while his attitudes are still being formed. It could be argued that the future citizen's attitudes towards self-responsibility, wholeness and sickness start at the level of the informal interaction at school. The stance of the health worker will affect the inexperienced child perhaps for life, however casual the contact may appear. Her awareness of this potential will dictate how she reacts to the child's presenting complaints. The following considerations may be useful in this context:

- The body, left to its own devices and given proper rest, warmth and nourishment, tends to be self-healing. Confidence in this natural power can either be strengthened or undermined by the response of the professional towards childish complaints. Will informed counselling be sufficient to counteract this immediate health hazard? Or are further scientific investigations needed?
- Much illness is self-limiting. What are the aims of intervention? To alleviate discomfort? To allay anxiety? To speed the healing process? Or just to be the line of least resistance to the child's or parents' demands?
- A child's discomfort canot be judged by any objective standards. The fear of exposure in front of classmates can be demeaning—whether it is caused by an epileptic seizure or by a forced admission of poverty. Disadvantages can be visible, such as a facial strawberry mark, or invisible such as enuresis, but either type can affect personality development, individual self-worth and even job prospects. The health worker who offers respect to every child whatever his physical or mental state will go far in building up his personal coping powers.

The Child and Physical Pain

The health worker in school will come into daily contact with the child's attitude to discomfort and pain. Adults can and do manipulate others to meet their demands by claiming attention for their physical needs. Children learn this technique of demanding very aptly, but they are seldom sufficiently adept at social skills actually to invent a need. The symptoms of the need may be misinterpreted—a complaint of a headache may really mean that the parents have had a row over breakfast—but the underlying need for help is genuine. Many children are unable to express their anxieties verbally, even to themselves, and far less to a powerful adult; so emotional and mental pain will often be subconsciously translated into a physical pain. Children are less keen than adults to appear to be deviant from their peers; so although one child may present with a stomach ache every time there is work to be done on the ropes in the gym, it will not be because he *wants not* to be able to handle them, or that he is deliberately lazy or cowardly. Without doubt every child *wants* to be as clever and as able as the best of his peers, so a need to do better is never concocted or artificial. Although the remedy may bring relief, it will also bring further anxiety because his inadequacy will be made more obvious to all. A complaining child always has a basis of complaint, although it may not be the same basis that he describes. He has not had the years of conditioning in which to develop antisocial subterfuge. It is easy to expect adult standards of dissimulation in children, but it is damaging to do so. The health worker should tend towards ready acceptance of each child's claim of need, while understanding that the real problem to be tackled may be something other than the one of which the child is complaining.

Dependence and Independence

Illness highlights the issues of role allocation, transfer of responsibility, the giving and receiving of gifts, and perceptions of pain. Disability, on the other hand, highlights the issues of dependency, independence and interdependence. In essence, *dependence* means 'hanging from'—to be in a state of continual suspense. Everyone is dependent to some degree upon something, but overdependency between helper and helped can result in an emotional tie that is negative and self-perpetuating. The one who is helped depends for the supply of his needs upon the helper, while the helper depends for her heroic role upon being able to help. This is a situation where any emotion can become intensified, either constructively or destructively. Love–hate is a powerful reality in which each aspect of dependency has a dual possibility; for instance, the comfort of being 'sheltered' can turn into 'deprivation of experience'. The health worker in school should be suspicious of the easy assumption that dependency should be converted as soon as possible into independence. There are many negative aspects to being dependent, but there is equally a real danger of dismissing the valuable positive aspects of dependency when it is replaced too officiously by independence (Table 4.2).

Table 4.2
Dependence—Its Dual Possibilities

Negative Aspects	
The Helper/Parent	**The Helped/Child**
Does everything her way, knows best.	Doesn't learn how to try, initiative quashed.
Frustrated by own inadequacy.	Anger at powerlessness.
Resentment at lack of choice, others' needs must be supplied.	Resentment at having to ask for supply of needs.
Self-righteous sacrifice, martyrdom.	Shame, belittled self-worth.
Power to demean the other.	Power to overload helper with demands made.
Intrusive, over-protective.	Interior self intruded upon, not able to build own privacy.
Tends to offer insufficient challenge.	Becomes bored, non-achieving.
Shields from exposure to stress.	Emotionally inexperienced, blunted.
Self-ostracising, 'no-one else really understands', social isolation.	Personal isolation, loneliness.
Pressure of needing to be always right (God image).	Self-responsibility taken away.

Positive Aspects

Sharing experience.
Acknowledging vulnerability.
Working problem out together.
Gift offering and receiving by each to other.
Warmth of acceptance, security.
Non-verbal communication, dignity in touch.
Growth of love, trust, commitment.

The supply of dependency needs *can* be the springboard from which self-worth and independence take off with vigour.

Independence is a priority in our present educational philosophy. The medical specialty of rehabilitation is built on the promotion of physical independence. While these efforts are emphasised, it should be remembered that independence involves separation, and separation from caring brings new dangers of aloneness. The proper personal pride and social dignity which develops from being independent are a universal goal: the long-term aim for the whole of society is, in fact, *interdependence*. Respect for each other and the double receiving and giving of benefits can lead to a strengthened sense of mutuality.

Who Benefits from Help?

Where the health worker takes her stand in the dependence/independence debate, will reflect how well she recognises her own dependency needs. On what do the satisfactions and rewards of her own job depend? Why is it that she wants to 'help'? Does it make her feel good? Does she, in fact, depend for her sense of worth on being able to help others? It may turn out that the cared for are supplying the needs of the carer in much the same way as the carer supplies the needs of the cared for. In other words, if I am being helped (to my reward) by helping him, who then is the helper?

It is revealing to note that a synonym for help is 'succour'; literally this means to run underneath, to reinforce. The health worker can provide 'succour' in several ways:

- Staff dealing with health care in school are in a special position for the exercise of empathy. Teachers and administrators are necessarily in a place of authority and control, whereas the stance of the carer can be 'alongside' that of the child.
- Help is often most acceptable at that point at which the child recognises that he needs it. If it is imposed while he denies he needs it, the result may be the exact opposite to that intended. Offers of help that are ill-timed, however well-meaning, may result in aggression and opposition.
- Some situations are made easier by using the direct approach: 'how about doing it like this?'; while others will improve by non-direct approach: 'your feet are very sore today, I wonder why that is?'

A timid child with asthma was overheard to say: 'I like doing my exercises with you because then I'm less frightened'. In this simple sentence, the child is expressing his own need as well as rewarding the health worker for the contribution she makes to his health.

Risk and Control

A further development of the stance of the health worker in school concerns her attitude towards *risk* and its parallel, the need to feel *in control*. Much of our striving in life is to prove to ourselves and to others that we can survive risk-taking, that we can handle our own lives, that we are masters in a shaky world. Many of the defensive techniques with which we protect our soft core are elaborately maintained in order to convince ourselves that we can't be taken unawares. In our society today, there is widespread difficulty in tolerating uncertainty; people who can give an instant correct answer are praised. In an educational establishment where the health worker is outside the environment in which she was trained, she will be questioned by disciplines that have different perspectives. For instance, she will meet difficult questions, such as whether a 13 year old boy who is subject to grand mal attacks should be encouraged to bicycle to school on his own. How far is it wise to allow risk-taking in order to offer opportunities for personal development? There will be many occasions when an absolute answer is not available—how much does she mind saying

'I don't know, I'll find out' to parents or teachers? Does she ever admit that no one really knows? How disturbed will she be at the uncertain outcome of much of her work? Two of the eight qualities quoted as being essential components of caring by Jean McFarlane (1982) are trust—letting go and taking risks—and courage, which makes risk-taking possible.The others are: knowledge, both general and specific; alternating rhythm of action and reflection; patience; honesty—openness and confrontation with self and with others; hope—commitment; and humanity—continuous learning.

All health workers must juggle with these ideas about health and illness, but only the individual can decide how to weigh one against another; the way in which she performs this balancing feat will depend upon her framework of values.

Models of Care and their Outcomes

The Medical Model of Health Care

Today there is a considerable amount of discussion surrounding the medical model of care. In fact this approach to medical problems has a long and deep tradition and has existed since the days of the Greek philosophers. Carthusian thinkers first described the human body as being made up of a number of parts. Those who hold this view contend that each part—whether it be an organ, a system or a function—can be examined separately and its specific faults repaired. This has been likened to the way in which an engineer sets out to mend a machine and has been called the 'mechanistic' approach (Black, 1979). This approach has developed along the following lines.

- The idea that the body is divisible into components means that each component can be examined separately.
- Each part has weaknesses of its own which can be discovered and repaired according to its individual failure.
- It is, therefore, necessary to separate out individuals from the general population to train as specialists in the discovery and repair of faults in each component of the machine.
- These specialists thus excel in their specialty and are invested with awe and authority.
- Information and decisionmaking are increasingly confined to the specialists. Although due to their separated position, the specialists can become distanced from the consequences of their decisions.
- Such authority necessitates a chain of command, each link unquestioningly taking directions from the link nearer the source of information. Strength is derived from the fact that each link replicates the previous link.
- Eventually, the person inhabiting the body with the problem is to do as he is told and all will be well.

This simplified picture will be familiar to health workers who trained in hospitals.

The Social Model of Health Care

Other models of care exist parallel to the medical model. The one most commonly articulated in the community is drawn from a much wider base and holds that disease and disorder are not just caused by bodily dysfunction, but are also caused by the effects of social conditions—bad housing, unemployment and insufficient opportunities for expressing vigour, enjoyment and creativity—as well as by dissatisfaction with personal relationships. Emphasis is laid on primary prevention; 'natural' factors in health promotion such as exercise, a whole food diet, health education and counselling are coupled with prophylactic intervention such as immunisation and screening. A basic necessity is seen as self-fulfilling engagement with work, family and community (Townsend, 1982). These are concerns that involve the whole population, ill or well, rather than concentrating on the few who ask for help from medicine.

The Environmental Model of Health Care

The supporters of the environmental or conservation ideals go further. They contend that pure air, water and ecological management of plants and animals have a part in the search for good health. Involvement with the developing nations, concern for the underprivileged, preservation of cultural traditions, all promote well-being among people. Legal systems and politics are as much responsible for the promotion of total well-being as are the systems of medical, social and educational organisation. Interdependence between all things is seen as a reality, not just an ideal.

The Philosophical Model of Health Care

There are also philosophical, psychoanalytical, behavioural and holistic models, and each religion has its own interpretation of the way in which humans should respond to the knocks that life brings. (The Buddhist, Hindu, Moslem, Tai-chi, Jewish and Christian doctrines, however, are too various to describe here.) As the following thumbnail sketches will show, underlying most of the ideas of this group is the conviction that discomfort, pain and disease are an inevitable part of life's rich pattern. These conditions can be used as opportunities to increase knowledge of oneself, to understand others' difficulties and to share common problems. Moral growth and spiritual wisdom evolve directly from the manner in which painful circumstances are met. The shaping power of emotional and physical pain cannot be denied; Utopia in this world will never be reached, but nonetheless prayer and worship combined with medical aid will bring meaning to the experience, and healing will often follow.

The Psychoanalytical Model of Health Care

Many of the troubles which beset an individual are related to emotional and/or physical trauma in childhood. Psychoanalysts often contend that if some of these early experiences can be uncovered and untangled, the fixations or 'hang-ups' attributed to them can be better comprehended. The desired result of analysis is a loosening of the fears which constrain personality growth and a liberation of natural coping powers. With increasing self-knowledge, the individual finds strength and competence to handle the pain and disorder which are part of all living.

The Behavioural Model of Health Care

In some contrast to this, the behavioural psychologist starts at the point the person has already reached. Ferreting out causes and triggers of certain difficult types of behaviour is too prolonged a process when problems have to be dealt with now. Given appropriately trained staff, each patient can have an individually tailored programme which employs specific stimuli to produce desired responses followed by agreed rewards. In this way people can be 'conditioned' to unlearn undesirable behaviour and to confirm desirable behaviour. The theory has been applied to therapeutic areas such as the medical management of children's problems, obesity, drug abuse, antisocial behaviour, classroom disruption and daily living skills. The principles of identification of goals, planning of short-term objectives, implementation and evaluation in a clear-cut plan have spread into many disciplines and have become accepted as one method of problem-solving.

The Holistic Model of Health Care

A reaction to the clarity of this approach, especially when it is universally applied, can be seen in the growing popularity of the holistic mode of thought. Where behaviourists reject 'fuzzies', that is, statements or ideas that are 'woolly', people who support holism are aware of the mystery in life and accept that many things are not plainly explicable. Since body, mind, spirit and soma are interwoven, and everything plays its part in the maintenance of the wholeness of the individual, the distinct separation of anything from its matrix can cause distortion. Well-being and enthusiasm for life are the result of proper valuing of each element in a person's make-up. Healing practices other than orthodox medicine are acceptable and thought-forms that are not scientifically proven also make their contribution.

Underlying all these models of care is one assumption that is seldom articulated. It is expressed in *The Health Care Dilemma* (OHE, 1975):

> The concept of the 'normal' human being which has been so firmly embodied in the teaching of medicine has done immeasurable harm. There is no such animal.

We are all imperfect; therefore, it is 'normal' to be imperfect. We just have to learn to compensate for each other's imperfections.

We are all inadequate; therefore, there is no place for a 'we' and 'them' or for difference between carers and cared for.

Models of Health and the School Health Worker

Authority, Accountability and Autonomy

How the health worker approaches her work will depend upon the model of health she adopts. For instance, in accepting that each of the models of care described is valid in itself, it is inevitable that questions about authority will arise. The school health worker is generally geographically outside her natural context in that her management is housed elsewhere; nevertheless direct authority exists although it comes from a different discipline. Furthermore, although she will be exposed to situations requiring decisions, she may have to do without instant confirmation of those decisions. In the light of these considerations, the following general observations can be made.

Authority is the proper vehicle for directions, information, support, legal cover and loyalty. It issues from top management, through to the workface and thereby reaches the client. It calls for appropriate response back up the line. In order to keep this two-way process intact, it is sometimes necessary for an isolated worker deliberately to make time to maintain regular contact with a busy and preoccupied source of authority which is elsewhere. Good management will normally make provision for this (Fig. 4.2).

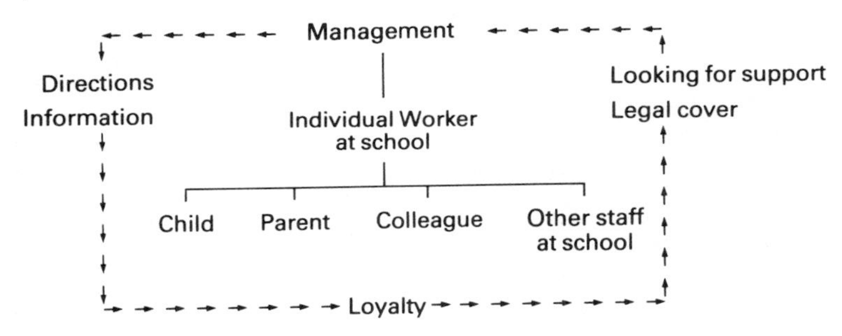

Fig. 4.2 Flow of authority.

The manner in which authority is expressed between any of these units can be that of imposition or suggestion, superiority or collegiate sharing. Some situations call for reassurance, while others respond more appropriately to discussion. The strength of authority is not diminished by listening to the other's viewpoint.

The school health worker collaborates with several disciplines, so their responses to a problem have to be taken into account. Accountability is due, at various times, to the headteacher, the school doctor, the classroom teacher, the paramedical staff, the parents and the child himself, as well as to nursing management. The worker will be primarily accountable to herself; the more she sees fit to take decisions into her own hands, the more accountable for her own behaviour she will have to be (Fig. 4.3).

Often the health worker in school will be unable to make instant reference to a higher authority for confirmation of her decision (unlike when working in a hospital or health centre). Some degree of autonomy is therefore necessary. The extent to which trust can be built up and autonomy increased will depend upon the personalities and circumstances and the agreed policies of employers. The responsibility she claims for herself may reflect the degree of responsibility she allows the child. Sometimes goals may have to be defined and mutually agreed upon by both management and worker, worker and other personnel, or worker and child.

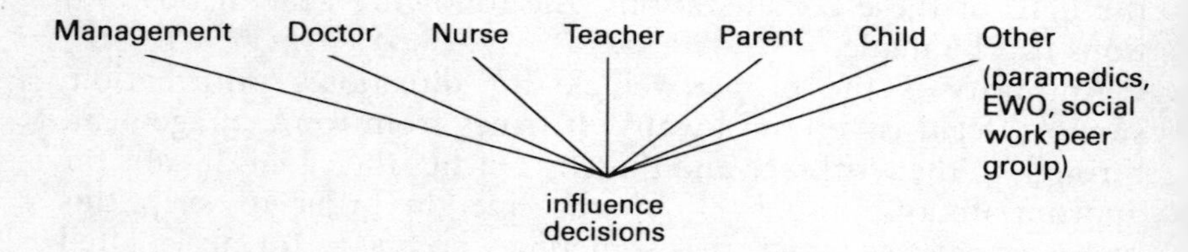

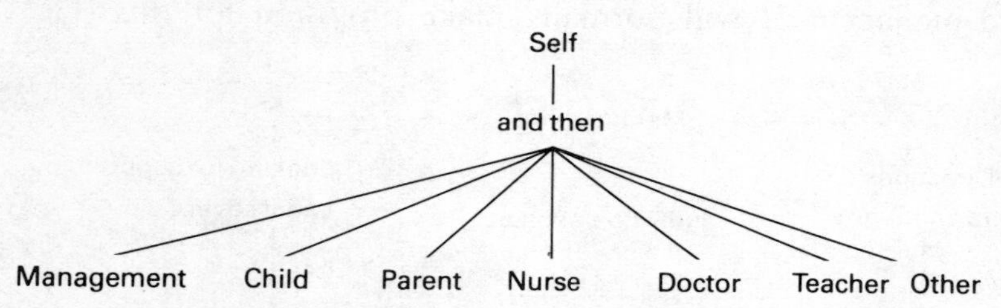

Fig. 4.3 Flow of accountability.

In Health Education

When the health worker at school is ready to carry responsibility for her own decisions and actions, she will transfer this attitude of self-empowerment to the children for whom she cares. Openness and acceptance on her part will be mirrored in the attitude the children adopt towards themselves, towards her and towards others. Personal and social development will expand among the new generation if they are in contact with people who demonstrate it in their own lives. Educating for wholeness may start at home, but the reinforcement it is given at school may well be crucial in the child's attitude formation for life.

The Search for Health Needs

The acceptance of personal autonomy will also be reflected in the conviction with which the health worker searches for unacknowledged needs in the school situation. She will realise that the referral of known health problems is an insufficient contribution to the development of the child and that there is also a responsibility to positively search out needs that she is in a position to supply. The habit of asking questions should lead her to discoveries that can explain a child's failure to thrive, his inattentiveness in class, his difficulties with peer relationships. Is he having sufficient sleep? Are the family in trouble? Is he conscious that his clothes are smelly? Does his mother understand his nutritional needs? Has he been taken to the doctor for his recurrent earache? Can he be worried about bed-wetting? Is there anxiety about his parents' marital relationship?

In addition to individual needs, there may be gaps in the provision for health in the school. For instance, the health worker may influence the hygiene requirements, such as sufficient privacy in the toilets and facilities to wash hands before meals. She may encourage regular dental inspection and create opportunities for first aid or life-saving courses. Health needs may be personal or institutional, but whether they are self-declared, acknowledged only by others or unrecognised, it is often up to the health professional to fill them.

Involving Agencies External to the School

The self-knowledge, professional awareness and interpersonal skills of the health worker should be used to the full in her dealings with people and facilities outside the school. Her enthusiasm may determine the extent to which parents and children explore the opportunities for health in the community, whether these be provided by the state, by commercial interests or by self-help groups. Indeed, this encouragement may be a key factor in the successful interaction of parents with other disciplines and community facilities.

Parents

Parents may well approach the school site with diffidence. Often they will have the memories of their own childhood difficulties to contend with and this may make them appear defensive. They can feel befriended by or alienated from the whole educational system depending on their first meeting with school staff. Professionals will not know what effort has gone into the establishment of a certain practice at home, and it may seem unjust to the parents to be asked to change it on the advice of an 'outsider'. Particular sensitivity is called for where parents have struggled with the management of a chronic condition in their child for years. The new nurse who states confidently 'That's not the way to do it. I'll show you the proper way' is intending to be constructive. However, the effect is more likely to be 'destructive'. It is important to establish a relationship of being alongside the parents, based on respect for their plans and ideas. Change should not be instigated until a real benefit can be seen by all parties—parents, child and worker alike. If a difficulty can be discussed during a home visit, the parents will be on familiar ground and therefore more likely to comply. Their perception of the worker's readiness to receive their ideas will help them to be more accepting of hers.

Other Disciplines

Other disciplines can be approached in an equally receptive manner. Sharing information, following-up the suggestions of others and keeping professional barriers as low as possible can all help towards mutual trust. Work-sharing and exchange of opinion is always creative. Case conferences need considerable communication skills if a minority view is to be presented at the right moment. The ease with which different agencies work together in a supportive manner may be a significant factor in their continuing interest in a case. Alienation or cooperation will be directly dependent on the attitude of the health worker herself. Interdisciplinary working and case conference behaviour are discussed further in Chapter 5.

Community Facilities

Services external to the school may be curative, preventive or promotional. The health worker who takes her stance in a wide framework can activate any or all of these. She will encourage parents to make full use of the family practitioner, health visitor, hospital, dental, paramedical, ophthalmic and child guidance services. The need may arise to contact the Educational Welfare Officer, the social services, the housing department or the local department of environmental health. Facilities in the community for the promotion of well-being grow daily. Opportunities for education and the use of leisure include those for sport and physical skills of all kinds: crafts, drama, art and music; Scouts, Guides and similar organisations; Church activities; community voluntary care; beauty and slimming groups; history re-enactment; and choirs, orchestras, bands and pop groups. Self-help groups abound; there is now one for nearly every identifiable serious condition. Extracurricular events at school may extend from drama after school hours to school journeys abroad. The professional health worker will have to consider how she should react to families who hold strong convictions about the benefits of alternative medicine. Is it her place to encourage or discourage herbal treatments or attendance at osteopathy, acupuncture or meditation centres? Should she remain neutral or claim ignorance? Or should she state her own views? Her first aim should be to understand the needs that are being relieved by these and why.

Summary

The worker for health in school comes into contact with a multitude of attitudes and ideas from people with widely differing baselines and goals. In order to make sense of health and wholeness for herself and the children she cares for, she must be sure of her own stance—her beliefs and professional objectives—and then be aware of those of others. The stance she takes will be both the result of her convictions and the source of her rewards.

5 The School Nurse: Roles and Tools

The Role

School staff who are concerned about the health of the child at school come from a range of backgrounds: their experience may be medical, educational, nursing or social welfare, and their training may be extensive or minimal. In previous chapters, this book has applied the term 'health care worker' to encompass all such staff. At this point, however, the book will focus on the nurse who works in school and on the roles and tools which are available to her.

The title 'school nurse' is itself ambiguous. Surveys of practice reveal that it is widely applied with vague connotations by people who have unclear expectations of staff with a variety of functions. This is demonstrated in Table 5.1. The bulk of Chapters 5 and 6 will relate to the school nurse who is employed by the District Health Authority, although it is hoped much of the discussion will be of interest to all nurses working in school.

National policy concerning the functioning of the school nurse in the United Kingdom is still very fluid and anomalies are common. Grades, duties, caseloads and conditions vary considerably. However, there is a growing professional cohesiveness amongst school nurses, an awareness of the potential they hold simply by being the only health employee in an educational establishment, and an increasing demand for further training. Expectations of the nurses themselves, and of those with whom they work, are high. The willingness of headteachers, paediatricians, educational psychologists and parents to utilise the skills of the nurse in the continuing care of the children in their charge has been frequently expressed at conferences and in published reports. These hopes are summed up in the often used description of the school nurse as 'the pivot of school health services of the future'. The Court Report (1978) is also often quoted:

Table 5.1
The Title 'School Nurse'

A. The title 'school nurse' should be properly limited to nurses
- who are *employed* by a District Health Authority to work in the NHS School Health Service as a member of the primary health care team.
- whose *training* is at least that equivalent of Registered General Nurse but who often has further nursing qualifications and, in particular, may have completed the school nursing course.
- whose *responsibility* is for anything between 100 and 20 000 school children, and whose duties include those that are statutory.

B. In practice, the title has been found to apply to workers
- who are *employed* by a Local Education Authority or by a governing body of independent/endowed schools.
- whose *training* may be Registered General Nurse, State Enrolled Nurse, Registered Sick Children's Nurse, Nursery Nurse Examination Board, or who may be unqualified.
- whose *responsibility* is for one named school and may include minor ailments, first aid, some pastoral care, 'miscellaneous' and clerical duties.

The strength of this last category of 'nurse' working with school children is that she is always in one school, knows all her children well and is known by all the staff. But she has no nursing management and usually little medical back-up.

> The role of the nurse in relation to education is of the utmost importance, and in the past it has tended to be overlooked and undervalued. The school nurse is required to be the representative of health in the everyday life of the school. It is she who mainly provides health surveillance of school children . . . and she is indispensable in the early recognition of sensory and other disorders. The school nurse will frequently be the first point of contact in the school on most health service matters, and she will be the person most concerned in maintaining continuous direct and regular contact with teachers over relevant health and family problems of individual children . . . she has a special contribution to make in individual health teaching and counselling of pupils.

Examples of good practice both in this country and abroad prove what can be achieved, but the necessary planning, financial resources and training are still patchy.

Approaching the Job

In our schools we have a captive population. Nearly every child in the land comes into contact with the school nurse. Opportunities exist which clamour for attention. For instance, the Black Report (1980) calls for revitalised school health care and emphasises three priority areas of national need. They are all areas in which the school nurse could be intimately involved. They are:

- to encourage good health by prevention and educational action.
- to give children a better start in life.
- to improve the quality of life of disabled people and as far as possible to reduce the need for institutional care.

While considering how to approach such large objectives, the school nurse will have the skeleton of her work provided by her statutory duties. But it will be up to her how to put flesh on the bare bones and how she develops her role. She can encourage high expectations of her services from children and parents and staff, or simply carry out her minimal responsibilities, according to the framework of values she has accepted. Her motives will probably depend on:

- the strength of conviction she holds concerning the opportunities of her work.
- the confidence she has in her own knowledge, competence and the support that is readily available to these.
- her belief that personal interaction can improve situations.
- her willingness to cope with situations that are unfolding and that require a constant shifting of priorities.

Anything that has to do with growing and developing is necessarily unpredictable. Children and conditions change constantly, and flexibility is of paramount importance to the school nurse. The demands made upon her personal and professional attributes will be of a different order to those met in clinical work. To highlight these issues, the nurse may want to ask herself the following questions:

> Am I dependent on an approach to work which is task-oriented, or can I adapt to doing things that can't always be measured or whose results cannot always be seen?
>
> Can I organise my own priorities instead of being told what to do?
>
> If I went in for nursing in order to nurture, how will I cope with surveillance?
>
> Since I have been trained largely in the medical model, can I relinquish some of the security and authority it gives me and become more flexible in response to other ideas?
>
> Can I give rein to my own ideas for health initiatives?
>
> Can I give the opinions of parents and other staff as much validity as I give to those I hold myself?

> Can I pass on an interesting problem and not mind not knowing the end result?

A positive answer to questions such as these will indicate the adaptability which is necessary for the nurse working in school. The conditions and equipment she meets may require imagination and a sense of humour in order to make the most of them; muddle and disorder will be part of her life, and it will be rare to find the clinical order of a hospital ward in the school. However, the openings for creativity are many, and the nurse is handed opportunities to design, initiate and develop new ways of doing things in which there is great satisfaction. The areas in which she may have influence are broadening to include more parental involvement, home visiting, health education, group work, oversight of disabled children and the promotion of self-care. Although a large part of her time may be taken up with regular surveillance and the monitoring of health problems, during the remainder of the time there will be valuable chances to be inventive and to cement personal relationships.

The work of the school nurse will be a mixture of being and doing. Figure 5.1 demonstrates the variety of her role. These are the possible opportunities that are available; it cannot be assumed that they all apply to every school nurse.

To Be a Nurturer

The verb 'to nurture' derives from the Latin word for nourishment. Metaphorically, it means to provide those elements which enable a growing thing to reach maturity—to feed, to foster and to cherish. From the sixteenth century, the people who applied these special skills to individuals who were particularly vulnerable, such as children and the sick, were called 'nurses'. In large medical institutions, 'to nurse' came to imply getting through the day's work by accomplishing a myriad of tasks—*doing* things *for* the patient. Properly applied, however, it means providing the nutrients essential to growth and then stepping back and allowing growth to happen—observing and enabling but letting the other do what he can for himself. This latter aspect of the word is particularly relevant to the nurse who is working in school. She has important advantages compared to other disciplines which she can use for the benefit of the child. (However, it is helpful, when exercising these advantages, to remember that she is a willing guest in foreign territory, just as a teacher would be who worked in a hospital ward.) The particular advantages of the nurturing role include the following.

She is available to every child in school and if she uses tact, she has access to every area in school and every member of staff. A nurse has many opportunities to get to know a child well at school. She can see him in class or at play, as well as during his visits to the

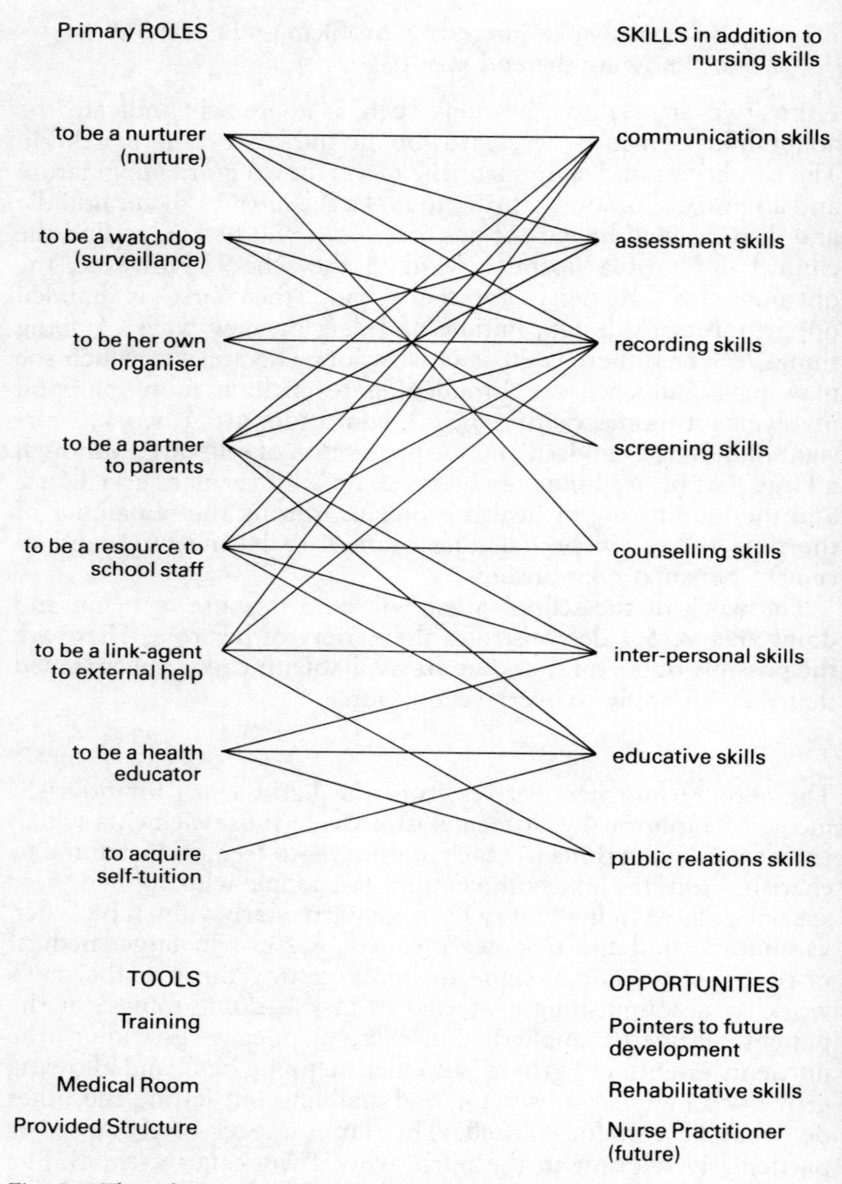

Fig. 5.1 The roles, tools, skills and opportunities of the school nurse.

medical room, so she can observe him both in his formal or informal behaviour. In particular, she can watch his interactions with his peers. She may make friends with him at the crucial bridge times of arriving at school and leaving for home. She can, if given the approval of the headteacher, offer chat-surgeries during which any child can share any difficulty—or pleasure—with her. He should be able to feel confident that since she is seldom directly involved in classroom behaviour, she can absorb incidental hostility or exasperation without necessarily reflecting it; her role may sometimes be as a buffer. The school nurse can also learn about the children from reports given her by teachers and care staff or from contacts with the aides, cooks, dinner ladies and escorts. From conversations held in the staff room, she may be able to deduce that a child who is labelled inattentive, stupid, sulky or isolated, may in fact be suffering from a physical disorder such as deafness, anaemia or diabetes and may need medical attention.

She is in a lateral position to all other disciplines. She is not in the hierarchy of the school, she cannot be promoted within the school, and she is neither competitive nor in a position of control. Since she has little to do with examinations, the marking of homework or the dispensing of discipline, she is not seen by the children as someone who has to be appeased. The advantage of being alongside authority but not always part of it is that, when appropriate, she can act as a child's advocate. She can put his point of view of the world as he sees it to his teacher, his parents or his medical overseers. If the nurse is seen around the school in non-medical situations as part of the staff team, she will be accepted by the children as part of their lives and not peripheral to them.

She can make use of touch as a means of communication where others cannot. Children cannot always interpret the meaning of words, but they are readily able to interpret the non-verbal communication conveyed by touch. Respect, reassurance or disapproval are implied—whether one is conscious of it or not—by the manner in which a hand is laid on the shoulder. Similarly, the way in which the nurse leads a child by the hand, helps him to undress or holds a hurt limb can transfer concern or

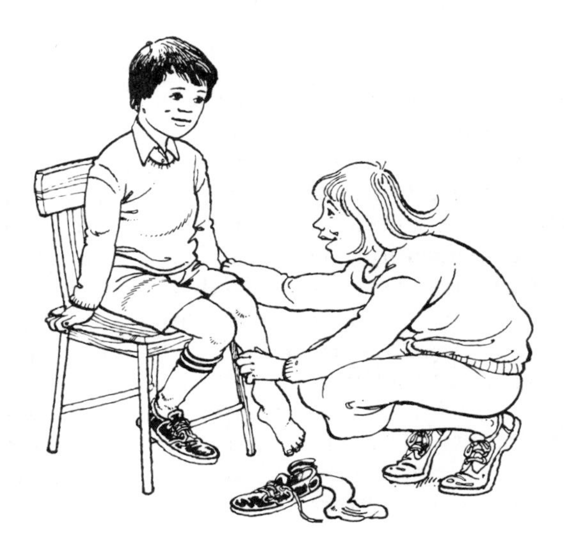

disinterest. Furthermore, the nurse is allowed by society to cope with damaged or 'bad', unsocial or 'private' and even 'shameful' places. The ways in which she manages these, whether the situation involves unhygienic underclothes, flea bites, incontinence, bruises or lice may affect permanently the child's feelings towards his body and his self-esteem. The use of touch is particularly important when caring for impairment; if the disabled or hurt part is handled with indifference, it will be difficult for the child to learn to treat it with care. Self-care has to be achieved with patience and dignity; if the nurse's hands are put on the affected part while she and the child work out its management together, the child will absorb the acceptance that she is demonstrating. Feelings of uselessness can be done away with. A disfigurement or a seizure, for example, may be seen by the child as a cause of rejection by his classmates; if the nurse holds him with composure and gentleness just as if it were 'normal', he will be less likely to see himself as anything else. Research has shown that if he then acts towards others with more self-confidence, it will improve others' confidence and liking of him.

She understands the variety of meanings that can apply to a complaint. Children are liable to make a physical complaint when they are unable to describe the source of their discomfiture accurately. A child saying 'I have a tummy-ache' may equally well mean 'I have a headache'. The same phrase could indicate a non-physical cause of anxiety, such as 'I can't get on with my teacher—the work is too much for me—I'm frightened Granny is dying—my friend has gone off me—Dad was angry with me last evening—my nightmares stop me sleeping—I promised not to tell about Mummy hitting me.'

Issues attached to nurture such as confidentiality, counselling and the conduct of health interviews will be commented upon at a later stage.

To be a Responsible Watchdog

Many of the statutory duties of the school nurse concern the oversight of large numbers of children. Her role in surveillance has been aptly described as that of a responsible watchdog (Thruston, 1980). She may have thousands of children of all ages in her care, or she may have a few hundred at one main school in her charge. Therefore, the translation into practical detail of her role in surveillance will vary from district to district. Health visitors and clinical assistants are also involved to different degrees. The law requires that the physical development of every child should be monitored as a right and free of charge, and the school nurse is responsible for much of this oversight. Monitoring will include a medical developmental assessment as the child enters primary school; vision screening every year until the child is in secondary school and thereafter every two years; hearing screening (audiometry) at school entry and thereafter follow-up of detected faults; regular immunisation; an annual check of health and hygiene of every primary school child; and medical interviews with the school doctor and the parents with any child having a suspected or recognised health problem—including learning or behavioural difficulties.

To be her Own Organiser

To combine these statutory obligations with the needs for nurture in the school demands considerable powers of organisation on the part of the school nurse. Ideally, child health surveillance can be seen as an ongoing process, not just as a series of jobs to complete. Continual monitoring, preventing, supporting and educating are all concurrent activities in the health care of each child. To keep the objectives of these various elements clear, while their performance is often linked, the nurse in school must be able to organise her own priorities and discriminate between the demands made upon her. The systems by which information reaches the school nurse and the sources from which it comes are not uniform. There will be requests channelled through her nursing officer, through the medical or health centre, through the headteacher, from the central data computer bank, from individual teachers or parents and from the children themselves. The assessment of priorities and the method with which she orders separate items will depend on the time that she has available, the immediacy of the task and the geographical area with which she deals. The unpredictable nature of much of her work has to be allowed for in her planning. Problems may develop during the day, relationships may unexpectedly need time spent on them or a simple enquiry may grow into a larger issue.

It may be sensible to organise her work into blocks of time such as the preparation for and completion of medical inspections with the school doctor. The degree of urgency that becomes attached to each errand will depend upon the nurse's own personal values and upon the experience she has built up of the ways in which other people react. Whether mothers are likely to respond better to an invitation that is written, telephoned or delivered in person on the doorstep will determine the design of the workload which precedes school medicals. Whether a particular secretary can be asked to send out letters or add notes to a school circular, will depend upon the cooperation of the headteacher and the relationship with the personnel involved. These things, in turn, depend on the stance taken and the interpersonal skills of the individual school nurse.

Goal-setting is a technique of organisation which can, with practice, become a frame of mind. Goals may have to be set not only daily, but weekly and termly. Table 5.2 is an example of the breakdown of one goal that is annual.

If goals are securely tied in with dates and times, they are more

Table 5.2
Goal Setting

Annual goal	Halt upward trend in glue-sniffing among pupils.
This term's goal	Assess the implication of glue-sniffing for the children who are in my care. Ask for cooperation of head-teacher, medical officer and manager. Suggest a series of three health education sessions with groups of 11 year olds to be held next term. Collaborate with the HE Department in the design of these sessions.
This month's goal	Collect ideas from colleagues, compare their experiences with glue-sniffing. Read topical and related items in the press. Formulate own policy and strategy.
This week's goal	Make appointment with your head, class teacher. Consider advisability of contacting parents about proposed course. Can they help? Can they come?
Today's goal	Visit HE Department. Sketch outline of one talk by me following a film. Discuss with manager and teachers.
Now	Get going!

likely to be achieved; good intentions can easily become dissipated in the comparatively unstructured life of the school nurse.

Consideration should also be given to the use of the *nursing process* in school. The principles of assessment, planning, implementation and evaluation can be applied in each of the following instances.

- The school where there may be a problem of dental ignorance or neglect.
- The class where there may be a problem of poor attendance. Is there a carrier of infection in the class? Is there a group of bullies? Are the conditions for seeing and hearing bad so that the children get bored?
- The family where there may be an unacceptably high level of stress. Are there children at risk?
- The child where there may be a problem of epilepsy.

A total programme could be devised for any of these examples.

Records should be kept efficiently and they should be succinct. They should ease the difficulties of workload and referral and not add to them.

The school nurse is seldom seen at work by other nurses. The advantage of not being in another's shadow is that she can put her own ideas to work and develop a certain degree of autonomy. However, in order not to become too idiosyncratic, it is important that she keep in close touch with her nursing colleagues and that she keep herself well-informed of current policy concerning school health, its research, development and practice.

To be a Resource for School Staff

Much of the above applies also to the relationship of the school nurse with other members of the school staff. A frequent request from planners, managers and educationalists is that she should be a resource. The school nurse is seen as a means of supplying a want by providing information or advice or action. This is sometimes taken to mean, for example, that a teacher who wants further information concerning a pupil's asthmatic attacks should seek out the nurse. But the school nurse can also take the initiative. Not only can she ask for and listen to comments from other members of staff. She can offer her own insights. Relationships within schools are seldom as hierarchical as in hospitals; instead they tend to be collegiate by comparison. The school nurse should remember that the informal sharing of ideas:

- provides a common core of interest upon which teamwork can be built.
- helps to identify the needs of the children.
- explains the attitudes and actions of the nurse to her colleagues.
- can encourage the assumption that her contribution is valid and worth promoting.

It will often be up to each individual school nurse to order her time in such a way that informal contact with teachers and other staff can be engineered. Meeting them in the cloakroom at the beginning or end of the day, spending time in the staffroom in a coffee break or lunch hour, and making sure that the outcome of any medical inspection is followed up with the appropriate teacher, are all important ways of maintaining contact. Too often teachers are heard to say that they do not know the school nurse, and that although it is they who are disturbed by a child being absent for a 'medical', they seldom hear why it was necessary or what happened. These are the opportunities which the nurse can use to build up trust by relaying details that are relevant to the child's learning. Mutual confidence will grow out of such contact; remaining distant only encourages indifference or suspicion.

Once a positive relationship is established, other openings will appear such as individual counselling, group work with children, cooperation in health education projects, involvement with case conferences, the planning of individual management of children with special needs, and attendance at leavers' meetings where future employment of those with a disability is being discussed. Some nurses are welcomed onto parent/staff committees or onto the board of school governors. Her role as a resource to the school will only be limited by the time and commitment.

An example of a programme for social education in the fifth year of a comprehensive school may be useful (Table 5.3). The items with black circles next to them are those where a school nurse may be asked, or she may feel it appropriate, to make a contribution:

Table 5.3
Example of Social Education Project

Family Life	Health Matters
• Adolescence Social skills and decision-making • Personal relationships and marriage Family planning (outside speaker) • Birth and infant care • Parenting • Growing old and the care of the elderly • Bereavement	• Safety and first aid • How to deal with stress • Drug abuse, including alcohol, nicotine and solvents • Abortion Venereal disease (outside speaker) Cancer care (outside speaker) • Handicapped children • How to deal with separation and loss
Community Caring Agencies (all outside speakers)	**Further Education and Careers**
Police Marriage Guidance Council Church and community Self-help organisations	Local sixth-form college Technical college Skilled crafts

It is not often that a school nurse is asked to regularly address a whole class. Her contribution in the above instances is more likely to take the form of suggesting ideas, saying where to get further information, participating in small group discussion or answering questions.

Table 5.4 is a summary of the ways in which a school nurse can be a resource to the different staff working in a school.

Case Conferences

School nurses are increasingly involved in case conferences. This is to be welcomed as school nurses can play a key role both as a resource within school and as a link between agents external to the school.

As yet, few nurses are trained in conference technique and some guidelines may prove useful. Working together as partners in a team is somewhat different from participating in a group which is considering a specific problem. In the former, each member has her own job to do which is reasonably clear-cut; in the latter, no decision has been made and each member offers their own experience and insights. Authority and defensiveness are both out of place, and the aim is to reach for collective wisdom.

Personal status has a significance which is not, theoretically, relevant to a collegiate case conference.

Case conference guidelines

1. The school nurse should make sure she understands the reasons for the conference being called. It may be to pool information, to

Table 5.4
The School Nurse as a Multiple Resource within School

She can be a resource to:	
The school doctor	— supplying information gleaned from teacher, parent, child, home visit, own observation. — ensuring that recommendations are carried out.
The teachers	— sharing information which concerns the child's learning environment and capabilities. — extending feedback from clinics and hospitals to the teachers. — cooperating in health education. — interpreting causes, symptoms, expectations, treatment of specific disabilities; discussing and explaining objectives of care and management.
The ancillaries	— overseeing management of physical care of children with special needs. — working out continuing development regime to suit each phase of care.
The school secretary	— in emergencies, when called. Some first aid, and as escort to hospital if necessary. — knowledge of NHS contacts in community. — advice on stocking of school tuck shop!
The Education Welfare Officer	— furthering the assessment of needs of individual children.
In addition, the school nurse acts as a resource to allied agencies outside school, such as:	
The child's parents	— explaining medical terms, demystifying test procedures and results, comparing experience with management, suggesting further sources of help.
The health visitor	— updating information, relating behaviour or symptoms to other members of the same family, confirming impressions of background.
School dental officer	— maintaining follow-up, cooperating with dental care, encouraging preventive practices.
Other clinical agencies	— liaising with enuresis, obesity, youth counselling clinics; physiotherapy, occupational therapy, speech therapy; mobility appliances; incontinence aids.
Others	— serving on parent/staff associations, school committees, etc.

work out a common policy concerning a difficulty, to sort out relationships between staff or between staff and child, or to allocate responsibility in different areas of a programme.

2. If the school nurse has been asked to prepare a definite contribution, she must be certain of the facts she is presenting. Clarity of presentation, especially in view of her non-medical hearers, is important; some comment will be expected on the significance of the various issues she introduces.

3. The school nurse must remain aware that each discipline has its own starting points and its own goals, all of which have a distinction of emphasis. The words of the other person must be listened to with his/her priorities in mind, not the imposition of one's own. Sensitivity to alternative approaches will make the nurse's personal comment both more acceptable and more valid.

4. In a round table conference, no one is the expert. Deference is due to everybody and in principle all can have their say, although not necessarily taking equal time.

5. Not everyone can be a coal-face worker. Sometimes authority and even concern have to be relinquished in order that one primary carer can carry out the concerted willingness of all. Possessiveness over a professional offer has to be handled with aptness—what is best for the child in the situation where he is?

6. Just as no one is entirely right, so the planned solution will not be entirely satisfactory to everyone. It must be tried out with goodwill and confidence.

Freire has summed up interpersonal interaction such as described above as 'a living and creative dialogue in which everyone knows something but is ignorant of something else, and all strive together to know something more'.

To be a Link Agent to External Help

Many of the principles of interdisciplinary working which have been looked at in the role of the school nurse as a resource also apply to her role as link agent with sources of help outside the school. The extent to which she is used as such will again depend upon the gradual process of building up professional trust. When it can be seen that the connections she makes are both suitable and well-timed, she will become increasingly relied upon for her liaison. She may need the skills of a diplomat, since over-zealous interference could earn her the reputation of being a nuisance. The strategy which should undergird any approach to another agent is:

Recognising—that external help may be needed.
Alerting —the nearest link in the chain of referral.
Facilitating —the advised treatment/management in school where possible.

The role of link agent has both positive and negative aspects.

1. The criteria upon which the nurse decides whether to take action or not lie in the basic question—will this help the child?

Positive	*Negative*
If change in the *status quo* seems desirable, will stirring the situation bring about improvement?	Change for the sake of a change may be stimulating to the worker, but not necessarily to the child who may grow out of the present phase anyway.

2. The tools with which to work for interdisciplinary cooperation are:

Positive	*Negative*
Appropriate: such as discretion, sharing, respect for the other opinion, follow-through and feedback concerning the decisions reached.	Inappropriate: such as aggression, possessiveness, coercion and defensiveness.

The lowering of territorial barriers does not mean that another can tramp all over the professional space; deference is still due to each one's unique expertise even when borders overlap.

3. Continuing communication is important, both between helpers and between helper and helped. Having triggered an intervention, the school nurse must follow it up by supporting the child and his parents.

Positive	*Negative*
Explanation of technical terms, of what is to happen and why, is often a part of this role.	If communication is clumsy or support inadequate, the child/parents may be left floundering and confused between agencies, and their second state be worse than the first.

4. When other services are involved in the care of a child:

Positive	*Negative*
They should be a resource from which the child can disengage when necessary.	They should not increase the child's or family's dependence.

One great advantage of the school nurse being accountable to several others is that, if a request for help from one source proves to be non-productive, it is often possible to re-route the request through another channel and gain a more acceptable result.

To be Engaged in Self-tuition

The effectiveness of the school nurse's role as link agent will largely be due to her commitment to self-tuition. For however much training she has had, the context of her work is such that there will always be gaps in her knowledge and she will always be touching on areas in which she can never be expert. Her competence in managing situations within her own limits and her consciousness of the need to refer those that may need further help, will be enhanced by keeping up-to-date with clinical, social, nursing and educational issues.

We are in an historic phase of the emergence of school nursing as a professional specialty of its own. All over the United Kingdom, school nurses are becoming aware of their cohesiveness as a group with common experience. There are many conferences and workshops organised by school nurses themselves, supported by their colleagues and providing stimulus and information concerning the subjects that they choose as important. Training, both voluntary and in-service, is still inadequate and responsibility for ensuring that knowledge is adequate rests with the individual nurse herself. It is up to her not only to maintain, but also to advance her professional knowledge and performance by self-tuition.

The Tools

> The school nursing service must be planned to develop and maintain the professional skills now required of the nurse so that she may contribute fully as a member of the school health team in meeting the complex health needs of children today.
>
> Review of the School Nursing Service, May 1980,
> Society of Area Nurses

Training

Training is the hallmark of professional authenticity. The professional body which offers a training seeks to provide a public guarantee of certain standards, standards of practice and behaviour which are based upon knowledge, skill and informed professional commitment.

In May 1980 the Society of Area Nurses (Child Health) set up a working party to review the School Nursing Service. The working party recommended further research into the nursing needs of the school child, the role of the school nurse, and the manpower requirements of the school nursing services. Because of the many changes in legislation, it pointed to the need for clarification of the basic statutory training requirements necessary for the practice of school nursing and recommended that Approved School Nurse Training Courses should receive statutory recognition. It further suggested that the title of 'School Nurse' be confined to the statutorily trained school nurse.

Many Colleges of Further Education have now established Approved Courses (lasting 12 weeks or its equivalent), but as yet they have not received statutory recognition.

The overall responsibility for nursing standards and nurse education rests with the United Kingdom Central Council for

Nursing (UKCC), and school nurses may address themselves to this body for a resolution of their professional difficulties, many of which are dependent upon a recognition of their role and the training requirements needed to ensure its fulfilment.

The Link with Health Visiting

Because of their common origin, the essential elements of training for both health visitors and school nurses are the same. The root of their practice lies in the understanding and recognition of what constitutes whole health, both for the individual and for society as a whole. The principles of search, recognition, intervention, counselling and education provide a common basis for training and for practice. But there is more. The health visitor is essentially community based; her work is centred upon the health needs of the community. The health needs of the child are perceived by her against the backcloth of family and community, within which the school plays an important part.

The work of the school nurse is essentially school based, and the health needs of the school child are perceived in relation to education and the school environment; as a member of the school team, the school nurse is the link person between school health, education and the community.

It is this difference in their roles and the settings in which they practise which dictates the difference in their training needs, although both rely upon the foundation of State Nurse Registration.

Approved School Nurse Courses

The current training course is based on a pattern of one-third practice to two-thirds theory. The syllabus received DHSS recognition in 1980. There are currently about 27 validated and approved courses in the UK, although their viability depends on the number of students enrolling and, therefore, on the support of the health authorities. The course aims to instil levels of competence in the following areas:

- A basic understanding of normal child development and behaviour, an ability to recognise any significant deviation, and knowledge of subsequent referral and action.
- An understanding of the importance of interpersonal relationships and communication.
- The development of the appropriate practical and organisational skills.

Syllabus subjects can be grouped under the following headings:

1. Child Development
2. Introduction to Sociology and Social Psychology
3. Social Policy related to the School Health Service
4. The School Health Service

5. The School Nurse—Role and Responsibilities
6. Care of Children with Special Needs

Practical training is an essential part of the course. It covers the range of general duties undertaken by school nurses. In addition to the preparation, organisation and management of sessions, it includes teaching and health education, record keeping and collection of statistics, participation in screening tests, and other relevant health procedures.

The Knowledge Base

There is an outstanding need for further research into the nursing needs of the school child and into the body of knowledge which can be identified as educational nursing. The present course provides a known minimum standard, but training should never be static and in the case of school nursing, it has to take account of changes in the education system. Some of these changes are:

- Comprehensive education which involves large numbers of children on the same campus, many of whom travel considerable distances from home.
- The move towards the integration of handicapped pupils into ordinary schools, and the resulting needs for constant professional advice and clinical nursing skills which were previously found mainly in special schools.
- The growing awareness of health education needs, and the effects of behaviour and attitude upon the health and education of the individual child. This presents both challenge and opportunity for the whole school team.

The Case for Further School Nurse Education

The role of the school nurse has undergone many changes of emphasis. The disease patterns of childhood have changed with the advancement of medicine and the greater awareness of environmental hazards. The separate strands of social, industrial and health legislation have come together to provide a safety net against adversity. Reduction of overcrowding, smaller families, programmes of immunisation, and more effective maternity and child health services have all contributed to the fall in the infant mortality rate and to the overall improvement in the health of children. We are better able to apprehend and provide for the needs of the child as a whole.

Educational disadvantage takes many forms. Today's challenges include the problems of congenital abnormality, non-accidental injury, socially related addictions such as alcohol, smoking, glue sniffing and drug-taking, stress and mental illness, sexually transmitted diseases, lead pollution, atopic syndromes and the hidden malnutrition of poor eating habits. These challenges require new knowledge and skills.

The school nurse of today is required to be the representative of health in the life of the school; she is the main provider of health surveillance and is often the first point of contact in the school on health matters. She is concerned with the health of children who are inadequately cared for at home, and she maintains direct and regular contact with teachers over the health and family problems of individual children. She has a special contribution to make in the curriculum planning and provision of health education and in individual health teaching and counselling of pupils. All these tasks require a high degree of self-motivation and the confidence which comes from knowledge, training and experience.

The content of a 12 week course must, of necessity, be limited, and there are few who would deny the need for further training. The syllabus provides the broad outlines of practice and a basis for ongoing programmes of professional education and development. Although we can point to individual examples of professional excellence which have developed from self-motivation, hard work and natural talent, these should not mask our recognition of the need for higher basic standards for the majority of school nurses. Instead they should be used as an example of what can yet be achieved. School nurses are poised to accept opportunities to further develop their skills and the effectiveness of their practice.

Ideally, approved courses could be *extended* to encompass the greater development of:

1. Advanced clinical skills.
2. Counselling skills, including home visiting.
3. Health education and practical teaching skills.

Reality compels us to recognise the increasingly high costs of training, but this must be measured against the benefits which accrue from a more highly competent work-force of school nurses. We need to consider:

1. How many children will be precluded from attending ordinary schools in the absence of suitably trained school nurses?
2. How many children are floundering for lack of sensitive and easily available advice and counselling in school?
3. How many schools have recourse to the services of health visitors in matters of health education and health teaching when the named school nurse could provide greater continuity, availability and expertise if she were trained to do so? How do we measure this in terms of health visiting time and the build-up of a resource within the school team?

Neither can it be said that a piecemeal approach to this problem is necessarily cheaper.

The Case for Statutory Recognition of Training

1. There is a recognised body of knowledge and practice which can be defined as Educational Nursing.

2. The role of the school nurse is no longer task orientated, but is targeted upon the needs of the whole child. This requires particular skills—to work effectively with children, parents and teachers and other members of the school health team.

3. The role and status of the school nurse as perceived by other disciplines has an effect upon their working relationships. The recognition of a known training and known skills provides a platform for cooperation and respect which must currently be earned by the majority of school nurses.

4. The demands made by modern school nursing require a high level of self-motivation. In an educational setting the school nurse must make her own decisions, organise her own pattern of work, and deal with health problems largely from a position of professional isolation. Her confidence, self-reliance and security of practice can only be assured by a recognised training.

5. The nursing profession has a responsibility to recognise the particular expertise required for school nursing, and to provide a satisfactory career structure within the context of nursing as a whole.

Labour Laws and Professional Organisations

Labour laws and professional organisations are among the school nurse's most important tools.

Labour Laws

The Contract of Employment Act of 1972 requires that all employees be given a statement or 'contract of employment' to include information concerning: terms and conditions of service, including grievance procedure and the period of notice to be served; rate or scale of remuneration; and frequency of payment. In addition it is reasonable for professional workers to request a job description and relevant details of the working structure, accountability and chain of command.

The Employment Protection Act of 1975 covers the principles governing dismissal, trade union rights, and other worker entitlements. Any nurse who feels that she has been unfairly dismissed or that the terms of her contract of employment have been breached should get in touch with her appropriate professional organisation or trade union.

The Health and Safety at Work Act of 1975 imposes wide-ranging general duties on employers and employees to ensure arrangements for: a safe working environment; equipment, including safety equipment, to be in good order; instruction and training for all staff concerning, for example, fire regulations and procedure; a written safety policy.

The Safety Representatives and Safety Regulations Act of 1978 enables recognised organisations and independent trades unions to appoint safety representatives and allow them day to day involvement in health and safety at their places of work. School nurses may be asked to act as health and safety representatives and serve on the local safety committee. Any nurse who has cause for concern in these matters should know how to contact the local representative for help and advice and should have a clear understanding of her responsibilities as an employee.

Professional Organisations for School Nurses

A professional organisation reflects the interests of the group which it represents. In particular it

- provides identity and a representative voice.
- provides a forum for professional discussion.
- correlates information.
- upholds standards of practice.
- provides legal advice and professional protection.
- provide resources, information and training.

The emerging identity of a new professional group is invariably heralded by the formation of such organisations and school nursing is no exception. There are currently three national groups:

The Health Visitors Association—School Nurses Group
The Royal College of Nursing—School Nurses Forum
The Amalgamated School Nurses Association

In addition there are a growing number of local and county-based groups. These can provide:

- local support for school nurses working in isolation.
- exchange of information on local practice.
- opportunities to develop and evaluate local projects.
- opportunities for discussion with colleagues from other groups and different disciplines.
- collective support and information for national groups.

In 1983 the total NHS nursing payroll totalled approximately 390 000. The still small voice of school nursing will be heard with greater clarity if, through their organisations, school nurses speak of their priorities with one voice.

6 The Skills

This chapter will concentrate on the skills which are needed by the school nurse as she cares for children, but which extend beyond the skills that she developed in her basic nursing training. Figure 6.1 demonstrates how each of these skills overlaps with others.

In this chapter each type of skill is given a set of general objectives which are specific to the school setting.

The *principles of the nursing process* support most functions of the school nurse; they are also applicable to the individual for whom she cares. The school nurse will be most effective when she assesses her aims; plans her priorities; allocates her time, effort and resources to the implementation of these plans; and evaluates the results of her work. She should try to keep level-headed as she organises the mass of demands on her as this will mean that her skills will be used for appropriate objectives and much time, energy and temper will be spared.

The bulk of the work of the school nurse is in preventive health. This is often described as having three layers:

1. Primary prevention—removing the causes of disease and disorder.
2. Secondary prevention—the early detection of disease before symptoms are clearly recognised.
3. Tertiary prevention—the curative and rehabilitative aspects of established disease.

Surveillance properly belongs to secondary prevention and involves the skills of both assessment and screening. In order to apportion work schedules suitably, school nurses need to realise that the aims and methods of these two skills are different. The temptation to 'bumble' should be avoided, as should the temptation to follow too closely a medical approach.

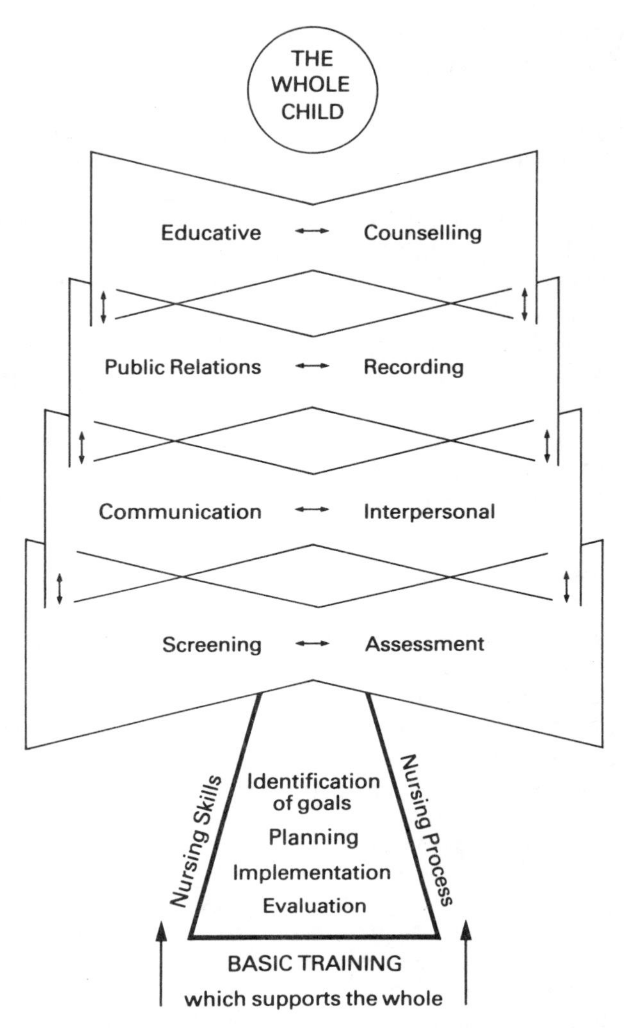

Fig. 6.1 Skills to be used by the school nurse for the well-being of the child.

Objectives in the Use of Assessment Skills by the Nurse in School

To notice, recognise and continually observe those factors in a child and in his environment that adversely affect his total well-being. To pay attention to these factors, and to form a judgement on what, if anything, should be done and who, if anyone, should be informed.

'*Assessment*' is a word that can trip off the tongue without the speaker being fully aware of the range of skills it covers. It involves the minute-to-minute perception, the total knowledge base, and the value framework of each practising nurse. *Assessment* is an act constantly in use in general life—what is there in the larder that will make a meal for today? What are the qualities in my neighbour which lead me to trust her as a good friend? The word itself derives from the old Latin of 'sitting beside', referring to the person who sat down to 'assess' a man's 'assets' prior to taxation. The gathering of information was an appraisal of his estate. In nursing terms, this becomes a listening, watching, and eliciting of facts in order to add up points of value or deficit in a person's condition.

These are often matters where subjective judgement plays a large part. If the decision to treat an obese girl depends upon how attractive the nurse finds her rather than upon how much she needs help, the nurse is allowing her personal reactions to count more heavily than clinical assessment. It is necessary, therefore, for the individual school nurse to be clear—to herself and to others—about how she is operating.

When a problem or a disorder presents itself to the nurse, she can use the technique commonly known as the *problem-solving process*. This is made up of:

- observation.
- collection of relevant information about the child and his condition.
- analysis of these factors: how do various needs balance?
- putting into order the issues which emerge.
- making a plan to deal with them.
- designing a series of small goals which lead successively towards a long-term aim.
- continual review of the progress of the problem and the effectiveness—or not—of the plan.
- support for all concerned.

Such assessment reflects the whole process of nursing. In school, it usually takes the form of an attitude towards work rather than a documented plan, as the borders to tasks are not as clearly defined as in hospital nursing. There is plenty of scope for the intuitive, creative side of nursing when dealing with children, but nonetheless an approach should be developed which insists on a clear awareness about the problems the school nurse tackles. The school nurse often has to think problems over again because she is constantly faced with the viewpoint of other disciplines.

When assessing the health status of any particular child, the following aspects should be borne in mind.

1. His present subjective complaint: this represents his own reality as he sees it and it must be accepted at his level. However, the school nurse must ask herself if it is accurate or whether it is the outcome of something related but different.
2. Have there been any indications from staff, family or peers which bear on this present complaint?
3. The pattern of his physical, emotional and intellectual development so far: is it within normal limits?

4. The observable state of his nutrition: does he seem pale, spotty, obese or skinny?
5. The condition of his hair and skin: is it neglected, damaged, bruised or below acceptable levels?
6. His self-concept: is he over-submissive or over-aggressive?
7. His teacher and peer reaction: does he feel sufficient approval?
8. His family background: is he allowed to feel that he is wanted? This may have an even more significant bearing on his health than size, financial status or marital position of his family.
9. His social background: is his behaviour congruent with his family's culture or ethnic expectation?
10. His use or abuse of nicotine, alcohol, drugs and inhalants: use and abuse can also be made of social status and possessions.
11. His coping powers: have they been sufficient or reliable up until now? What, if anything, is different?

Any of these factors can influence the child's health, his concept of his own life and his self-esteem. They may also affect the attitudes that others have towards him. The school nurse herself may be affected in her like or dislike of a particular child and she should be aware that her behaviour towards him should not reflect such leanings. Human elements in relationships should be taken into account in assessment, but the heart and the head have to live together, neither dominating the other.

Having assessed the position of the child, the school nurse must then assess what is to be done. Should she keep quiet or should she intervene? Are there obstacles or stresses that can be removed? Should she trigger other people to take action—the medical officer, the teacher or the parent? What is her part in helping the child?

Objectives in the Use of Screening Skills

To undertake screening procedures in such a way that physical difficulties which affect a child's learning or impede his development to the least degree are detected as early as possible and referred for appropriate treatment. To manage these procedures with minimum disruption of the class or of the child's general equilibrium.

Screening involves collecting one aspect of information concerning a large number of children at a time. This is different from assessment which involves the gathering of a large amount of information concerning one child at a time.

Screening is task-oriented, and because of this the nurse must ensure that the quality of her relationship with each child and teacher is not secondary to the quantity of testing to be undertaken. Different parts and functions of a child can be checked and the results ticked in a little box or recorded on a form, but it must always be remembered that an individual is more than a series of ticks in boxes. Furthermore, each task is one of a series and together they form a valuable string of experiences which make up a relationship between child and nurse.

The rationale of screening and the details of what, when and how are dealt with in Chapter 9. This chapter looks instead at more general aspects of screening skills from the point of view of the different people concerned—the administrator, the nurse, the teacher and most important of all, the child.

From the Point of View of the Administrator

From the administrator's viewpoint, the school nurse must be scrupulous in her blanket coverage of all children in the category being tested. Frequently the details of names and ages of children who are due for a particular investigation will be sent to her from a central data collection base; this data may have been assembled by computer and should be checked with the nurse's personal knowledge. Accuracy and promptness are required to keep records up to date. From the mass of details collected, statisticians can ensure that policy requirements are being fulfilled and epidemiologists can trace past and future trends in health care and behaviour. In some sense, all large scale preventive measures owe their financing to the proof of success held in records, so the nurse's role in keeping them accurate is important.

From the Point of View of the School Nurse

In order to encompass the demands made upon her by such administrators and to comply with that part of her job description, the school nurse will need to systematise her screening procedures. She should plan the work in such a way that movements of children and equipment are streamlined and time and resources are used effectively. If the least possible energy is laid out in the mechanics of ushering children and recording results, there will be more to spare for the children as people; even a few seconds given to friendliness will make the child feel that he can return at a better moment with his real worry. A short explanation of the procedure may have to be repeated to each child, but if the nurse uses skill in slightly altering the words and adapting them to the personality in front of her, she can keep up her interest and that of the child. Boredom and monotony have an unfortunate way of transferring themselves and it is more difficult to extract accurate responses from a child who 'catches' apathy from the nurse.

The instant recording of results is important, particularly if the nurse is trying to hold a conversation with the child at the same time. When results have been obtained, those that deviate from the norm should receive further attention. The exact procedure of referring to the school doctor, the local clinic, the general practitioner and the parent will depend on the set pattern of the district health policy. This must be followed carefully and any case of special difficulty brought to the attention of the head teacher. Those children whose results are borderline should be followed up at monthly intervals when the degree of deviance can be reviewed with the class teacher. Classroom behaviour such as inattentiveness or constant demands for attention can bear significantly on the ultimate diagnosis, and the nurse's comments can help the teacher decide the proper position in class for a child who has difficulties in hearing or seeing.

From the Point of View of the Teacher

Cooperation between nurse and teacher is central to all screening procedures. From the teacher's viewpoint, all intrusions into the regular running of the classroom are a nuisance, and care must be taken to consult with her beforehand about the best way to manage the programme. An orderly, quiet and calm approach will always be welcomed, whereas confusion and disturbance will create anxiety and furnish anecdotes for the staff room for some time to come.

From the Point of View of the Child

It is sometimes difficult for the person who operates screening procedures to hold in her mind the viewpoint of the child. Although some measures become almost automatic to the nurse, the experience may be unique to the child. He may not have completely understood the explanation offered to him or he may be confused by the interruption to his routine or bewildered by the instructions being given him. The child may, for instance have a longstanding hidden dread of going blind—like his pet did just before he had to be 'put down'—or he may be acting with bravado in response to a dare from a friend that he can put one over the nurse and kid her that he is blind. He might even fancy himself in glasses as an attention-seeking ploy. Each individual who passes through will have his own fears and fancies, and stereotyping will not produce good results or build future relationships.

Immunisation and dental screening both have a surprisingly high 'cringe-factor', even in this generation when television violence is commonplace. Careful explanation and reassurance will never be outdated. A repeated reminder that the school nurse is available for further chat at a particular time is usually appreciated.

Many of the skills necessary to the school nurse in her screening duties cannot be learnt from the printed page; they must be 'caught' by watching her fellow practitioners. But how to make mass procedures personal will have to come from her own imagination and understanding.

Objectives of Interpersonal Skills

To establish and maintain personal relationships in such a way that trust, understanding and information may flow easily between individuals. To underline and reinforce the other's worth and build mutual respect. To exercise her role as link agent in a manner that encourages continued interest.

Interpersonal relationships involve balance, togetherness and the interchange of offering and receiving. They involve giving others their due and accepting theirs in return. Relationships and 'relating' are happening all the time; we are constantly putting out messages, whether they are intended consciously or not. However, if we *are* aware of what is happening, it is more likely that we can make this mutual exchange as productive as possible.

The following is a simplified description of the interpersonal skills used by the nurse in school. Taking five questions, this section looks at some of the factors in those relationships.

- How do I recognise me (my space, shape, image)?
- What happens when I meet you?
- What is in the space between you and me?
- Can we negotiate in this space?
- Can the risks be taken on board and the likely outcomes be predicted?

The terms I and me apply to the working school nurse, and the term you represents the other, whether the other is a child, parent, teacher, doctor, nurse manager or external helping agent.

How Do I Recognise Me?

Basic to the business of relating is my conception of myself. I have to start where I am. How I behave towards others will be determined by my understanding of my use and abuse of my personal influence, opinion or power and my conviction of my own worth, acceptance or vulnerability. This is shown in Fig. 6.2.

When I meet you, there is instantly an interaction. This consists of nuances, intonations, eye-activity, interlocking glances, subtleties of facial movement and body gestures, all of which either confirm or negate the words that are actually spoken.

What Happens When I Meet You?

Each of us transmits, knowingly and unknowingly, hints and clues about how we feel at that precise moment about ourselves and about the other person. Sometimes I give away more than I intend by non-verbal means, but equally sometimes I can translate more signals than you convey in your words. At the same time, there is a continual testing of each other and weighing up of the integrity of the person and the consequences of the relating. The indicators of good or ill, and the devices we use for influencing it, are as follows:

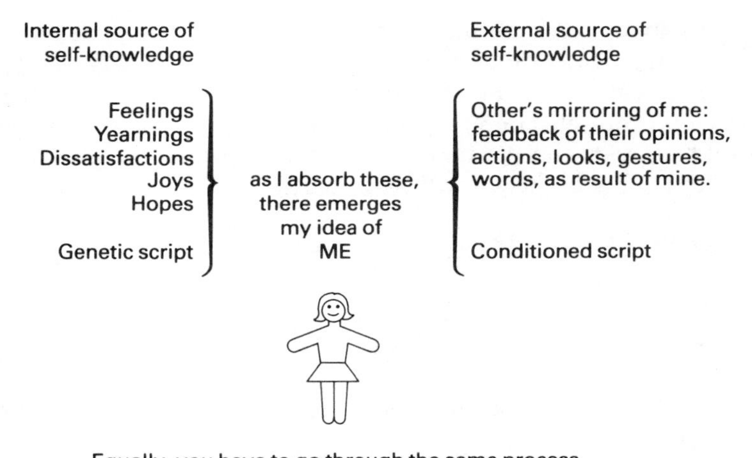

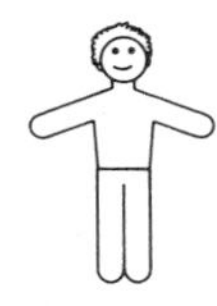

Fig. 6.2 How do I recognise myself?

- Eyes — open or shielded? gaze direct or guarded? contact maintained or avoided? aggressive or defensive?
- Facial expression — warm or grim? interested or bored? concerned or switched off?
- Voice — free or strictured? verbal cadences and tone in agreement with words, or are they flat? emotion controlled or uncontrolled? innuendoes voiced or implied?
- Silence — companionable, reflective, astonished or hostile?
- Hands — restless and nervous? clenched, still or open?
- Posture — apathetic or alert? submissive or assertive? embarrassed or condescending?
- Body — rigid or relaxed? wanting to get away or happy to stay?
- Hair / Clothes / Grooming — casual or formal? fastidious or careless? status-seeking or neglected?

What happens as a result of this exchange of signals is that impressions of each other are established. Unfortunately, often an imbalance is struck and maintained after the initial contact due to insufficient thought being given to the relationship. It is only possible to create the right balance by giving proper weight to each individual. This is shown in Figure 6.3.

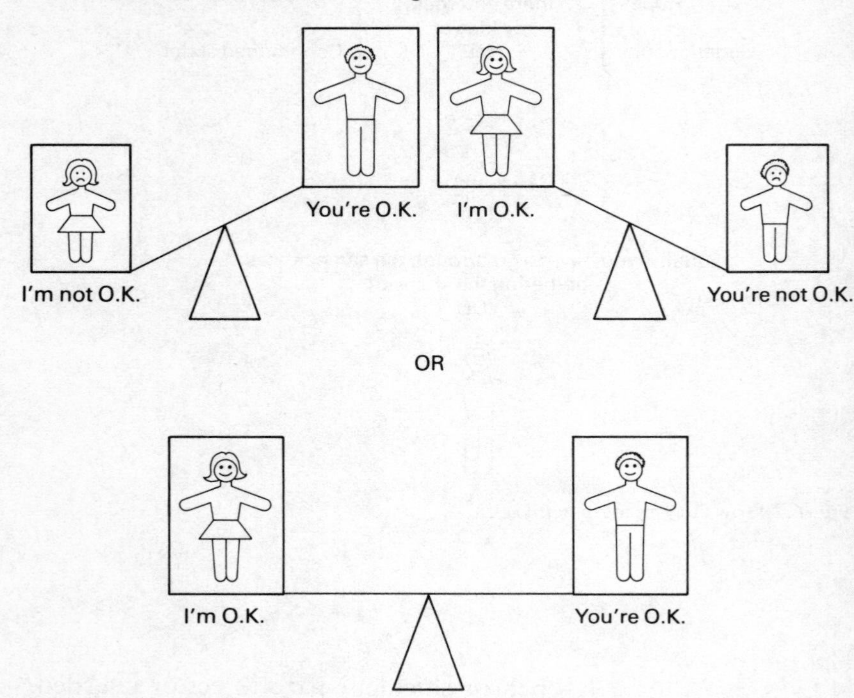

Fig. 6.3 (Above) an imbalance is created. (Below) the right balance.

What is in the Space between You and Me?

Generations of interpersonal activity have created stylised behaviours. Generally accepted rules have given rise to common courtesy as well as to the elaborate codes of doctor/patient, teacher/pupil and manager/nurse relationships. These codes have been followed almost without question for years, but in modern times many individuals are preferring to choose their own way of relating to others. For instance, the myriad formalities of who I should greet and how and when I should do it are now kept more loosely. Nurses talk to doctors in the corridors and even strangers sometimes smile at each other. This freedom of personal behaviour, however, also brings extra risk: although I can now begin to know you better, unprotected by social convention, I rarely receive full information about your innermost feelings, so I know you only in part. And I show you myself only in part. There can be further complexities of inaccuracies, misrepresentation and false assumptions. The space between people may be filled with threat instead of warmth and security (see Fig. 6.4). If I am perceptive, I can gather more about your attitude towards me and towards the subject we are discussing from your body language than from your words. For example, if you say 'I am happy and I am going out' when in fact, tears are running down your face and you are taking your coat off, then the language of your body is more convincing than your words.

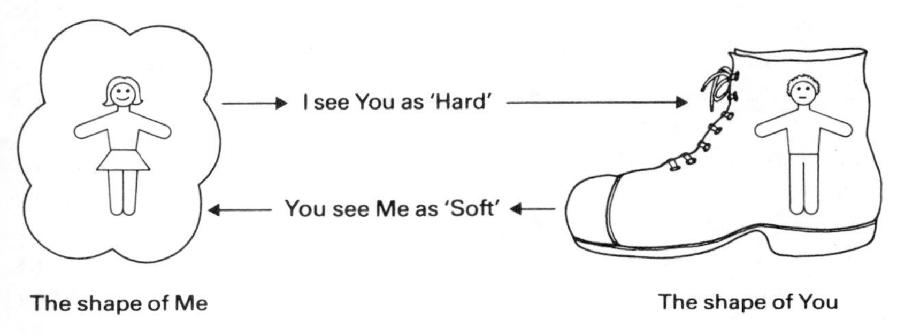

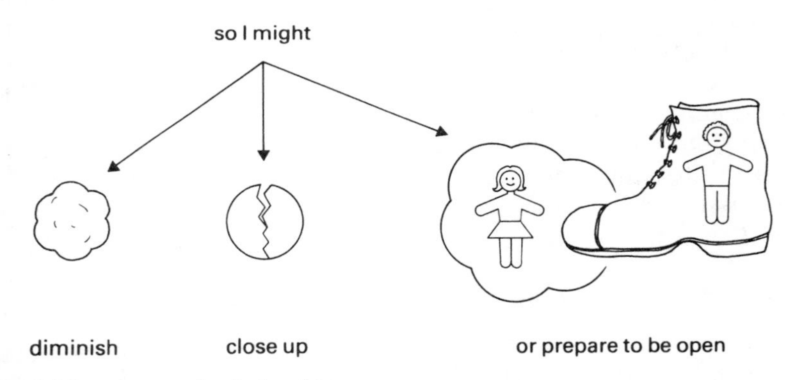

Fig. 6.4 Interpersonal relationships.

In the space between people, therefore, there is both verbal and non-verbal language which must be interpreted in the light of social rules—conventions—to which we may or may not conform. From this interplay of facts, intuition and observations, meaning has to be extracted. There are two important guidelines to finding the correct meaning.

- I must attend to you with an empty ear—empty of preconceived ideas about what I think I will hear. If my ears are full of what you might be going to say, I will not be listening to what you are saying in fact.
- I must reflect on what you say before I act. I can do this by asking: 'do I understand you to say . . . ?'; or by imagining what

you mean by those words (and not what *I* mean by those words). Then I can act with more relevance.

Can we Negotiate in this Space?

If I make a grab at something that is rightly yours, you may well be angry. If I make a grab for your favourite chair and I am bigger and more powerful than you, you may appear submissive but you would be covering up resentment and a sense of injustice. If I acknowledge that it is your chair and ask politely if I may use it, you will in all likelihood share it willingly. So it is with interpersonal relations. If my attributes and territory are acknowledged, and I feel I get that which is due to me through them, I will be less possessive and more open with them.

The process of recognising the other's weight and shape and deferring to them when appropriate has been described in many ways. It has been called 'offering positive regard' or 'stroking' or 'prizing' the other person. In our society we have worked out minute details of deference and proper demeanour, delineating when it is all right to encroach upon another's space and when it is not. Bumping into a stranger accidentally on the pavement can produce confusion and apology—his body has not been hurt, but his space has been intruded. My shape is mine, and until I offer to share it with another it is private, and when I do soften my edges and let you in, it will not be the whole of me you see and you may not push in further than you are invited. Similarly, if you give me an opening into your shape, you must be able to trust me not to encroach too far. The offering of privacy and proper dues are the basic issues with which to negotiate interpersonal relationships (Fig. 6.5).

Can these Negotiations Ensure a Desirable Outcome?

Human reactions can never be guaranteed. But if the school nurse is generous with her own territory, it increases the likelihood that others will be generous with theirs. If she can disarm the suspicions of others—by preserving their sense of worth and respecting their integrity—they will have no need to be guarded. If her openness and warmth is neither feigned nor exaggerated and if she can convince others that she believes that their truth is as true to them as her truth is true to her, then relationships will be mutually rewarding. Trust engenders confidence and confidence is a gift to be cherished above all. The goals are positive support for personal worth, personal truth and personal wholeness.

Objectives in the Use of Counselling Skills

To produce a situation in which a child can explore his own feelings in safety, in order to discover connections for himself and to determine his own way of facing life. To foster his sense of what is worthwhile and help him find a positive path ahead.

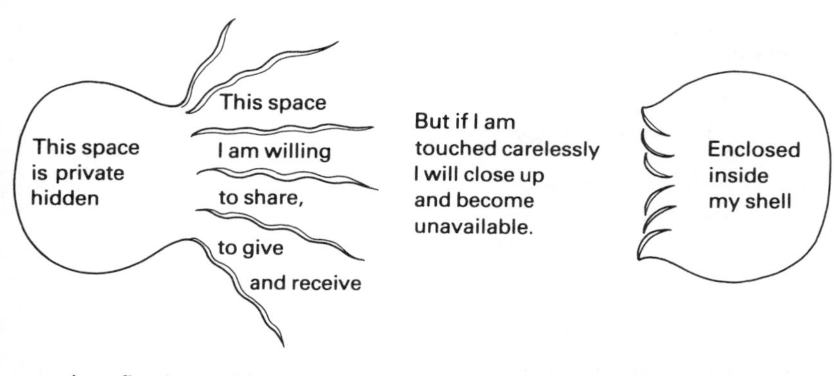

Fig. 6.5 Interpersonal space.

The word 'counselling' can be a misleading term. Spelt with a small 'c', it is sometimes equated with befriending, but that is not what it means. Spelt with a large 'C', it is sometimes used to describe a skill that is learnt by people who have attended short courses in counselling, but this is also inaccurate. There is also the professional counsellor who is a person with extensive experience of psychotherapy—her role should not be claimed by anyone else. However, there are people who have an innate ability to listen with objectivity, warmth and understanding; there are others in whom the qualities of tolerance, patience and empathy can be developed with even limited training. Among these people are school nurses who feel an urgency to relieve the enormous stress that is experienced by many young people today. They are keen to offer help that is easily accessible within the student's own environment. Many educationalists, psychologists and sociologists are pressing head teachers to make room in the school timetable for boys and girls to voice their anxieties in private. The developing role of the school nurse may lead to her increasing involvement within this process—if she has the qualities that are suitable.

It is imperative that any person taking on the counselling role should have a strong prior desire to do so; it is not a function to be urged upon someone who feels that her strengths lie elsewhere. The practice of counselling skills brings rewards, but only sometimes, and there is always the risk of mismanagement.

Being open to the personal worries of other people is a tricky matter. It requires knowledge of one's own interior dynamics and not just sympathy towards those of another. Sometimes a listening ear will be sufficient to trigger a child's exposure of his troubles and this may happen spontaneously; but on the whole, the nurse who intends to build up a listening service—perhaps a 'chat surgery'—will need to take positive steps to adapt her working conditions in order to do so. The following comments are offered as no more than *guidelines* to school nurses who want to take up counselling.

Creating the Situation which will Foster Confidentiality

Careful and thoughtful preparation will allow better communication. The anxious child will approach the appointment with some trepidation. His need is to find a someone who he can trust and who will accept him and his view of life 'warts and all'. He will need to reassure himself that he has selected the right counsellor—one who is relaxed, unpreoccupied and interested in him. To make it easier for him, the nurse will have to make sure that the practical arrangements are adequate beforehand. This will mean that she has to find:

1. a specific place which is warm and comfortable.
2. a specific time, when she can be unhurried. This time must be set within definite limits and understood by the child. (Usually the time and space will have been agreed upon beforehand.)
3. absence of interruption by people or by distracting noise. A notice on the door may prove helpful, although some children cannot relax behind a door that is closed tightly.
4. two chairs: the desk can be beside them but it should not be a barrier between them. If the chairs are placed at right angles to each other rather than directly opposite, the nurse and the child may look at each other periodically, but the intensity of continuous appraisal is avoided.
5. conditions whereby the eyes of child and nurse can be kept at about the same level. If there are no chairs suitable, the nurse should not tower over the child. If necessary, the nurse can perch on a table or squat beside a wheelchair. When looking at the child, the nurse should look at his eyes, but not all the time. Eye contact can show empathy, but a child who is frightened may be unable to maintain it constantly.

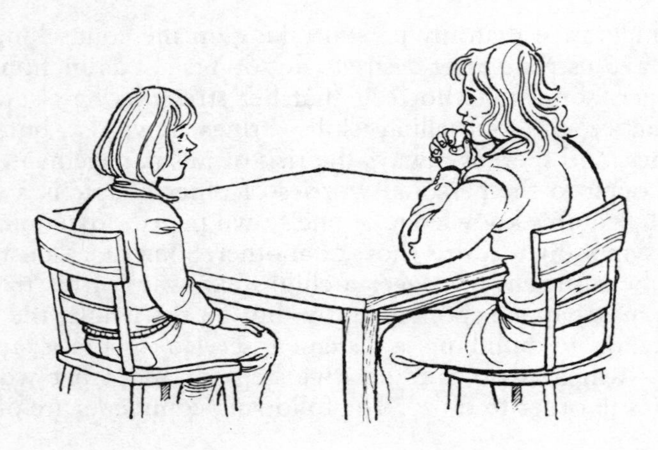

Reaction of the Counsellor

It is a first principle of counselling that when the counsellor hears the client's anxieties, she should resist over-reacting. There should be no sign of shock or outrage, no matter how disturbed the counsellor may feel and no matter how hard the child might try to test the limits of the counsellor.

It may be useful for the counsellor to see herself as either a receptacle into which used up emotions can be thrown and thereby got rid of—or as a tray upon which confused emotions can be laid out and sorted. She herself may not need to say anything positive, but just offer occasional monosyllables or noises that encourage him to continue. She may be able to see related themes between his worries and lead him to trace these connections himself. For instance, she may be able to guide him to realise that his mother's recent unfriendliness and tearfulness are because there is less money in the house and not because she has stopped loving him. Or she may enable him to untie some knots that are wrongly placed; the fact that he was 'naughty' one day was not the cause of his Granny's accident the next day.

It is important that she reflect his feelings, not add her own. She can say: 'You say what happened makes you feel angry?', but not 'What you say makes me feel angry'. The therapeutic interview is for him to ventilate his feelings, not for her to air hers. The counselling situation is fundamentally different from the befriending situation. The purpose of the first is to ventilate the specific problem of the client; it is in the second that concerns are shared.

Unless she is directly asked, the nurse is not in a position to offer positive advice. She can nudge him into seeing a solution for himself when necessary; instead of saying the words 'you must...', she can ask 'had you thought of...?'

If possible, it should be made easy for the child to reverse his ideas without his losing face or inviting undue comment.

Sometimes it may be helpful to offer to act as the child's advocate—to put his point of view to parents or staff whom he thinks of as being too powerful to confront—but only if he asks for it. He should be encouraged to manage the problem with the counsellor's support and not necessarily with her participation.

Disengagement tactics are essential for the nurse as well as the child. Generally children are able to free themselves more easily than an adult when the need for close contact is no longer necessary. Most school nurses are too busy to allow themselves to cling to the helping role after it is no longer necessary. A well-known story illustrates this principle well: a wealthy Arab died leaving 17 camels. His will stipulated that his eldest son should inherit half his camels, his second son a third, and his young daughter a ninth of the total. Consternation followed the reading of the will, jealousy and panic—how could his wishes be carried out? A wise neighbour intervened with the offer of one of his camels, making the total 18. This enabled the son to have half the total (9), the second son a third (6) and the daughter a ninth (2). Having settled the problem, the neighbour withdrew his own camel, and was none the poorer. In such a way, a wise counsellor steps in to enable others to solve their difficulties, and steps back when his work is done.

Confidentiality is a matter of perennial concern. At the first stage, it is the confidence that the child feels in the listener which enables him to be secure enough to let out his feelings. Once he is so exposed, his own confidence in himself will have to be rebuilt. But what if the confidences that he has shared with the listener need to be introduced to other people if the problem is to be solved? How much is confidence confidential? When this becomes a difficulty for the nurse working in school, the following criteria may be useful.

- As soon as the listener feels out of her depth, uncomfortable or inadequate in any way about her coping power, she should consider referring the child to someone else. Battling on to see the situation through is in no one's interest, and it is at this point that mishandling could compound the problem.
- At this stage there are four options open to the listener:
  1. suggest to the child that he might like to approach someone else (either a specific professional or an appropriate significant other), but do nothing herself, keep quiet about the whole incident.
  2. suggest to the child that he might like to approach that other person, but communicate with that person herself without telling the child.
  3. suggest to the child that he might like to approach the other person, but make sure a little later that contact has been made and has been successful.
  4. suggest to the child that she approaches the other person herself with the child's permission, or indeed that they go together.
- On the rare occasions where the ultimate physical or moral *safety* of the child is in question, the school nurse can share the trouble with a senior colleague—school doctor or head teacher as seems most relevant to the case—whether or not she has the child's permission. The counsellor will have to decide, in this instance, whether telling the child of her intention will relieve either his burden of responsibility in the matter or his anxiety about the other agent's reaction. Where relief is unlikely, the nurse may have to leave her verbally expressed intentions vague. On no account must she 'promise not to tell', and then do just that. In gross cases such as repeated incest, where she promised

secrecy as the condition upon which to draw the confidence of the child, she may be able to indicate to an appropriate colleague that there is a matter that needs further investigation. There can be no hard rules; each circumstance and each individual will need a different and sensitive management.

These comments on the skills of counselling may appear too constrictive to the well-intentioned reader. But discipline of one's own emotions is necessary when caring for developing children. Each child has a shape of his own. They each need to explore the world around them and grow at their own rate. They put out tentative tendrils that can become bruised or twisted among obstacles that distort their shape. Sometimes they need to be disentangled or helped away from directions that are harmful. Warmth, encouragement and watchful care are needed—not heat, pressure or clumsy pruning. The school nurse can provide just such an environment, but she must be fully aware of what she is doing.

Objectives in the Use of Communication Skills

To employ techniques whereby intentions and meanings can be conveyed which otherwise would be unavailable or lost. These techniques may be used one-way, but the messages are shared and mutually understood.

Communication is achieved by a combination of process and skills. This section concentrates on the technical aspects of communication such as language, the framing of the message and the reception of the message.

The skills of the speaker/initiator lie in three areas:

1. In being able to give *full attention* to the recipient—

   what can *he* understand?
   what is *his* level of receptivity?
   can he use words as tools to convey *his* meaning?
   do his formed words match his mental capacity?
   to what extent does my meaning match his meaning?

   The initiator makes this assessment whether the recipient is a 'normal child', a child with special needs, a parent or another member of staff.
2. In being able to *continually adjust* to the needs of the recipient. To do this, the speaker will choose an appropriate language style. It can range from the simple, non-elaborated, restricted vocabulary type to the expert, elaborated, wide-ranging usage already familiar to her.
3. In being able to choose how the message is conveyed. It can, for example, be conveyed by personal contact, the 'unseen' spoken word, the 'unheard' spoken word and/or the written word.

Language

It is fundamental to good communication that words are chosen according to the understanding of the receiver, rather than according to the understanding of the speaker. I, the speaker, must choose words, signs and codes that match the level of understanding of the child or adult to whom I am speaking, and this involves care and expertise on my part. But at the same time I must accept from the recipient whatever he can offer, whether it is expert or inexpert, appropriate or inappropriate, and I must work to understand what he *means* to say. The reply that he gives will depend on his experience, his powers of sensory perception, his muscular control and his level of verbal development at this stage. These same principles apply whether I am dealing with a child with speech difficulties or whether I am telephoning a colleague or writing to a parent.

There are certain forms of words that are unsuitable to use in certain situations; for instance, although children use the latest slang amongst themselves, it is not often fitting that the nurse should use such phrases when writing to a parent. Similarly certain medical jargon can be used as an efficient professional shorthand between medical staff, but it would be inappropriate to expect other disciplines to understand it. This difference in meaning can apply to quite simple terms and phrases; for example, the question 'did he perform well?' will refer to totally separate functions when put to a teacher concerning a child's test results, to a critic concerning a pianist, to a parent concerning school cricket or to a nurse concerning a constipated child. Meaning becomes even more open to misunderstanding when complicated phrases are used between people with differing levels of education and training. The Mad Hatter was right when he said that it is as difficult to claim that 'I say what I mean' as it is to say 'I eat what I see'.

The Message

There are several principles involved in sending an effective message. These principles may appear elementary, but it is surprising how often they are neglected. These main principles are:

1. identification of the person for whom the message is intended—for example,

   Hello, Mrs Smith...
   Good morning, Mr Jones...
   Please ask Jo Green...

2. identification of the speaker—for example,

   It's the school nurse, Mrs Brown speaking.
   My name is Mrs Brown, I'm the school nurse.
   ...from me, Mrs Brown—and remind him I'm the school nurse—if he could...

3. the use of words that are clear and accurate as interpreted by the recipient, including date and/or time as applicable.
4. the use of as few words as is necessary to attain this end.

5. the establishment of goodwill—for example,
   I hope you're well...
   I'm glad to see you...
   ...please...

The Recipient with Special Needs

These principles are particularly important when choosing words for use with a child whose vocabulary is restricted. Each word must be telling. Many techniques have been devised for communicating with people whose ability in speaking, seeing, hearing, reading or comprehension is partial. Such schemes are increasingly found in the ordinary school and although it is unlikely that the peripatetic school nurse will be called upon to be expert in such special skills, she should be familiar with their general management.

Children with Immature Speech

This group would include young children, new immigrants or those with problems of comprehension. Simplicity and clarity are the keynotes to communicating with people whose level of verbal development is immature. If the wording or the message is too complicated, the recipient may pretend to understand in order to gain the approval of the speaker. It is important to be sure that the meaning of a sentence has been understood before launching into a new one. If the expected response does not come, repeat the same words slowly and clearly, as long as those are words known to be recognisable by the child. The following are pointers to bear in mind:

- Avoid tension, disapproval, confrontation, confusion, complexity or haste.
- Encourage a relaxed attitude in both speaker and child; light-heartedness should be encouraged, especially when mistakes are made (but never ridicule the child).
- Encourage play; 'can you copy me?'
- Aim for one stimulus and one effort at a time. Distraction by too many simultaneous demands is counterproductive.
- Reassure the speaker: mistakes do not matter, try again.
- Reward the speaker for success; this should be offered instantly, not delayed until later. The reward can be a pleased nod, a smile, a counter, a sweet or a hug.
- Reinforce the correct response; repeat the correct sound, whether it came by accident or on purpose. All desirable efforts should be confirmed—undesirable sounds and behaviour should be ignored in the hope that they will fade. An impression given of strong disapproval may 'fix' the unwanted word in the child's mind and it will inhibit his further attempts to try something new.
- Have patience and an interest that is real and maintained.

Children with Limited Sight

Verbal contact with children who are partially sighted is usually excellent. The exception is the child who has been blind since birth. Due to his condition, he will not know some of the non-verbal signals which accompany speech; facial expressions cannot be learnt by young children who are unable to see them. These children do not give feedback to the speaker—above all, the subtle movements of muscles around the eyes and mouth, which are part of the language armoury of the sighted person, tend not to occur. This may result in facial expressions that are inappropriate to the speech used, but they do not represent inappropriate meanings.

It is important for the speaker to place herself in front of the child with limited sight and look directly at him. His acute hearing will detect whether her head is turned to one side. If he can feel that he is not receiving the speaker's full attention, he cannot be expected to respond with total interest.

Written communication with partially sighted people is usually by means of books prepared with large print or using the Braille alphabet. Typewriters are available in school, although arrangements to avoid distraction for the other children, due to their 'clacking' noise, may have to be made. The list of books available, both with large print or in Braille is extensive and growing all the time.

Children with Limited Hearing

Deafness has been called the hidden handicap. It does not call out for sympathy because its signs are not visible. If a child cannot hear well, he cannot know what it is he should have heard. This simple fact often leads to false assumptions; the child with poor hearing may appear to be slow or even stupid because he is not aware that there is anything to which he should respond. Communication with the child who has been diagnosed as having a hearing loss, whether it is temporary, partial or profound, is based on three techniques:

1. *Lip reading*—Considerable concentration by the child is required and anything that could be distracting should be eliminated.

   The speaker should:

   —enunciate deliberately, but not in an unnatural or exaggerated fashion.

   —look directly at the child and avoid turning her head or distracting the child by gesticulating with hands or arms.

   —resist the temptation to raise her voice. This is usually pointless and can appear to be shouting or a display of anger to the deaf child and his classmates.

Lip reading may be accompanied by the use of cued speech—that is hand movements on the part of the trained speaker which indicate the pitch and tone of sounds and the differences between mouthed consonants.

2. *The use of mechanical hearing aids*—These systems may be of three types:
   —a small amplifier worn behind the affected ear(s). These post-aural aids can scarcely be seen, but their controls are difficult for young children and their power is restricted.
   —an earphone may be connected to an amplifier with easier controls and more power, which is attached by means of braid straps to the child's chest or worn on a belt at the waist. This device can include separately designed amplification for each ear if necessary. It can also incorporate a microphone to pick up the child's own voice and/or environmental sounds. It may have a receiver for the teacher's voice.
   —a microphone and transmitter may be worn by the teacher herself—signals from this can be sent without further wires across a room, a large gym or even a field.

   The nurse in school may be required to clean the ear-moulds of these aids, using mild soap and water but not spirit-based solvents. The equipment should not be allowed to become too damp and must be removed before swimming or bathing. Changing the batteries may be the nurse's task. There may also be a recharging stack within the school where phonic ear systems are left overnight. The nurse in school should check the child's ears for wax or infection when necessary.

3. *The use of sign language*—Children who have been deaf since birth or who have a profound acquired deafness may need to rely solely on signing with their hands. This inevitably tends to isolate them in auditory speech situations. However, children who are skilled in silently 'talking' in sign language take enormous delight in it. The closeness and comradeship within a group busily signing to each other is something to be prized.

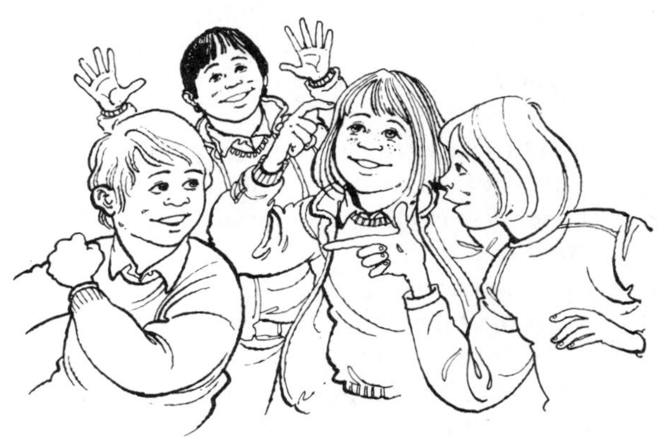

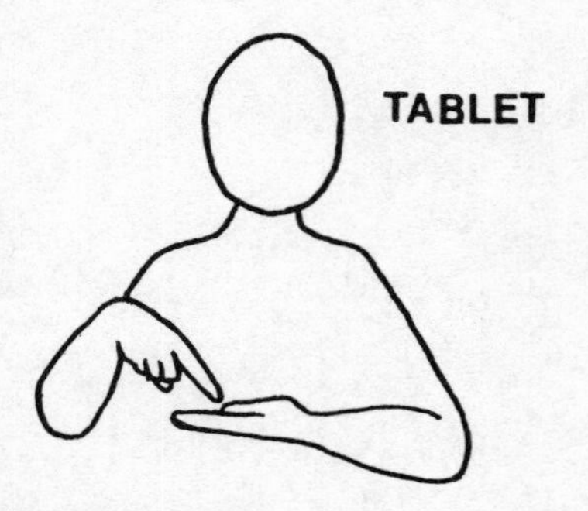

index finger draws small circle on other palm

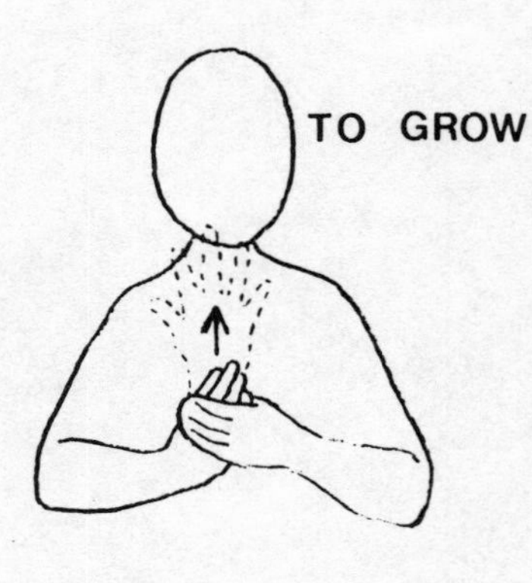

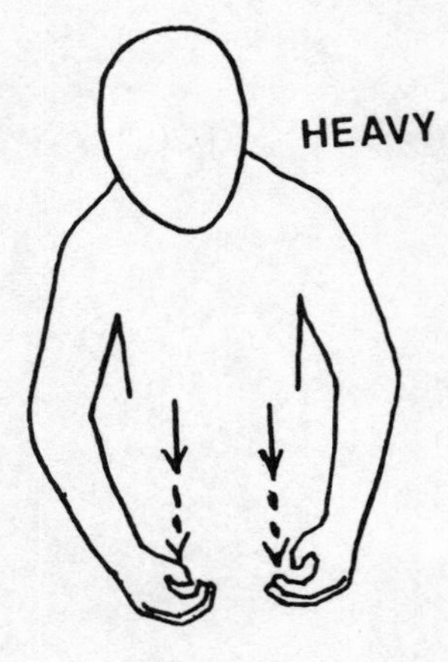

Fig. 6.6 Examples of Makaton words. Reprinted with permission from Margaret Walker, Makaton Vocabulary Development Project.

Children with Limited Speech

The process of converting images held in the mind into neurological stimuli which mobilise the larynx, pharynx, tongue, cheeks and lips is extraordinarily complex. Any obstacle at any specific stage can result in a difficulty in speaking. The ensuing aphasia may be due to a problem of conceiving the initial idea, of expressing it in speech, of hearing the message or of interpreting its meaning. The causes of language disorder include social deprivation, congenital impairment such as harelip, neoplasm, psychological trauma, mental retardation, brain damage due to accident or violence, or perinatal neurological damage such as spasticity. Within these causes, effects can be mixed: restricted neurological or muscular control may affect a child with normal or above average intelligence and impose a speech problem; alternatively, a child with normal musculature may have restricted intelligence and yet present a similar speech difficulty. Occasionally a child with disabilities in all these areas may have symptoms producing the same problem. In practice, the school nurse meeting a child with obvious language difficulty in ordinary school should never presume that he has limited intelligence; the two conditions must not be confused.

There are two further considerations: first, an otherwise healthy child can have immature language due to social deprivation. If he does not have sufficient experience of words or of living, he will not have the tools with which to speak fluently nor the ideas to speak about. Second, there are dramatic cases where a child can speak, but he prefers not to—for reasons that may be conscious or unconscious. Usually these children have become withdrawn due to fear, repression or a sense that they themselves are only able to add harm to a situation. Neither intimidation nor cajolery can 'force' these children to speak; what is needed is warmth, security and the confirmation that they are of value for themselves. Fortunately these cases are rare and they are usually referred for child guidance.

Since language disability has so many and various causes, a number of substitute means of communication have been created. The most commonly used at present are:

1. remedial techniques with a speech therapist.
2. the finger alphabet. This is still perhaps the commonest sign language in use; however its users must have a fluent knowledge of normal spelling.
3. Makaton sign language (Fig. 6.6). In this language symbolic gestures and movements are attached to complete words or phrases. For instance, 'drinking' is expressed with an action that is recognised around the world—lifting a cup to the mouth and tilting it. Abstract symbols are also included in the vocabulary, and

the imaginative user can invent his own strategies of meaning. It is therefore a system with flexibility and reward.
4. less well-known signing techniques are the Paget Gorman for intelligent aphasics and the Amarind system.
5. methods which need external equipment are Blissymbolics, Possum operated type-outs and more recently, synthesised voices. All these need specialist teaching, although they can be 'read' easily by the listener. If the nurse comes into contact with any of them in an ordinary school, they will be operated by children who can hear, so her main responsibility will be to spend time with them, to speak to them directly and to 'stay with it' while they work out their response.
6. techniques of emotional release as guided by a child psychologist.

Children with Limited Mobility

The essence of working with these children is to go to them where they are without expecting them to come to you. It is useful to establish level eye contact—the school nurse can make herself their height instead of making them crane their necks to contact her. The teacher has to be seen to stand up straight in front of her class; it is easier for the nurse to be more informal and sit or squat or kneel next to a wheelchair or a short child in calipers. If appropriate, she can hold or touch the arm or hand or shoulder of the child while he is speaking—reassurance can be given in this way, especially to a child whose image of his own body is distorted, unbalanced and perhaps, therefore, difficult to accept. In this the nurse has a great advantage over school staff whose roles require them to retain more distance.

Summary

Communicating with others is an exacting task; it demands patience and empathy, although the aim is always to make it appear easy and flowing. A non-verbal element such as facial expression, which is approving or disapproving, can make the difference between a child opening up or closing down his personality. Whatever methods are used and whatever responses are obtained, communicating is the vital link between the child's interior world and the wide exterior world. The caring adult acts as mediator.

Objectives in the Use of Educative Skills

To make an informed contribution to both the learning environment and the actual learning of the schoolchild. To develop his awareness of his own responsibility in health care and to encourage apt decision-making in his own personal and social growth.

Education should be a process of discovery. It is a two-way process between learner and learning, and those who teach may identify themselves with one or the other. From the standpoint of the nurse, education enables children in her care to acquire facts, methods and meanings about maintaining their own full health. If conditions are right, the school nurse can both extend her skills and help to expand the student's appreciation of wellness.

The nurse who is working in an educational establishment but who is rarely trained as an educator herself will have to become truly aware of what is meant by the 'optimum learning environment'. Looked at negatively, a child's learning capacity will obviously be reduced if he is unwell, cold, hurt (physically or emotionally), frightened, or bored. Therefore anything the nurse can do to better the situation will make learning easier for the child.

The skills which the nurse needs when she considers her own teaching capabilities will depend upon the style and circumstances she prefers. Does she prefer one-to-one instruction, taking part in groups or talking to a whole class? She may incline towards working with one child so that content can be tailored exactly to needs. Relating to a group, on the other hand, will provide greater stimulation, interchange and a variety of opinions or solutions. The third option, taking on a whole class, calls for skill in the control of numbers and the ability to handle unexpected questions from a position at the head of the room. In preparing her teaching activities, she will have to take into account:

- the number of students involved.
- their stage of physical and academic development.
- their degree of maturity.
- their commonly used vocabulary.
- their cultural background.
- the attention span that can be reasonably expected from a particular group of pupils and their capacity for absorbing new information.

There will be times when a student will be particularly receptive to learning and others when he has to tread water in order to consolidate what he has learnt. There will be cycles in his mental activity, and after a forward leap he may need to come back to what has been said before. The amount of stimulation put into one session has to be carefully assessed; an overwhelming display of knowledge can reduce concentration in children and blunt their attentiveness, just as an impoverished presentation can produce boredom. Audiovisual aids are useful as tools, but they are only an aid to teaching and not the teaching itself; they will need the back-up of discussion—either on the same occasion or at a future date.

Working with teachers to create a learning environment, the school nurse will come across different theories of learning and different styles of teaching. These will reflect the various temperaments and experiences of the teachers and the various personalities and inclinations of the children. Some will prefer the giving and receiving of formal, proved facts and some will respond better to shared exploration.

This is not the place to enlarge on educational techniques, but some comments may be useful.

- It is good, where possible, to allow others to learn out of their own interest and curiosity—because they *want* to construct their own meanings out of confusion. When there is a gap in our understanding, we all feel the need to fill it and we all enjoy the pleasure and relief of being able to do so. If the gap is instantly plugged by someone else, we are denied this satisfaction. It is then that the instruction can become boring and valueless.
- Similarly, if learning is something to be got through in order to appease an adult, the excitement of discovery will be taken away.
- It is all too easy for an adult to use the fears natural to childhood to reinforce her own position. For instance, a child's anxiety of being shown up when wrong, of not conforming to 'normal' behaviour, or of not pleasing the person in authority are powerful inhibitors and should not be manipulated. Similarly, if spontaneity and originality are to be encouraged, mistakes cannot be looked upon as failures, but rather as episodes which can be learnt from.
- Adults may have to relinquish the position of being always right. Even the position of being seen to be in control of information may not always be appropriate. Open-endedness can be more helpful in allowing pupils to work things out for themselves.
- Stress, frustration and tension often act as precursors of some new insight; they are not necessarily states to be avoided. Before a shift in position can occur, the extra energy needed to deal with the change has to be mobilised. Pressure from within or without may be an acceptable precondition which triggers off this new charge of energy or motivation. The various dimensions of educating young people are shown in Fig. 6.7.
- We tend to educate our children in the collecting of right answers. But often there is no right answer, just a selection of alternatives from which to choose. Choices and decisions are major concerns of education and the ability to adapt to changing circumstances is a major outcome of education. This process of problem-solving includes both thinking and behaviour; it embraces intellectual cleverness—which is made up of accurate memory, efficient recall and an ability to order factors so that they form connections—as well as the development of responsibility towards oneself and the community.

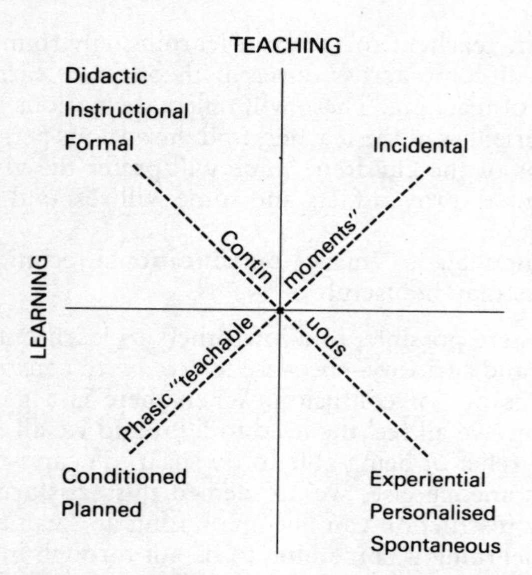

Fig. 6.7 Dimensions of educating.

- Some would contend that the people best able to cope with life are those who have learnt to think for themselves and adapt to changing situations as they arise.
- Risk and uncertainty surround us in the adult world. Those who have learned that breaking apart and reordering are in the nature of things become less disturbed by this uncertainty. Change and further change are integral parts of growth and development and dynamism.

The most desirable assets with which to leave school can be summarised as:

- An ability to make friends, to trust and to remain unthreatened by pretended power.
- A capacity to live with uncertainty in an ever-changing world.
- Creativity and the courage and faith to carry through ideas.
- Curiosity which is continually and confidently looking for a greater understanding of the people and things around us.
- Wonder which results from an acceptance that there are no absolute answers.

Together these constitute a large measure of *wholeness*.

Further discussion of education can be found elsewhere (see bibliography). However, it should be noted that there is a growing movement to include in schools more teaching that is directly relevant to daily living. This teaching emphasises the qualities which help people to enjoy life and get along together such as self-reliance, initiative, kindness, spontaneity, courage, creativity, responsibility and wonder—rather than the qualities which focus

Table 6.1
Methods of Learning

Precepts of Conventional Learning	*Aims of Expanded Learning*
Accepted and formal methods	Natural, spontaneous, self-discovery methods.
Authoritarian, hierarchical style	Collegiate style, each teacher and student respecting the other, in the round. Autonomy not quashed.
Primary reliance on didactic instruction	Discussion and experiment welcomed. Exploration of facts, ideas, relationships encouraged. Creativity, includes guessing and spontaneity.
Compliance by student, acceptance and recounting of given 'correct' answers	No right answers—each can find own solution which may agree with others or may not. Agree to disagree when necessary.
Emphasis on content and on proved material	Emphasis on questioning, providing for oneself, searching for connectedness, creating coherence and significance which is real to the individual.
Discipline imposed by fear of sanctions	Self-discipline confirmed by approval.
Learning has a product; the desired outcome is 'good' exam results and 'good' paid work	Learning is a progress, journey never completed.
Uniform instruction—same numbers, time, place	Variety and balance in gregariousness/privacy, exuberance/quiet.
Education is contained mainly within the classroom	Community and the environment are part of matrix of education. Family's values are important, as is the responsible use of resources.
Schooling is seen as a limited period spent in legally assigned places to inculcate minimum knowledge and social skills to hold on to a productive job	Schooling is seen as lifelong process, the desire for which is whetted during childhood development and part of which takes place in established school sites.

upon success in a job-orientated world. Such alternative educational aims seem sensible as children face a future in which there is likely to be more leisure and less work.

Principles and methods of learning are under much discussion at present. Some of those that are current are summarised in Table 6.1.

Objectives in the Use of Recording Skills

To document information that is relevant to a child's health, safety and physical development in a form that encourages continuity. To build a record that is readily retrievable to those professionals whose concern it is to coordinate services for the well-being of the child.

Today the quantity of information is so large that the problems of what to record and how to do it are as never before. But what does recording entail? The verb 'to record' encompasses several ideas:

- To *register*, literally to carry forward, particulars that are entered systematically in a register: e.g. weight and height measurements.
- To *represent* in a permanent form knowledge that is authentic and worth preserving: e.g. perinatal data, congenital abnormality.
- To set down for *remembrance* facts that could be distorted if committed to memory only: e.g. health behaviour patterns such as falling down in playground, asthmatic attacks and school absences.
- To set down for *reference*, providing an attributable source to look back upon: e.g. the first time the child complained of headaches, the dates he was found to have bruises, the last time his vision was checked.

The word 'record' comes from the Latin to bring again to the heart, to think over or to be mindful of, but this connotation forms a paradox in modern recording. Records that are permanent are not the proper place for subjectivity or personal opinion, especially when accountability and possible litigation are taken into account. However, there are instances when the manner in which facts are recorded has to be reflected upon with extra care.

When the essential qualities of permanency, accuracy, authenticity, accountability and legibility are taken on board, it is understandable that there should be a natural reluctance to make a record of anything other than measurements. The following comments provide guidelines for nurses and others who find the task somewhat daunting.

Why Record?

The reasons for recording are strong. The organisation of health findings and measurements into one document can be pivotal in the treatment or management of a child. Not all children attend health centres, GP surgeries or hospital clinics regularly, but almost all children do attend school regularly. The school health record is, therefore, a tool for interdisciplinary cooperation; it is an accurate record of fact should any question arise; it is an instant aid for new members of staff and for relief workers should regular staff be absent. Impressionistic knowledge has its value, but where there is need for the transfer of duties, only objective data is acceptable. In these terms, the child's health record can be viewed as an instrument of communication.

How to Record?

Three methods of recording are presented here. In practice, however, different arrangements are found in different schools and it is the responsibility of each school nurse to ensure that her recording procedure is adequate for the fulfilling of her responsibilities as outlined in her job description. If the nurse inherits a position in which it is difficult to do this, it is up to her to ask her management for the space and equipment which will enable her to discharge her duties efficiently.

It is worth noting here a detail that applies to all recording: only brief measurements or notes should be put down when the mother, father or child is present. Lengthy and silent writing can alienate confidence and create barriers—'what's she writing down about me now?'

Example 1 The usual five year old developmental health examination is undertaken at the medical centre a few months before school entry when the children are around four-and-a-half years old. At this examination, the children who will soon be starting at 'big' school can get to know each other, and the mothers can meet the school nurse with the health visitor whom they already know. Child health records can be discussed together and the relevant details copied by the school nurse for her use at school. In some districts, mothers are encouraged to keep the booklet containing their child's health record themselves and to bring it to school for updating at each screening session or medical examination. The progress of physical development, illness and immunisations can all be kept in the one booklet.

Example 2 In some schools, the health visitor prefers to visit the school nurse a few weeks after the entry of the children in their patch. Relevant details can then be transferred onto the 10M forms supplemented by the 10(B)M which is kept at school. These may be stored in the medical room or in the headmaster's office, depending upon the facilities available.

Example 3 If the child's previous history is not known, the school nurse can contact the mother for his health information when she visits school early in the term of her child's entry. Some nurses design a questionnaire to glean the necessary facts themselves, and when this has been duplicated and approved by the head teacher, it is sent home via the children. Some nurses meet the mothers by interview or at a parents' meeting or as the parents deliver their children at the school gate.

In summary then, the collected information can be kept in:

- the child's own health record booklet.
- 10M charts kept at school.
- other card indexes kept by the nurse at each school.
- records kept by the school nurse in filing cabinets at a central clinic.
- records kept in a computer bank by lay administrators.
- computerised total child health register which collates neonatal discharge data, infant and preschool immunisation, significant diagnoses and treatment, medical personnel attending, school screening results and appointment clinics.

Easy access to stored information and ready retrieval of exact wanted facts should be high priorities in the chosen system of storage.

What to Store?

The problems of *how* and *where* to store records will often reflect the difficulties of *what* to store. *What* needs to be stored is usually clear and generally includes information of birth date, position in family, preventive health care in infancy and childhood, infections, chronic illnesses or disabilities, effects of treatment, allergies, dietary needs, regular medical records and results of screening procedures.

Questions often arise about what to do with information that does not fall into a clear category. The school nurse will meet many potentially tragic situations—some of which can be made worse by officious intrusion—and she may have to pause to consider the outcome of further enquiry before recording information. The school nurse is often the first professional who is contacted, and she will have to decide whether a hint is a veiled cry for help or simply an indication of a difficulty which will resolve if left alone. This is where the *assessment of probabilities* may have to be discussed with a respected colleague—if possible avoiding proper names if confidentiality is involved. These sensitive areas include:

- Indications of marital distress as reflected in the child.
- Alcohol abuse in the home background.
- Reports of hidden physical bullying at school.

- Parental criminal record as it affects the child.
- Suspicion of non-accidental injury to the child.
- Suspicion of sexual abuse.
- Incest.
- Self-inflicted violence.
- Emotional maladjustment.

Satisfactory guidelines for these situations have yet to be devised. The following pointers may help:

- The drama or novelty of any situation should be resisted. When possible, a pause is advisable so that reactions can settle down and the real threats can be assessed before action or public recording is undertaken.
- Only factual evidence and not suppositions should be recorded. In some circumstances phrases such as 'the class teacher expressed concern . . .' may be seen as a 'fact'.
- Beware of adding heat to a situation; a problem that is merely smouldering can become inflamed if it is stirred.
- Where possible, the agreement of the client should be obtained before a confidence is told to a colleague.

What Goes into the Records

The content of the records is largely defined by who has access to them. They will always be available to the school doctor, the head teacher and the nursing manager. Class teachers should be kept in touch with health information relevant to the child's learning capabilities.

Who is to Share Information?

As more children with special needs are admitted to ordinary schools, more staff in different disciplines will be concerned with their care. How to extend such care and yet avoid duplicating it depends largely upon a central school medical record which can be seen by and added to by all staff concerned. There are moves to allow parents to see records, but this is not common policy yet. It is usually acceptable for statisticians and epidemiologists to see the records. In future a system may develop whereby each class teacher is automatically given a slip describing the outcome of the medical examination of a child in her class if time does not permit direct personal contact. Such good practice is rare at present.

The cooperation of the school secretary is often crucial to the smooth working of the peripatetic school nurse as she will be the carrier of messages, the key to access of information and a fund of clues about recording. Friendship and good relations between the school secretary and nurse will directly add to the welfare of the school child.

In the fluid situation of the present time, it is still not possible to lay down correct procedures in these matters. Through all circumstances, each school nurse will be responsible for her own integrity regarding records and for carrying out common policy.

Objectives in the Use of Public Relations Skills

To establish means whereby the work of the school nurse may be better understood and better used by the population she seeks to serve.

The value of developing skills in public relations may not be immediately obvious to the nurse working in school. However, the fact is that if the benefits she offers are not sufficiently publicised, some of them will remain unknown and underused. As the potential of the school nurse gradually gains proper acknowledgement, it is important that each school nurse ensures there is wide understanding of her contribution to the total well-being of the children in her care. There are many public relations opportunities of which she can take advantage. Publicity can be gained through writing or speaking, in person or through the media, in surroundings that are familiar or unfamiliar.

These activities can be enjoyable as well as rewarding.

- The exercise of public relations skills can be through *writing*: short articles in the school paper, notes in the school newsletter circulated to parents, letters to the local paper or to the national nursing press and/or articles in various journals. It is important that each school have a simple leaflet describing the prevention and promotion measures offered to the children by the school health service. Some districts have such leaflets already designed which are distributed in all their schools. Some head teachers prefer to have their own policy document tailored to their schools' needs. The services of the school nurse can be highlighted in these leaflets. Some nurses prepare their own introductory sheet, which is then duplicated. Any of this publicity material can be given to the parents of new entrants, each member of staff and all interested visitors.
- The exercise of public relations skills can be through *speaking*. Short talks can be given to parents if the head teacher approves. Groups of professional colleagues often appreciate some description and clarification of the work of the nurse in school. Interdisciplinary staff meetings at school and informal meetings of colleagues in the community are all welcome opportunities for increasing understanding. Meetings outside school of school governors, community nurse trainees, GP trainees, or voluntary organisations can provide a forum where the work of the nurse can be discussed. When a request is received for a talk to be given, whether inside or outside the school, it should not be difficult to obtain the necessary approval from nursing manage-

ment although the nurse may like to put out 'feelers' to test the reaction before a definite commitment is made.

The success of speaking engagements will depend largely on the commitment of the hearers to attend and to listen as well as upon the willingness of the speaker to prepare her material well. The manner in which she presents herself is important for both the credibility of what she has to say as well as for the regard in which she and her profession are held thereafter.

- On occasion, there might be a request to exercise the public relations skills of the school nurse on the *visual media*, especially where a training programme is being reported or a particular event described. The school nurse should not be shy of showing her presence in such instances; the public should be made more aware of her involvement.

The purpose of any public relations activity is ultimately the good of the child. By defining her role and by encouraging the interest of others in the needs of children the school nurse can extend the concern for their welfare.

7 The Sessions

This section is written with the needs of both teachers and school nurses in mind.

> The role of the school nurse in relation to education is of the utmost importance, and in the past it tended to be overlooked and undervalued.
>
> Court Report, 1976

School Nurse Sessions—a Means to an End

The sessions in which school nurses are involved form part of an overall programme designed to protect, promote and improve the health of the child in order that he may derive the maximum benefit from the educational opportunities available to him. Formal education is in itself a means to this end, and both health and education services have undergone many changes in pursuance of it.

The way in which a service is planned, programmed and presented plays a crucial part in the measure of its success; the uptake of services and the motivation and efficiency of staff are to a large extent dependent upon these factors.

Traditionally the tasks associated with the school nurse have been predominantly overshadowed by the image of hygiene inspections and the control of infestation. Indeed the College of Heraldry might most appropriately have produced a School Nurse Coat of Arms based on a Snellen Eye Chart quartered with a Fine Tooth Comb, and topped by a female Dragon—but times have changed. Many of the health objectives of the past have largely been achieved: the old environmental hazards relating to impure water supplies and poor sanitation are now subject to social and industrial legislation; advances in medical science and programmes of immunisation have brought many childhood diseases under control; and the mystery which surrounded the diseases of the past has disappeared. In its place there is a greater public awareness of the current health issues and a greater willingness and desire on the part of the individual to be responsible for his own health.

Health visitors and school nurses can rightly take pride in the part which their colleagues have played to bring about these changes—changes which have effected shifts of emphasis and altered working practices within the school health service. The arbitrary pattern of routine school medical examinations has given way to the following system:

1. Medical examination and assessment of every child at the time of his entry into full-time education.
2. Programmes of immunisation and serial screening for vision, hearing, growth and development.
3. Subsequent medical examinations can be carried out on a selective basis.
4. At secondary school level there is a further medical examination or health interview for every child at about the age of 13.
5. Children are screened with a view to employment opportunities, and advised against unsuitable employment.

The effectiveness of this system is dependent upon:

1. The continuity, availability and expertise of the named school nurse in the school.
2. Efficient methods of health surveillance.
3. The vigilance of teachers.
4. Relationships of trust and understanding between the teachers, the nurse and the doctor, and regular opportunities for discussion and consultation.
5. A shared responsibility to encourage children as they get older to refer themselves to the school doctor or nurse.

Although the aims of the health and education services remain the same, the scene is set for a change in the methods by which we achieve them. Many health and education authorities are seeking to establish a pattern of work for school nurses which takes account of these issues. Two priorities emerge:

1. The need for early discovery of any disorder or deviation from normal which may affect the child's well-being or his ability to learn.
2. A policy of collaboration throughout the school between teachers and school nurses which is concerned with the whole development of the child, the state of his health, his perception of the combined efforts being made to keep his health under surveillance, and programmes designed to promote the awareness of health values and individual responsibility for health.

With these aims in mind, some health authorities have introduced school nurse programmes of annual health surveillance which include serial screening procedures. These yearly interviews provide a comprehensive oversight of the general health development of each child and the opportunity for individual health education and counselling—thus replacing the outdated image of the task-orientated school nurse and allowing her to use her professional judgement, her skills and her training to much better effect.

Under this system a personal health record card for each child is kept by the school nurse, and if at any time during his school life a child seems to be failing to thrive, the teacher may be confident of the services of a school nurse who, as part of the educational team, can provide a link with the school doctor or any other agencies who might usefully be involved.

The arguments in favour of such an approach can be summarised as follows:

1. *The use of a named school nurse* as an integral part of the educational team, and available on a regular basis, fosters good working relationships, improved communications, and a full appreciation and use of the school health service.
2. *The child's response to health care* is affected by the way in which health care services are delivered. There is, for example, a subtle difference between caring for the eyesight of a child and caring for the child and his eyesight. The child who is waiting his turn for vision testing is hardly likely to regard this as an opportunity to discuss anything other than his eyes, and in the presence of his classmates he may be inhibited even from this, exposed as he is to publicity, the pressure of time, and the awareness of being processed. His response to the privacy of a health surveillance interview, where his eyesight is screened as a part of general health care, may be quite different. He is aware that this is his interview, concerning his health care, and that it is of sufficient importance to merit individual and undivided attention.
3. *Professional responsibility and motivation*: the health care of children should be regarded as an aspect of education in which there is team involvement. Task-orientated sessions are apt to be seen as sporadic and disruptive visits from outside the education service, rather than integral to the whole needs of the child. In these circumstances it is hardly surprising that some school nurses are overlooked and undervalued, and constrained by their isolation and working conditions from carrying out their full professional duties. Moreover the sheer repetition of mass screening sessions can lead to diminishing returns in terms of efficiency and self-motivation.
4. *Research, record-keeping and evaluation of services*: the evidence of the Isle of Wight Study indicated that during their childhood as many as one in six children might suffer from a permanent or temporary disability liable to affect normal growth development or adjustment to life. There is a great deal of disturbed behaviour in children of all ages; it is suggested that between 5 and 10% of children have disorders of sufficient severity to handicap them considerably in everyday life, and for many the duration and severity of the disturbance leads to family distress, personal unhappiness and educational underachievement.

Given well-designed school nurse records, the application of the *nursing process* could be an effective tool in providing a comprehensive health plan for the child which would encompass his parents and teachers, and provide for his individual needs. The child would be encouraged to participate in self-care and to understand his own health needs, and make appropriate use of more formal health education programmes.

In the absence of sufficient collected data, it is difficult to measure or evaluate the cost-effectiveness of the school health service, particularly in terms of prevention. The available evidence points overwhelmingly to improvements in nurse/teacher cooperation, greater parental involvement, and a high degree of professional motivation among nurses engaged in work schemes similar to those recommended by the Court Report. More research is needed into the value of this approach.

As far as the present situation of health cuts is concerned, no growth should not mean no action—it does mean, however, that we should concentrate the mind in order to make the best of what we have.

The computerisation of health records is underway, and it behoves the nursing profession to ensure that staff are adequately trained in these techniques, and that the tool does not become the master.

The recording of information based on programmes of immunisation and health screening involves the processing of large numbers of children. While the computer may inform us that 20 children have slipped through the screening net, it cannot always tell us why this should be so, because much of the personal and sensitive information regarding the child and his family may never be recorded; nor can the computer teach us how best to repair these omissions. The provision of health data is a tool; the final health outcome relies, and will always rely, upon the skill with which the tool is used.

The principle of GIGO (garbage in—garbage out) must be sufficiently understood by all school nurses, so that the service while becoming more efficient in its processing of information, will consistently provide the essential elements of personal care.

Do school nurse records provide a comprehensive profile of individual health needs? How can they be used in the best interests of the child? The collection and analysis of data could supply the answer to these questions, and provide the blueprint for plans and health aims for the future.

Health Accommodation

The system of individual annual screening requires adequate facilities in school. These can be termed *health accommodation.*

Under the NHS Reorganisation Act of 1973, local education

authorities have a duty to make 'accommodation available' for medical and dental inspections; this is no longer an acceptable minimum standard. Implementation of the Education Act 1981 and modern methods of school health care necessitate fresh planning, a new approach to the health needs of children in school, and reappraisal of health accommodation to ensure its suitability.

The provision of medical examinations carried out on a selective basis has increased the need for a named school nurse with an established health base within the school. Teachers, children, parents and doctors are better able to contact the school nurse if she is available at known times and in a known place within the school. A leaflet explaining the school health programme and the times at which the nurse is available can be distributed to the parents of all new entrants, and displayed upon the school notice board.

Many schools do not contain purpose-built medical or dental accommodation and, where school populations are falling, consideration should be given to the reallocation of rooms to encompass the plans of health and education authorities, and to provide for the following needs:

1. A school nurse room suitable for carrying out health surveillance and screening procedures.
2. Special facilities which may be needed for the health care of children with handicapping conditions.
3. Medical/dental accommodation for routine examinations.
4. Changing room/waiting room/rest room facilities.
5. First aid facilities.

School Nurse Room or Health Base

This needs to be situated in a quiet part of the school with easy access to toilets. It should contain a desk, a few chairs, lockable filing space for school nurse records, lockable storage facilities, a telephone and a wash handbasin. It should be large enough and sufficiently well lit to enable vision screening to take place satisfactorily, and a soundproofed area is necessary for hearing testing. Health is a happy state, and its achievement is greatly to be desired. A room which is too clinical and does not provide comfortable seating for its visitors does not encourage the confidence and relaxation which is needed for health promotion and health care. A smile, a bowl of flowers, children's pictures or an attractive poster may do more for a child than any direct advice or education; it may also serve to lift the spirits of the nurse when life proves tiring.

This should be the room where, in addition to health surveillance, teachers and nurses can discuss health plans and programmes. The room should serve as a health resource centre within the school, and reference material should be available. It should provide a place where children, parents and working colleagues can come for information, advice and counselling, and where partnership in education and health care is forged between children, their parents and the educational team.

Special Facilities

Under current legislation, the option to attend ordinary school should become available to an increasing number of children with special needs. Much depends on the way in which educational provision is planned by the education and health authorities, and the resources which are available to them. Some authorities have already earmarked one school at each age level which will be able to provide for children with disabilities. The quality of nursing care and support in these schools is crucial to the well-being of the child, and the extent to which he is able to benefit from education. In all our dealings we should recognise and respect each child's bodily territory as his own. The child must be able to regard special nursing and toileting rooms as places where you do rather than are done to, and learning to cope should take place with *privacy* and dignity.

For some children toilets with wide doors, hand rails and space to accommodate a wheelchair may be sufficient, but for others special help may be required. Children may need to be taught the skills of self-care, management of bowel and bladder functions, stoma care, self-catheterisation, the application of appliances, skin care, the measurement and self-administration of drugs, and these skills must be developed mindful of home conditions. Parents as well as children may need the help of the school nurse and school facilities in order to ensure continuity of training, and practice of everyday care under supervision at home and at school.

There must be adequate facilities for the disposal of used dressings and syringes. Where nursing procedures are undertaken regularly a *nursing record* should be kept. It should contain comprehensive information regarding treatment, drugs and the general care of each child, so that in the absence of the regular school nurse, her locum replacement is adequately informed.

Storage and supervision of drugs: Drugs should be kept in a securely locked cupboard. They are the property of the child for whom they are prescribed, and the nurse should obtain directions in writing from the parents. The drugs should be personal, clearly labelled, and kept in the containers issued by the pharmacy. In no circumstances should nurses issue prescribed drugs from stock bottles, or dispense supplies to parents or teachers in spare containers. A prescription for two separate supplies may be needed in order that a supply may be kept at home and at school.

A record should be kept of all drugs as soon as they are dispensed, and teachers should be advised if drugs or drug dosages are changed, so that they can be alert to any behavioural changes or other effects which they may notice in the classroom.

Medical/Dental Accommodation

It is important that the room is suitable and adequately equipped to fulfil the purposes of the examination by the doctor or the dentist. Screening procedures and measurements of height and weight can be carried out at the time of the medical examination—as a general rule, it is less disruptive of school activities. In addition, this allows for full discussion between parents, doctors, teachers and the school nurse, and it is more economic of time. There should be sufficient allocation of space for the doctor and nurse to work independently of each other, but in close proximity; if the existing health room provides the facilities for screening, then it may be possible to allocate a suitable room nearby where the medical examination can take place; such a room would require hand washing facilities, adequate equipment for examination purposes, and the necessary privacy. Alternatively, if the health base is used as a medical room, then quiet, well-lit space will be needed close to it with adequate facilities to conduct and record the results of prescribed screening tests.

Rest Room/Waiting Room/Changing Room/First Aid Facilities

In every school there should be a place where first aid can be administered and where an ill child can lie down. Arrangements will differ according to the type of school and the personnel involved, but the room allocated for this purpose must be quiet and easily accessible, so that the nurse, school matron, school secretary or other responsible person delegated for these duties can keep the child under observation. Such a room might also usefully serve as a changing room, or waiting room, and could possibly be made suitable for the carrying out of hearing tests.

A Safety Net of Surveillance

The sessions now described present a possible pattern of school nurse work and health surveillance (Table 7.1). While it is recognised that there are many different ways of achieving the same ends, the search for the best way is the cornerstone of community health philosophy.

Preparing for School

Going to school is an important event in the life of children and their parents. It marks the end of one pattern of living and the beginning of another. Not every five year old child has developed the social maturity to meet new situations with confidence, and some are overwhelmed by unfamiliar faces and the strangeness of new surroundings. For the mother also it can be an anxious time: she knows that her child must cope with this new routine alone, and she may be worried about handing over the care of her child to teachers whom she does not know and who may not understand his reactions to it.

If parents are to establish their new role as partners in the education of their child, they need to build a relationship of trust

Table 7.1
Format of School Nurse Surveillance

Surveillance effected by:	
1. Pre-school preparation	(a) parents
	(b) health visitors
2. First health interview—signs of good/poor health	
	(a) weight and height
	(b) posture
	(c) vision
	(d) nose, throat and lungs
	(e) dental health
	(f) communication
	—adjustment
	—speech
	—hearing
	(g) skin and personal hygiene
	(h) hair and scalp
	(i) clothing and cleanliness
	(j) self-help skills performance
General follow-up and recording	
3. On-going surveillance	(a) dyslexia
	(b) scoliosis and lordosis
	(c) systemic analysis
	(d) screening priorities
4. Parent/school sessions	
5. Puberty and adolescence	(a) the middle years
	(b) adolescence
6. 13+ health interview.	

and confidence in the school; both parents and children need to know the school and be known by it before admission takes place.

Many schools arrange *pre-admission programmes* for parents and next term's new school entrants, and the children are introduced to school activities while their parents meet members of staff and get to know each other. Sessions such as these provide an excellent opportunity for parents to meet the school nurse as part of the school team, and to discuss the general care and well-being of their children. It is important that the discussion is allowed to develop informally so that the parents can ask questions and gain information, and become aware of the support and care which is available, and the teamwork which exists between health and education services.

As an example of a way to encourage discussion among mothers, a school nurse and head teacher from Southampton

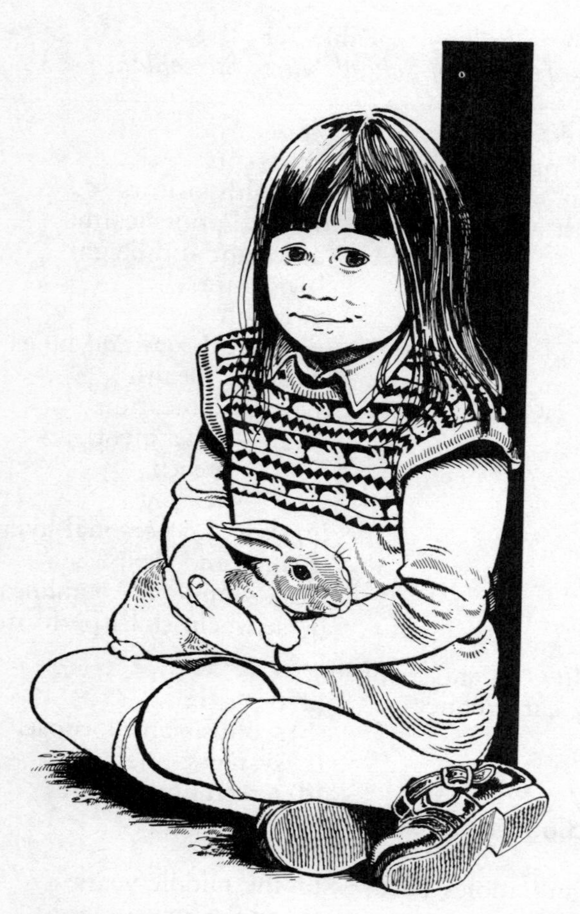

devised a set of slides which show children in typical situations and which cover the topics most commonly raised by mothers. They include social skills such as doing up buttons and coping with shoe laces, the need to manage taps and toilet handles, problems with food and eating habits. Will he be forced to eat everything up? Is he a slow eater? Will he be given time to finish? What happens in a school if a child is ill or has an accident? The topics also cover the school health and dental services, care of ears and eyes, hair and hygiene, immunisation, road safety and coping with children's quarrels and jealousies.

The introduction of pre-school sessions enables the school nurse to make contact with the appropriate health visitor. When a child enters school, it is important that information concerning his health and care is readily available to the school nurse. Many problems may already have been brought to the attention of the health visitor who has a continuing responsibility for family health care. When the case-loads of health visitors are related to specific family doctor practices, it is not easy to devise a system of communication which ensures that relevant information is shared.

Health visitors may carry out pre-school surveillance at day nurseries, nursery schools and classes, and child health clinics, as well as at home.

Not all parents will be able to avail themselves of pre-school sessions, and the school nurse should make a special effort to inform herself regarding these families, in order that their children receive the care and reassurance which is needed when first they go to 'big school'.

The School Entrant

Health surveillance in school forms part of an ongoing process which begins during the antenatal period and is continued throughout the pre-school years. Parents, health visitors, child health doctors and family practitioners will all have information and opinions concerning the health and well-being of the child.

Lists of new school entrants are usually issued to school nurses the term before school entry. When the health visitor receives information that a child will attend a particular school she transfers the records of health and developmental screening to the school medical folder together with a summary of her work with the family. Not all children on the school lists will be known to the health visitor, and records may have to be sought from other authorities when children have recently moved into the area. Similarly some children will attend schools elsewhere, and their records will be sent to the appropriate district health authority. Some authorities offer a full medical examination immediately prior to school entry, whereas others prefer to delay it until the first or second term at school, in order to give the child time to settle into the new routine and to assess his response to it.

First health interview: Emphasis has been laid upon the way in which the health interview is conducted, and on the ability to recognise signs of ill-health and to appreciate their significance. The practice of specific screening procedures is covered in outline rather than in detail.

The school nurse will compile a *personal health record card* for each new entrant, based initially on information which she obtains from pre-school records. Before commencing her survey, she should make a note of absences from school which are related to ill-health. In this way a profile of the child and his first school health surveillance will be of great value to the school doctor when the child is medically examined. Approximately 15 minutes may be needed for each interview, but this may vary with the age of the child and his ability to cooperate. The more quickly the child is put at his ease, the more confident will be his response; time spent in creating a cheerful and encouraging atmosphere will be time well spent.

Effective health surveillance depends upon meticulous application of the right techniques, adequate conditions in which to apply them, and a two-way exchange of information; having assured herself that the conditions and equipment are satisfactory, the trained school nurse must consider her relationship with the child. Am I doing something for him? To him? Or with him? And is he given room to do something for me? These are the ingredients which constitute normality in the building of a fruitful relationship.

One of the ways in which the school nurse can educate others is by doing her work as well as she is able in every respect, both technically and in her approach to children, teachers, parents and colleagues. Children absorb their values. If we are cold in manner so will they be, they notice how we treat each other, and how we relate to other children; they pick up cues from us. If the cues they pick up are socially acceptable they succeed, and success is reinforcement; so their confidence grows, and they are not afraid to try out new things and extend their knowledge and experience.

Each successive interview provides an opportunity to offer the guidelines that he needs and to present them in a way which he can accept. Signs of good health are:

1. Bright eyes, a good colour and a clear skin.
2. An upright posture and firm well developed muscles.
3. Height and weight within normal limits.
4. Good appetite and normal bowel function.
5. Breathing through the nose, mouth closed.
6. Sleeps well.
7. Normal progress and development.
8. General confidence and alertness.
9. Interest and curiosity in surroundings.
10. Understanding and ability to communicate.

Signs of subnormal health are:

1. Pallor, dull eyes and hair, dry or blotchy skin.
2. Drooping stance and flabby muscles.
3. Height and weight outside normal limits.
4. Poor appetite and constipation.
5. Mouth breathing and frequent colds.
6. Poor sleeping habits.
7. Delay in maturity and general development.
8. General apathy and lack of social competence.
9. Inability to communicate.

Some of these signs will be apparent on sight, others will show themselves as the interview progresses; their significance needs to be assessed against the background of information which is available. All the facts should be carefully noted in the school nurse record so that the general direction and pattern of health can be seen in context, and adequate measures taken to halt a downward trend. Frequent absences from school should also be noted so that the record is complete. Some children are sent back to school before they are fully fit; the administration of antibiotics for childhood illnesses may halt the disease but delay the development of natural immunity, and this may result in children exhibiting signs of chronic ill-health and succumbing to yet more minor infections.

Procedure

After checking the identity of the child with his health record, and making sure that he understands the reasons for the interview, it is best to start with a procedure with which he is familiar. Weighing and measuring could be a sensible choice.

Weight and Height

Sequential records of weight and height provide a valuable pointer to the child's general growth and development. Nutritional problems and early indications of obesity are more quickly recognised. These records can also provide the supplementary evidence which is needed for effective action in cases of deprivation and child neglect.

For the record to be valid, scales must be checked and serviced regularly, and the same amount of clothing worn by the child at each weighing. Height measures must also be checked to ensure that the headpiece is firm and at right-angles to the upright frame. There are a variety of *standard charts* available, and the instructions for their use must be accurately followed. The charts are laid out with 'centile' lines which indicate the accepted range of normality for the age of each child, and although his measurements may be above or below the average, they will generally be expected to follow the centile line on which they started. If any marked deviations occur, they should be discussed with the doctor and reasons for the deviation should be sought.

Posture and Muscle Tone

The nurse will have noticed the child's posture as he entered the room, and general slouching and round shoulders may be observed also. Poor gait, protruding shoulder blades, bow legs, knock knees and flat feet may be more easily observed from behind the child as he walks. Specific comment should be made on these aspects in the school nurse record, and the physical education teacher can be asked to observe the child's activities and the way in which he performs over a period of time. This will not only provide the school doctor with additional information, but remedial measures can be taken to rectify bad habits before they become too ingrained, and the treatment of underlying causes can be commenced.

Poor posture is not an independent problem. Fatigue, malnutrition, obesity, recent illness, visual defects, uncomfortable or inappropriate clothing, for example, tight shoes or high heels, are among the more common causes, and children will not attain the best mechanical use of their body unless they are given an interest in good posture, and helped to attain it.

Vision

Defective vision is of special concern at school as it is one of the common causes of reading disability and is frequently connected with learning delay. Inattentiveness, lack of concentration, and lack of interest in class may all be associated with visual defect. Signs to watch for are:

- Children who rub their eyes and blink frequently; they may be trying to brush away the blur.
- Holding a book very close to the face.
- Screwing up the face when looking at distant objects.
- Shutting or covering one eye.
- Tilting the head on one side.
- Frequent headaches.
- Local signs such as styes; swollen, inflamed and encrusted lids; reddened conjunctiva; watery eyes or discharges.

Screening tests carried out by the school nurse are designed to indicate the effective visual range and are in no sense an eye examination; eye defects such as squint and astigmatism are detected by other means. Any child who consistently exhibits symptoms of visual disturbance should be referred for eye examination regardless of the result of visual screening tests.

Ideally every child should be tested annually, but this is not always possible; it is therefore important to recognise the children who are most likely to develop defects and screen them more frequently. The following groups should be borne in mind:

- Children with a family history of eye defects.
- Children with other defects or handicaps, for example, Downs syndrome, heart disorder or brain damage.
- Children experiencing a growth spurt, particularly at puberty.

Vision Testing

Whichever system of testing is in use, it is essential that the school nurse understands and is thoroughly trained in its application. Reliable results depend upon:

- The choice of test, the performance of which is within the child's ability and comprehension.
- Conditions suitable for its administration.
- Meticulous application of the instructions given for each test.

Unless all these conditions are completely fulfilled, the test cannot be considered as valid, and it would be better that it were not performed at all.

Stycar Vision Tests are generally used for children between the ages of 4 and 7 years, and the choice of near and distance screening tests is dependent upon the age and maturity of the child. Most normal school entrants from 5 years can be tested satisfactorily using the Stycar 9 Letter Chart over a distance of 20 feet (6 metres). The more mature children will be happy to sound or name the letters as they are indicated by the school nurse. Children who are not familiar with the names of letters can be provided with a 9 Letter Key Card, and asked to recognise and match the letter which is being indicated. In some schools 20 feet of floor space is not available; it is also extremely difficult to keep the attention of a young child over this distance. There are two alternatives which can be used:

1. Testing at 10 feet (3 metres) with the use of a mirror fixed to one wall of the school nurse room. The child sits at a measured 10 feet from the mirror and is provided with a 7 letter key card of reversible letters. The tester remains alongside the child and shows single letters in the mirror for the child to identify on his card.
2. Testing at 10 feet (3 metres) without a mirror. This system uses cards with half-sized letters which are the optical equivalent of those used in the tests conducted over 20 feet.

For children over the age of 7 years, material that is less easily memorised is required, and Snellen Charts which give longer lines of letters are used. Some authorities use the Keystone Vision Tester or the Master Vision Screener. These are designed to cope with the difficulties of lighting and space which are encountered in many schools. The essentials of good practice are as follows:

- Check in advance that the appropriate equipment is available and is in good order.
- To ensure accurate measurement, keep a piece of unstretchable string which is knotted along its length at 3 metres and 6 metres, and a piece of chalk to mark the floor at the correct distance for testing.
- Make sure that the child understands the test and is able to carry out efficiently the procedures asked of him.
- Effective occlusion of one eye while the other is tested is essential.
- If a card or wooden spoon is used, make certain that the child cannot peep round it. Plastic eye covers must be well-fitting. The occluder should not exert pressure on the eyeball. Bearing in mind the risk of eye infections, whichever method of occlusion is adopted, the materials used must be disposable, or capable of disinfection.
- A standardised routine avoids confusion and facilitates recording. If a child wears glasses, test first without them. Before testing with his glasses, they should be checked for cleanliness, scratched lens and well-fitting frames. Note whether the lens are shatterproof; these are safer if the glasses are worn during

sporting activities. In order to minimise the chance of inaccurate recording, always test the right eye first and record the result immediately.

Strabismus (or squint) is caused by a lack of balance of the eye muscles, which results in the deviation of one of the eyes from its proper direction. Initially the defect causes double vision, and in order to remedy this, the brain disregards the image formed by the squinting eye, and the sight of that eye is soon lost.

Diagnosis should be made before the age of two years, and the earlier treatment is initiated, the greater is the likelihood of success. Parents are understandably reluctant to submit their child to surgery or other treatment at a very young age, and they may mistakenly assume that it will be equally effective when the child is older; it is important that this aspect of deterioration is thoroughly explained to them so that they can cooperate fully in the treatment. The school nurse must always make sure that every possible case of squint is investigated at the earliest opportunity.

Methods of treatment include the wearing of glasses, exercises to train the eyes to work together, occluding the good eye for a period in order to exercise the lazy eye, and eye muscle surgery. In some cases where the sight of the eye has already been lost, surgery can be carried out for cosmetic reasons.

Colour Vision

Abnormalities of colour vision are hereditary and sex-linked. They can occur in approximately 5% of boys, but are rarely found in girls. The inability to distinguish red from green is the most common form of partial colour blindness, and it is important that it is detected early for three main reasons.

- The need for teachers to modify teaching methods; for example, colour matched materials are sometimes used in the teaching of early mathematical concepts.
- The need for parents to be aware of the condition so that they understand its practical implications. Green and red are the colours most commonly used to represent safety and danger in everyday living. Because the child appears to see normally, some parents find difficulty in comprehending and accepting the nature of the defect. This can best be overcome by showing them the test materials.
- The need for both the child and his parents to be aware of the possible limitations to future employment, so that useful plans are made.

The Ishihara Colour Vision Test is generally used. This tests the child's ability to distinguish dots of one colour on a background of dots of another colour, and he is asked to trace or name the outline which is formed.

The test should be carried out in good daylight, as artificial light may distort the colour shades. A selection of different colour plates is used, and they should not be left exposed to strong sunlight as the colours will deteriorate. Any defect which is found should be referred to the school doctor for further investigation.

Referral and Follow-up

Any child exhibiting possible squint or other signs of visual disturbance should be referred to the school doctor, as should any defects found by any of the visual screening tests. Distance vision is recorded as a fraction, and any child with 6/9 vision or worse in one or both eyes, or whose recorded vision with glasses shows deterioration, should also be referred. If the school doctor considers that further investigation and referral are necessary, and the parent was not present at the time when the test took place, the school nurse may be asked to make a home visit in order to explain the situation to the parents and to obtain the necessary written parental consent to referral.

A child who attends the children's eye clinic is seen by the ophthalmologist who will diagnose and prescribe treatment. If glasses are prescribed, they will be fitted by the ophthalmic or dispensing optician. Two pairs of glasses may be prescribed free of charge for school children, provided that National Health frames are used. Replacements and repairs are also free, with the exception of safety lenses. The additional cost of these must be paid by the parents, unless the child is suffering from a severely handicapping condition.

Failure to attend the eye clinic should be followed up so that another suitable appointment can be made. Some parents prefer to make their own arrangements for diagnosis and treatment and choose not to attend the eye clinic.

Management of Spectacles

The need to wear glasses is not popular with all children; their concerns should be listened to and should receive understanding. It is important that the glasses fit well and are comfortable, so that the child gets used to them quickly and appreciates the advantage of improved vision. He should be taught how to clean and look after them and to make sure that glasses kept at school are marked with his name and are clearly identifiable. Teachers should be made aware of the implications of any loss of sight and the reasons why glasses have been prescribed. For some children special lighting may be needed in the classroom. Children undergoing treatment for strabismus need particular care; the child who has been prescribed glasses may suffer from double vision again as the condition improves, and may resist wearing them unless he understands and is encouraged to persevere. The teacher should also be aware that it is the good eye which is occluded during treatment and that the child is reliant upon the sight of the lazy eye which may already be impaired. Information of this nature should be given in writing so that it is available to all members of the teaching staff. The standard national record form 10(B)M is a subsidiary school medical record kept so that day-to-day matters such as this can be recorded and made available to the teacher. In schools where this system is not in use, the school nurse should devise her own means of written communication, which is known and approved by her nurse manager, and by the school teaching staff.

Nose, Throat and Lungs

Colds and throat infections account for the majority of school absences in young children. Note any evidence of catarrh, nasal speech, colds or coughs. If there are any signs of wheeziness, ask the child how often and when it occurs, and check the school attendance record for absences caused by chest conditions. Inflammation of the throat and enlarged glands should be noted and a history of repeated sore throats should also be recorded.

Dental Health

The general responsibilities of the Health Authority include the provision of a School Dental Service which offers inspection and treatment. Section 10 of the 1973 NHS Reorganisation Act requires health authorities and local authorities to cooperate in this. When a child is deemed to be in need of dental care and treatment, parents are free to make their own arrangements through the General Dental Practitioner Service or to use the school dental service. Four aspects to be considered are as follows:

- Condition of teeth—dental caries and crowding of teeth and malocclusion.
- Presence of gingivitis and bleeding gums.
- Dental hygiene—correct and regular brushing of teeth and gum stimulation.
- Eating of sugar—particularly at night and between meals.

Bacterial plaque is responsible for the occurrence of periodontal disease and dental decay. In the presence of frequent exposure to sugar, acids attack the tooth enamel beneath the plaque and initiate tooth decay. When plaque is in contact with the gums, the bacterial action within it causes gingivitis, and this can lead to destruction of periodontal tissue. A correct method of brushing the teeth at regular intervals provides gum stimulation and inhibits the build-up of plaque. Limitation of sugar intake inhibits acid formation.

Establishing sound habits of dental hygiene is an important part of health education. Using a jumbo-sized brush and a set of teeth, children can be shown how teeth should be cleaned and can practise their skills. Many subjects can usefully be discussed: how much pocket money is spent on sweets and when they are eaten; the times when teeth should be brushed; the last visit to the dentist; strong even teeth are good for chewing; and this leads into the subject of eating habits and daily food. Many young children suffer from tummy upsets. Sometimes these are linked with emotional disturbance, but equally they may be caused by poor diet, constipation or inefficient mastication caused by malocclusion and dental caries.

Families which place a low priority on dental hygiene have a tendency to avoid the dentist unless they are in trouble; this means that the children who would benefit most from conservative procedures such as fluoride coating, early fillings and orthodontic care are less likely to receive them.

The value of school dental examinations is greatly increased where there is a planned follow-up programme. The school nurse should make herself known to the school dentist and seek his cooperation in the development of dental health projects for children and their parents.

Communication, Hearing Loss, Speech and Maladjustment

Every child is deserving of 100% of our care. If by a miracle, however, it were possible for us to give 110%, then there are two groups of children who should receive it: children with communication deficits such as speech and hearing loss, and those who we call maladjusted. These are children for whom we may inwardly weep, and for whom our inward weeping must be turned into practical help and professional compassion. They are children who hunger to communicate, and who hunger to understand and be understood, and for them we should strive utterly to believe in miracles.

A child with emotional and behavioural difficulties may not always be noticed as showing signs of serious maladjustment until he has been at school for some time. There may be many causes and many reasons for these disorders:

- adverse home conditions.
- standards of behaviour learned and accepted at home, but at variance with those accepted at school.

These can set up a hurdle of confusion and uncertainty which a child cannot surmount unless he is helped to do so with sensitivity and understanding, and unless he is given the hope and encouragement to persevere and the time which he needs to effect a reconciliation of his views. His difficulties may be exacerbated by factors within the school, perhaps by its organisation, lack of resource or expertise, or lack of personal qualities in the staff. What is it that the child cannot adjust to? This question should be asked whenever the nurse or teacher encounters a child who is consistently withdrawn or whose behaviour is difficult to control or understand. How can we provide a lifeline which will prevent him from drifting further and further out of range of meaningful communication? The answer lies in the quality of *our* communication with him.

We should consider the feelings aroused in us by particula children and their behaviour. Our relationship and dealings wit each of them must be firmly based on total and unswervin acceptance of the child; this is the lifeline which we must continu to offer him in the hope that he will recognise and grasp it. Ou rejection of unacceptable behaviour must be recognisable by hin as a firm and considered rejection of his actions, and not o himself; every display by us of negative, personal emotion cut away a strand of the lifeline by closing the door on communication.

We must be alert to receive and encourage any attempt t communicate. If we hope to engage a child in conversation, w must choose our words carefully and watch for signs of interest we must take care to laugh with a child and not at him; above al we must sense when he is ready to make a gesture of approach t us and know when to be silent.

Even if humans had never learned to speak, they would stil have found ways to communicate. The child with hearing loss speech difficulties or emotional problems can still perceiv situations, sense attitudes, see gestures and facial expressions often with heightened awareness; and buried in all of us is a nee to be accepted by touch. All these factors should come to our ai and we should use them to the full. They are the strands whic make up the lifeline.

Never believe that no apparent response means no inne progress. Seeds are slow to germinate, and for some children th road to understanding is a long and difficult one. A 'blank' fac may be the result of not knowing how to respond.

A child who is not making progress or whose behaviour canno be contained at school may be referred to the educationa psychologist for assessment and special help. The child guidanc service may be asked to work with the whole family. Som children may need special educational provision on a daily basis o by attending a residential school. A small number of children ma need hospital care. The sooner their alienation is recognised, th greater is the opportunity to bridge the gap; the health base ma provide the time-out haven of relaxation needed to see hin through the day.

Language, Speech and Hearing Impairment

Individual health surveillance provides an opportunity to listen t a child's speech and gauge the level of his language development There is a difference between the child who has poor speech an the child whose language development is deficient.

Failure to develop communicable language may involv physical, emotional and environmental factors, and these must b identified before a remedial plan of action can be made. Th process of identification should always include a medical examination and a hearing test, in order to eliminate such physical conditions as:

- Permanent hearing loss
- Periodic hearing loss due to wax in the ears, enlarged adenoids, or catarrhal conditions affecting the middle ear, such as partially treated otitis media.
- Mental retardation
- Autism
- Cerebral palsy
- Malformation of palate or teeth

Environmental and emotional factors include:

- General shyness and immaturity.
- An over-indulgent home where the child's needs are anticipated so that he does not need to communicate. This may also occur when he is the youngest of a large family or a twin.
- Parents of low intelligence or of limited language ability.
- Deaf parents who do not talk to their child.
- Mixed language families.
- A background lacking in nurture and stimulation. The child who is bathed in language, encouraged to listen and communicate, and stimulated in imaginative play will make progress in the development of inner language.
- An unstable or unhappy home background; emotional deprivation, lack of parental affection; or unsatisfactory fostering or child minding.
- Unsettling separation from home.
- Illness or accident.
- History of non-accidental injury.

A child with purely articulatory difficulties may have normal development of inner language but suffer from defects in the speech mechanisms; and he may require expert help and advice, and regular speech therapy sessions. Speech or language deficit may be due to a combination of factors. Particular examples should be borne in mind. Children who suffer from Downs syndrome are frequently subject to colds and middle ear infections. Never assume that poor speech is necessarily due to mental retardation; it may be the result of intermittent deafness. Children who suffer from any degree of deafness may have poor speech, poor language development, and be slow to respond. There have been many instances of misdiagnosis and consequent delay in treatment. Never assume that a child is mentally retarded because his responses are slow; it may be that his deafness has passed unrecognised.

Whenever we encounter a child with difficult speech, we should observe the following golden rules:

1. Take time to listen and help the child to know that he can succeed if he perseveres.
2. Do not hurry him or snatch the words out of his mouth; our patience is his educational opportunity.
3. Accept a child's verbal contribution uncritically, and then if it is necessary rephrase and give back to him the correct version.
4. Confident children may unwittingly monopolise the conversation; make sure that the less confident children are afforded the opportunity and encouraged to communicate.
5. Create opportunities and encourage participation in every aspect of school life. The child who feels different or excluded may show his unhappiness by withdrawal or aggressive behaviour.
6. Personality development is an essential part of growing up and confidence increases with successful practice.

It is estimated that 5% of school children suffer from some degree of hearing loss. Signs of hearing difficulty are often wrongly interpreted, and the child may be thought of as shy, quietly insubordinate, stupid or difficult. The child himself will not tell us that he cannot hear well, as he has no means of knowing that he hears less than other children; he will know, however, that he is not succeeding, and he will feel discouraged and misunderstood. Common signs of possible hearing loss include:

- Frequent colds and earaches, discharging ears, mouth breathing.
- Failure to respond to speech unless facing the speaker.
- Frequently asking for comments to be repeated.
- Inattentiveness and failure to concentrate.
- Listening with the head turned to one side.
- Talking too loudly.
- Faulty enunciation of words or consonants.
- Unusual pitch of voice.
- Complaints of buzzing and popping in the ears.
- Tendency to ignore the drift of general conversation and to make irrelevant comments.
- General apathy; withdrawn or aggressive, attention-seeking behaviour.
- Hearing loss may be permanent or intermittent, and one or both ears may be affected.

Hearing Tests

These can be described in two categories: *screening tests* which are designed to identify children whose hearing is below normal levels, and *diagnostic procedures* which are used to define more accurately the nature and extent of suspected hearing loss.

It is essential that all testers are thoroughly trained in the techniques which are to be used and that their own range of hearing is normal. It is also essential that the child is of the right age and maturity, and is capable of cooperating fully; reasonably quiet conditions should be available for all screening tests.

Sound is the result of vibration, and the difference in vibration frequencies accounts for variations in pitch. Speech sounds can be grouped together in frequencies and can be measured in cycles per second. The loudness of sound depends upon the power which causes the vibration, and it is measured in decibels.

The screening of very young children is based on behavioural response to sound, including speech sounds. Young children in school may be asked to repeat specific words or sentences which test the hearing of high frequency consonants and low frequency vowels, which is essential for speech discrimination. The tester covers his mouth to prevent lipreading and stands 3 metres from the child. The child should hear a quiet conversational voice at this distance. These tests are not reliable for use with children whose vocabulary is poor or for children who cannot imitate.

The audiometer tests the ability to hear pure tone sounds over a range of frequencies and measures the level of decibels at which the sounds are heard. Each ear is tested separately, and the results are charted on an audiogram. The resultant graph gives a clear picture of the degree and type of hearing loss.

In school the sweep check screening method uses a simple portable audiometer designed to identify children who may require more accurate testing. It is important that the equipment is regularly checked and serviced to ensure accurate readings. The volume is set at 20–25 decibels and sounds at different frequencies are presented; the test is dependent upon the child indicating each time a sound is heard. It is therefore essential that the child understands his part in the procedure, and that he is willing to cooperate and capable of doing so.

A doubtful response should always be regarded as a failure, although it may only be due to a cold in the head. A further test is carried out after two weeks, and if there is a second failure the child should be referred for specialist investigation. A full sound threshold test will be carried out under soundproof conditions.

Personal Hygiene

Children absorb their standards and learn by imitation. It is much easier to be clean and self-reliant if good habits are learnt young and become automatic in the course of daily living. For the young child, training in personal hygiene should include a daily bath or all-over wash; handwashing before eating and after using the lavatory or playing with pets; regular nail cleaning and trimming; cleaning the teeth before going to bed and after meals; washing the hair every week, and daily brushing and combing; covering the nose and mouth when sneezing and coughing, and careful disposal of tissues; and a daily change of underwear. Not all children have been trained in this way, and children do not always understand or completely believe in organisms which they cannot see. A white tissue with a little white flour folded into it produces a display of 'hidden germs' when it is shaken over a dark surface. This second demonstration provides an unexpected and convincing entertainment and may live long in the child's memory because of its visual impact.

Children should not be wholly undressed without written parental permission, but the uncovered parts can be inspected.

The general condition of the skin should be noted and the hands, feet and limbs should be examined for signs of infection or infestation, eczema or insect bites. Complaints of itching may indicate that there could be bites, patches of eczema or scabies on the body. Look for warts on the hands, evidence of scabies on the wrists and arms and between the fingers, and notice the condition of the fingernails.

The general condition of the feet should be noted, particularly the spacing of the toes. Tight socks and shoes that are too small or too narrow in fitting may cause permanent foot deformities. The feet should be inspected on the soles for plantar warts and between the toes for athlete's foot. Ringworm may occur on the skin and nails as well as on the scalp.

Hair and Scalp

The condition of the hair will often reflect a person's state of health. Patches of alopecia or baldness may be symptomatic of emotional stress, malnutrition and poor general health, but must not be confused with ringworm of the scalp. Diagnosis of ringworm can be made by Wood's lamp. Dandruff may be caused by insufficient rinsing, harsh shampoo or soap, but it can also be an indication of poor general health and poor diet.

Having almost completed our survey, we come to that very small part of the school nurse's duty—inspection for head infestation. Health authorities have made it clear that routine inspection of hair is the responsibility of parents. The stigma and outdated attitudes to this problem will increasingly be removed if health education time is allotted to it.

There are many popular misconceptions concerning head lice, but it is now regarded as a nuisance rather than a threat. Treatment with lotions which contain the insecticides malathion or carbaryl are extremely effective. They can be purchased by parents without prescription or obtained free from school clinics. The difficulty lies not in the treatment of head lice but in their detection. Anyone can catch head lice—they are transmitted from head to head regardless of whether the head is clean or dirty.

The following advice and information should be given about the prevention of head lice:

- If a louse is injured, it lacks the ability to recover; for this reason, twice daily combing of the hair from roots to tip and regular washing with normal shampoo are excellent preventive measures.
- Insecticidal shampoo should not be used as a preventive measure as this could lead to the development of resistant lice.
- Parents should be advised to inspect their children's hair weekly and look carefully for nits at the hair roots.
- If one member of the family is discovered to have head lice, then every member of the family and their friends should be checked.

If all parents were to adopt these measures, the incidence of infestation would be considerably reduced.

Some health authorities have introduced a system of simultaneous checking of all the schools in a particular neighbourhood, in order to ascertain and control the level of infestation and provide appropriate follow-up measures. Individual episodes of infestation may derive greater benefit from the school nurse's advice and assistance, and her time is more profitably spent if it is directed in this way.

Clothing and Cleanliness

Inappropriate clothing or clothes in poor condition may or may not be pointers to the attitudes of parents. The prohibitive cost of children's clothing, and in particular children's shoes, may compel the parents of larger families to hand down to younger children clothes which may not have been of good quality in the first place. Furthermore, they may be ill-fitting and inappropriate for the time of the year. Whereas lack of cleanliness and good personal hygiene have implications for health protection and the spread and control of infection, poor clothing militates against the self-worth and personal health of the child and his family, and it is important to make this distinction. Being a poorly dressed child in a comparatively affluent community is something which a child may have to live with, and human dignity may compel him to adopt an apparently uncaring front. We cannot provide effective help in this situation unless we are aware of the true reasons for it; and in every circumstance help and care should be given according to the needs of the child.

The health authority has a duty to ensure the cleanliness of school children. Medical officers and nurses working in the school health service are the authorised persons for this purpose. When a child is found to be seriously infested or in a foul condition, he can be legally excluded from school in the interests of other pupils. Normally an informal home visit is made by the school nurse or health visitor and cleansing procedures are explained to the parents. If a child is persistently verminous, a written report will be sent to the principal school medical officer and compulsory cleansing instructions may be given. The school nurse must be fully aware of the particular procedures that are in force in her own health district.

Teachers sometimes ask for help and advice when a child is smelly. Careful enquiries need to be made in order to discover the reasons for this situation:

- Parents and/or children may need general advice on cleanliness.
- Poor families may lack adequate laundering facilities or hot water for bathing.
- The child may not possess sufficient changes of underwear.
- The child may have problems of enuresis or soiling, because he is shy and unable to cope with school routine and toileting facilities.

Guidelines for procedure:

- Check the child's personal health record and the school absence record for recent indisposition.
- Contact the health visitor. She may be able to provide information concerning the family before a home visit is made.
- When parents are consulted, they must be approached in a spirit of cooperation so that the true reasons are uncovered.
- Provision of facilities and clothing: some families are unaware of their financial entitlements. Help may be available through social security and social service departments. Voluntary organisations may be able to help with provision of laundry equipment or clothing. Some schools have clothing shops run by parents.

Adopt a quiet, matter-of-fact approach when talking to the child:

- Assume that he is unaware that he smells unpleasant and explain this clearly and simply to him.
- Discuss the possible problems with him and agree on practical solutions.
- Tell him what you intend to do about the circumstances outside his control.
- Agree to an ongoing plan of action with him.
- Always arrange a follow-up interview; he needs to be assured of encouragement and support; the school-based nurse who is known to the children can offer this more easily.
- Report the arrangements to the child's teacher, and check with her the adequacy of the school health education programme at all age levels.
- Enlist the cooperation and appropriate support from parents.

General Health Information

The child's medical record should be checked, including the history of illnesses, hospital attendances and the state of immunisation. If the child is known to suffer from any complaint which necessitates the administration of medicines or treatment at school, then the daily arrangements can be discussed to ensure that the child is confident and accepts health care as a natural part of being at school.

There may be aspects of the survey which need further investigation, discussion with teachers, or written information and discussion with parents. As a general rule this should be explained to the child before he is sent on his way back to class.

Recording and Action

Health surveillance record cards are confidential and are exclusively for the use of the school nurse. It is important to complete each individual record card at the time of the check and to list all matters which require further action.

All information which is required prior to medical examination should be transferred to the Main Medical Record Form 10M and there should be a system of recording whereby teachers have access to information and advice relevant to the child's educational needs. Some health authorities use the subsidiary Medical Record Form 10(B)M for this purpose, while others have devised their own forms. Overall statistical returns are also required by the DHSS.

Well-designed and accurately completed returns provide an overall picture of the work being carried out, and a breakdown of figures will allow comparison between schools. Quality and listening cannot be quantified, but the figures can be used by the individual nurse to evaluate the effectiveness of her own working methods and to formulate plans for the future. If further investigations are indicated the correct information or referral forms should be used.

The school nurse may need to make personal contact with appropriate agencies. It may be necessary to arrange a meeting with the teacher, health visitor or social worker, or to contact the school doctor, or make a home visit. Make a clear note of the items to be discussed and the information which is to be given or obtained, so that time is not wasted on misunderstandings. Make a note also of any action which is agreed as a result of the meeting, so that results can be checked and recorded.

Ongoing Health Surveillance

As the child grows, the safety net must increase in strength and flexibility. The recorded observations provided by regular school nurse surveillance plot the state of a child's health: his growth, development and progress towards maturity.

Every stage bring fresh responsibilities and new opportunities to influence the pattern of his progress by early preventive awareness, and by appropriate and effective health education. The extent to which different screening techniques are employed varies from one health authority to another. Once a basic pattern of surveillance is established, the school nurse may herself collect data from within her practice which lends credence to national research findings, and may encourage the health and education authorities to introduce further measures to improve their current health programmes. The school nurse can formulate an overall health programme which sets out clearly the scope of health work, the observation, screening and health education which is appropriate to each age group, and additional procedures can be built into the work pattern.

Developmental Dyslexia

This is a neurological condition in which the child has difficulty in learning to read. The results of a three-year study of orthoptic investigation suggest that stable ocular motor dominance is necessary for reading and that orthoptic screening followed by treatment techniques designed to develop a 'leading eye' for reading can successfully be employed; this procedure is most effective if it is carried out before the age of seven years, but can also be used for older children.

Scoliosis and Lordosis

Without careful screening most children with progressive scoliosis (or abnormal curvature of the spine) remain undetected, and may present in later life with permanent disability; at least 10% of cases of child scoliosis are progressive.

In 1977, when Nottingham Health Authority introduced their scheme of school health surveillance, a pilot study involving 'one minute school screening' of scoliosis and lordosis was included at the request of the University Hospital and Medical School in Nottingham. It covered children between the ages of 8 and 12 years. In other authorities, initial screening is undertaken by physical education teachers in conjunction with school nurses. The early identification and treatment of these conditions may prevent children from undergoing a spinal fusion operation.

Blood Pressure, Urinalysis and Blood Analysis

There is considerable discussion at present concerning the prevalence in later life of kidney disease and coronary heart disease, and the controllable factors whch lead up to it. In a limited number of places screening for deviant blood pressure and urinalysis is carried out for specific age groups. The relationship between levels of folic acid in the blood and the incidence of spina bifida is an area of current research which could affect the screening of girls at the age of puberty.

Screening Priorities

One of the significant considerations concerning new practices of screening—in addition to those of time, staff and cost—concerns the ability of the NHS to provide the resources which would be required to deal with the number of deviations discovered. The selection of screening procedures must take these factors into account in order to give priority to the screening of serious degenerative conditions and those which may impose permanent health disadvantage.

Ethnic Considerations

Nurses working in schools with children from ethnic groups who have recently entered the country, or who have recently returned from a visit to their country of origin, must be on the alert for particular health risks. These include:

- Conditions which may have been contracted abroad, for example, malaria, tuberculosis, intestinal worms.
- Conditions attributable to dietary deficiencies, for example, anaemia and rickets.

Parent/School Sessions

Playing an active part in school activities provides an opportunity for parents, children, teachers and nurses to establish good communication. Many schools have established Parent–Teacher Associations, and meetings may provide a useful forum for discussion of health issues, and health information and education sessions can be arranged.

School open evenings are designed to give parents advice and information concerning their child's educational progress. If health and education are genuinely regarded as aspects of a common task, then it is essential that the school nurse is available at these sessions, so that parents are given the opportunity to discuss any concerns that they may have for the health of their child.

Puberty and Adolescence

The transition from childhood to adolescence involves both intellectual and physiological change. It is imperative that through their training school nurses are given an understanding and insight into these processes. Each child is born with his own developmental path, and his progress towards physical maturity is controlled by his own biological clock. In Britain the age of puberty is tending to get younger. Sexual characteristics may begin to appear in girls from 10 years, and the average age of menstruation is 13 years. Sexual changes in boys take place between the ages of 12·5 and 15 years. For each child the arrival of puberty is a different experience; its effect upon them is influenced by factors over which they have little control, and making sense of the changes that occur is a personal part of the process of growing up.

The middle years: the child between 7 and 11 years can structure his thoughts concerning things which he can see, hear and touch; during these years of preparation for puberty and adolescence there are three important elements of understanding which are related to sexual maturity:

- The information which he is given and the way in which it is presented bear directly upon his responses to a changing situation.

- His scope for independent action is growing, and with it his opportunities for decision-making and self-discipline. The child who learns early to make decisions which are within his competence develops an inner security and self-reliance, and the choices which confront him in adolescence will be easier to make.
- Children at school are bombarded with auditory and visual learning opportunities: chalk and talk, radio, tape and television. The knowledge which they absorb through touch is rarely considered. They experience the rough and tumble of the playground, the push of rejection, the jostle of the cloakroom. Yet how often for them, in their daily lives, is touch linked with the simple giving and receiving of affection?

The child who has absorbed this knowledge through his own experience will later be better equipped to discriminate between a relationship based on sexual desire, and one which uses the touching of sex to express a oneness of personal feeling.

Adolescence: the ongoing developmental process of adolescence may take years to complete. For girls and boys the onset of puberty brings with it the need to adapt to body changes, and to adjust the mental image of their bodies. Each one experiences:

- A growing awareness of the capacity to produce children.
- A growing realisation of future adult responsibilities, and the urge to relinquish adult care and become self-responsible.
- An increased ability to develop abstract ideas, and the need to establish his own fundamental beliefs and his own conscience.

Many children can take these changes in their stride, but—to quote a Croydon school nurse—'some adolescent children are drowning in problems'. Problems that occur are often related to:

- Displays of behaviour which are unacceptable to parents, teachers, or society as a whole.
- The need to establish a sexual identity.
- Depression, moodiness and feelings of isolation.
- Seeking after new inner experiences and heightened creative understanding.

The adolescent is neither a child nor an adult; the working effectiveness of his beliefs must be hammered out by him and tested in society; in this way he can discover the source of his own integrity of character.

Experience of school health surveillance programmes in Croydon suggested that children soon learned that the nurse was an available and informed person who would try to deal with problems in a sympathetic and confidential manner (Croydon DHA, 1979–80).

The 13+ Health Interview

This session provides the young person with an opportunity to consider the state of his health and to identify any problems on which he may need advice or guidance. Although his parents will be informed of the interview, they need not be present except at the request of the child.

- The following procedures should be included:
  Vision testing.
  Measurement of height and weight.
  Posture—screening for lordosis and scoliosis may be included.
  Immunisation—in addition to polio and tetanus boosters, BCG vaccine and rubella protection are offered in this year. Separate sessions may be arranged for immunisation or it may be carried out on an individual basis.
- The general health record and health reasons for absence should be checked. Children often use minor health complaints as a means of seeking advice for other more pressing worries; it is important to elicit by informal discussion the child's own views on his state of health, his interests and progress at school and elsewhere.
- Note the general appearance and be alert to signs which would indicate addictive behaviour such as glue-sniffing, alcohol or drug-taking.
- Record the stage of sexual maturity and the commencement of menstruation. With girls, problems concerning menstrual pains, personal hygiene, growth and development should be discussed. Girls are frequently preoccupied with diet as a means to control 'puppy fat' and because they are finding it difficult to 'recognise' and accept themselves in a changed body. They often neglect to take adequate exercise and it may be useful to link the two aspects when giving advice on diet.

  Boys are all too often neglected because their problems are less obvious. Programmes of health education should include more opportunities for boys to seek individual advice and information as they mature.

  Both boys and girls may have need for contraceptive advice and guidance and may occasionally contract venereal diseases. Any soreness of the vagina or penis or complaints of discharge should be referred for medical advice.

  Some school nurses are trained in family planning and counselling and may play a specific part in health education programmes and give individual advice. Young people may not wish to consult their family doctor and may prefer to seek help from the adolescent advisory clinic. The school nurse should know of the local facilities available to young people, and the referral procedure which should be followed.
- Parents and children: children whose behaviour is causing family upheaval and parental trauma may frequently adopt an

intransigent attitude. This may be completely at variance with their true feelings for their parents, and inwardly they may be deeply anxious and concerned. Parents also are torn between their feelings for the child and the challenge of his insubordination. When this situation arises, the solution would seem to rely upon a genuine exchange of views and beliefs between the parents and the child. Sometimes this can be accomplished with the help of a third person who is trusted by both. The child with his half-considered beliefs is unable to explain his views clearly when confronted with upset and adamant parents. The parents need to be reassured of their child's concern before they are able to review and reconsider their own long-held beliefs. The school nurse may be able to represent the child's views and feelings to his parents, and facilitate constructive discussion between them, so that better understanding and sensible compromises may emerge.

This system of school nurse health surveillance ensures that health education goes hand in hand with school practice and individual care. For the safety net to be effective, it requires close cooperation and support from the school doctor, backed up by NHS facilities.

School Medical Examinations

These may be classified as follows:

1. New entrant.
2. Selective—children identified for further review by the doctor at the new entrant medical; or by school nurses as a result of annual health checks; or by requests from parents, teachers or children themselves.
3. Assessment of special educational need—this examination must fulfil existing statutory requirements.
4. Secondary school 13+ health interview or examination—to include assessment for suitable/unsuitable employment as guidance to children, parents and careers officers. Special documentation is completed for normal and handicapped children.
5. Special examinations:
   (a) 13+—fitness for part-time employment.
   (b) Fitness to participate in schemes which require mental and physical endurance, for example, outward bound and nautical courses.
   (c) Fitness for school trips abroad and consideration of the supporting arrangements required.
   (d) Special recuperative holidays, free milk or special diet, or special travel arrangements.
   (e) Infectious diseases—following exclusion from school, or on admission or return to boarding school.

(f) Research—occasionally with the parents' consent, to collect data.
(g) Visiting consultants—ongoing examination of children in special schools or units.

Guidelines for Preparation and Procedure

1. Written parental consent to examination must be obtained and arrangements made for parents to be present.
2. It is important that the doctor is provided with all the available background information, and that the documentation is up to date and correctly recorded.
3. Teachers and the school secretary should be consulted concerning the procedural arrangements so that disruption of classes is kept to a minimum, and so that teachers who wish to speak to the doctor have the opportunity to do so.
4. The room must be suitable for examination purposes and arranged and prepared in advance.
5. The nurse should check that the essential equipment is provided and is in good order. Essential equipment will include:
   (a) Stationery—to include a complete range of school health documentation and referral forms.
   (b) Weighing scales, height measure and standard growth charts.
   (c) Vision screening equipment for distance, near and colour vision testing.
   (d) Stethoscope, auroscope, torch and tongue depressors.
   (e) For young children, Stycar developmental testing materials may be required.
   (f) When immunisation is to be offered, a surgical tray must be prepared in advance and the procedure for disposing of used syringes and needles must be followed.
   (g) Hand washing and drying equipment.
6. Ensure that there is a reasonable degree of privacy for the doctor, parents and children.
7. Routine administration must be organised to allow time for discussion between the doctor, parents and children: unhurried and courteous treatment of children and their parents, and absence of rush and confusion are the hallmarks of a well-run session.
8. Time must always be allowed for discussion between the doctor, nurse and teacher, so that any action which is taken will be clearly understood.
9. Check that medical records and referral forms are accurately completed, and that necessary parental consent forms have been signed for referral or immunisation.
10. As the session proceeds make a list of follow-up actions:

Parents—home visits to give advice and information or to obtain consent for further action.
Teachers—information, advice and health education planning.
Children—health surveillance follow-up, health care and education.
Contacting other agencies—health visitor, education welfare officer, social worker, nurse administrator, etc.
Doctor—special requests.

School Clinics

When a child is discovered to have particular problems, these clinics supplement or provide an alternative service to that of the family doctor or hospital outpatient clinic. Provision varies throughout the country according to local needs and may cover a wide range of health disorders such as: asthma and allergies; enuresis; obesity; skin conditions; visual defects; ear, nose and throat, orthopaedic and foot complaints; and conditions relating to particular ethnic groups. In addition some authorities have established special family clinics where mothers and children can come for health advice. In some districts clinic nurses are appointed, but in others school nurses may be called upon to participate in these sessions. They may be held in health centres or child health clinics. Advantages include:

- The provision of time and opportunity for more detailed discussion and advice in a relaxed and informal setting.
- In some areas local clinic facilities are more accessible and less time-consuming for working parents.

Family planning, speech therapy and school dental clinics may also be held at health centres and child health clinics. Their value is enhanced when an efficient system of communication exists to provide school staff with information and expert advice.

Environmental Health and Communicable Diseases

> The environmental health department of the local authority is responsible for the control of communicable diseases. It receives medical advice from the designated medical officer for environmental health, and its procedures are based on guidelines laid down by the DHSS and the DES.
> DHSS and DES. Memorandum on the Control of Infectious Diseases in School, HMSO, 1977

In addition to the national list of notifiable diseases, children may suffer from a number of other communicable conditions which could necessitate their exclusion from school. Contacts of those infected may need to be traced, and occasionally a whole school may be closed. Procedural instructions, which include a chart to indicate the incubation and exclusion periods for the more common diseases, should be available in every school. The school nurse is involved with the following responsibilities:

1. Drawing attention to environmental deficiencies; to the lack of general cleanliness, inadequate provision of toileting facilities and unsatisfactory rubbish disposal; to the need for organisation and encouragement of personal hygiene; to deficiencies in storage, serving and disposal of food; and to unsatisfactory arrangements for keeping and caring for school pets.
2. Identification of infection through health surveys.
3. Tracing and inspection of contacts.
4. Obtaining nose and throat swabs.
5. Home visits and advice to parents.
6. General oversight of children on their return to school.
7. Staff occupational health programmes, for example, rubella vaccination.

8 Health Education in School

People are obstinate. They tend to go their own way whatever good advice is available to them. In 1474 a regimen for good health was devised which, over the next four centuries, was translated into every European language and reached 240 editions. Its recipe for keeping healthy was:

1. Avoid great changes and thoughts and cares (anxiety).
2. Eschew anger.
3. Eat and drink soberly (sensibly, in moderation).
4. Take a light meal in the evening.
5. Walk moderately after meals.
6. Avoid sleeping immediately after meals.

Rule of Health of Salerno, 1474

Five centuries after this early effort at health education, the public at large is still neglecting this wisdom. Indeed it has been claimed that we are now living in a society that too often damages rather than promotes health. In recent times it has proved easier to persuade people to take additional (therapeutic) drugs than to give up excesses of food or social drugs such as alcohol and tobacco. The debate over health is particularly heated today as the differing interests of curative methods, caring services and preventive measures compete for limited resources. There are several main arguments in the health debate and they highlight the need for health education in school.

It makes greater economic sense to prevent ill health, than it does to spend vast sums on cure.

Many public health measures are undertaken from this viewpoint. However, two significant principles are involved. First, where is the borderline between public responsibility and individual responsibility? The general good health of the population depends on clean air, pure water, refuse disposal, control of environmental contaminants, and the inspection of fresh food for sale. Should the same logic be extended to mass fluoridation of water? Or the imposition of high fibre bread? Or the withdrawal of cigarettes? These are issues of personal choice, and many people would see these measures as an assault on their freedom.

A second principle is also a practical fact. Where there is pain to be relieved *now*, it will always take precedence over pain that *might be*. The child needing a liver transplant now will receive more attention and financial response than research into how such a situation could have been avoided. The theory of prevention may have many rational arguments, but it will always have to compete with the insistence of distress that is happening at this moment.

The population is made up of individuals, each of whom decide what to eat, drink, smoke and enjoy, and how to exercise, relax and cope with their lives. Therefore all efforts to establish good health habits should be directed at the individual level.

Each individual has to make personal decisions concerning his own health behaviour; but those decisions are always influenced by something or someone else. For instance, a child may decide to choose an apple to eat at break instead of a toffee-bar—because his mother told him to, because his dentist advised it, because his favourite TV serial was interrupted by an advertisement for apples, or because the school tuck shop had been removed as a matter of school policy. Should health education therefore be directed at the child, his mother, the professionals who advise him, the media or at changing environmental policies?

There is no hard and fast rule. Unfortunately this can result in health education that is diffuse with its effectiveness restricted by lack of cohesion and distinct purpose. Health education has few boundaries—it overlaps personal, political, social, moral, medical and intellectual areas. This means that the allocation of responsibility for the delivery of health education becomes complicated. The definition of target populations and decisions about how to persuade individuals to alter their health behaviour are practical issues that inevitably become bound up with ethics.

Health education should be directed at children, since wise health choices will then extend into a healthy, productive, adult generation.

It is generally accepted that children should be encouraged in the development of self-responsibility at school as well as at home. However, in the attempt to influence children who are inexperienced and impressionable, various factors have to be considered:

- All sides to any question should be given without bias. Fair presentation is difficult and time-consuming.

- There must be sensitivity to other influences in the child's life. His parents may smoke, eat unwisely or have other poor health habits. If health education becomes too ponderous or judgemental, it may cause reactions which run counter to its aims.
- Children's responses are often unpredictable; they may range from a defensiveness about the behaviour they recognise, to a daredevilry which challenges advice. Attempting to influence these children's health behaviour involves risk.

Some schools hesitate to question health behaviour. Is it the parents' or the schools' responsibility to broach these matters? Cooperation between the two is the goal.

School is the proper place for educating children for health.

Given an ideal world, perhaps all parents could be relied upon to instil beneficial attitudes in their children; but children do not always listen to parents, and parents do not always have adequate information. In an ideal society, environmental conditions would be such that the need for specific education concerning health choices would be minimal. If policies on a national, regional and local level were coordinated to supply clean air and water, good schools, homes and hospitals, pollution-free industry, adequate disease prevention, conservation of natural resources, absence of extravagant media advertising, sufficient leisure and transport facilities, freedom from undue stress, and opportunities for creativity—then, and only then, would the role of the school in health education become less significant. Meanwhile, schools remain the most appropriate place for children to learn about health and personal development.

Health Education in School

The promotion of health education at school carries its own problems.

- The school is a community of specialists. At secondary level in particular, each teacher is an enthusiast in a separate subject. Personal growth of the children is the concern of all, and the speciality of none, so it is understandable that health education has a struggle to gain a strong foothold.
- There is no measurement of 'success' in the teaching of healthy living. There is no regular written examination to give the subject structure, sequence, and respectability in the criteria for promotion. Some far-sighted schools have devised their own CSE Mode 3 for use in their own schools, but as yet these models are not transferable to other schools.
- Where it has been possible to appoint a coordinator for health

education in a school, personal assessment records of the children's progress have been made. Further education institutions and future employers have not always been receptive to the degree of input these records represent, and they have not as yet gained widespread approval.
- Even where the head teacher supports the efforts of the health education coordinator, it is a difficult task for him to persuade specialist teachers to give up some of their curriculum time to a subject that is so general. With these constraints in mind, the nurse in school has a very significant role to play.

The Development of Health Education as a School Subject

During the early half of this century, one of the greatest threats to health was *infection*. Much of what is now thought of as education for health came under the auspices of either *public health* or personal hygiene. In broad terms, the Ministry of Health undertook the responsibility of the former, while the Ministry of Education was responsible for the teaching of the latter. Up until the middle of the century, many teacher training colleges included in their courses a component dealing with how to teach children to keep clean. The voluntary organisations, such as the Scouts and Guides, the Boys' Brigade and the Girls' Friendly Society flourished on the image of keeping clean—in thought, word and deed as well as body. It is worth noting that this phraseology is seldom met today. As the major threatening infections of polio, tuberculosis, scarlet fever and other childhood illnesses came under control, so the emphasis on cleanliness and hygiene decreased. Teachers gradually took less professional interest in the matter and by 1974, when the health monitoring of children was firmly in the hands of the NHS, the term 'hygiene inspection' had become virtually synonymous with the search for head lice.

During the decade of 1970–79, there was an increasing awareness among both theorists and practitioners that health education in school covered a much wider base than personal hygiene. The disease patterns of childhood had changed: illness resulting from infections had decreased, but illnesses due to misused affluence and self-induced or stress-related behaviour were on the increase.

In the table on p. 168 it can be seen that while much of the distress implied in the left-hand column was due to attacks from outside a person, much of the distress implied in the right-hand column could be controlled by strengths from within a person.

It has now become obvious that clean habits are no longer enough to ensure good health. Greater affluence has brought with it greater competitiveness and stress; more leisure has brought greater exposure to media persuasion. A number of professional surveys have demanded that more attention should be given to socially related behaviour in school. These have included:

proper nutrition
use and abuse of social drugs such as nicotine and alcohol
sexually transmitted diseases
stress and conflict
personal relationships
affluence disorders
parenthood

Gradually a new emphasis in school health education has evolved which tackles motivation and attitude formation *before* harmful health habits are established. The new emphasis looks at how to stimulate awareness and deliberate choices in the growing child.

Early Twentieth Century	*Middle and Late Twentieth Century*
Polio	Congenital malformation
Tuberculosis	Perinatal brain damage
Scarlet fever	Allergies
Rheumatic fever	Obesity
Pneumonia	Dental disease
↓	Phobias
	Addiction
	VD
Decreased due to improved infection control	Truancy and vandalism
	Depression
	Road traffic accidents
	↓
	Increased due to improved environmental factors such as medical advances, greater affluence and more leisure

How Health-learning takes Place

Related to this new emphasis is the important question of how health behaviour is learnt. Studies undertaken in the fields of sociology, psychology and education point out that information alone does not establish a healthy life-style. It is when *knowledge* is *accompanied by a relationship* and confirmed by an *attitude* within favourable *circumstances* that behaviour is influenced.

Taking the example of a child being offered glue to sniff, this is how the model would work in practice.

Knowledge	+ **Relationships**	= **Attitude**
Glue-sniffing can lead to addiction.	My parents don't know about it.	I'd rather not but I'm not sure.
Glue-sniffing can put me on a high.	My friends do it.	
Glue-sniffing has resulted in deaths.	Teacher says don't.	

Attitude	+ **Relationships**	= **Behaviour**
I'd rather not but I'm not sure.	I don't want to show my parents up.	No thanks.
	I'm sorry Bobby and Bill got sick.	
	I like my teacher.	

Behaviour	+ **Relationships**	= **Health maintained.**
No thanks.	No hassle.	
	I like myself better.	
	Well done.	

This model can be applied to most behaviour that threatens health; it emphasises the contribution of each component—enhancement of any one by itself is not enough. Relationships are the thread which connects knowledge and experience and forms attitudes and behaviour (Fig. 8.1).

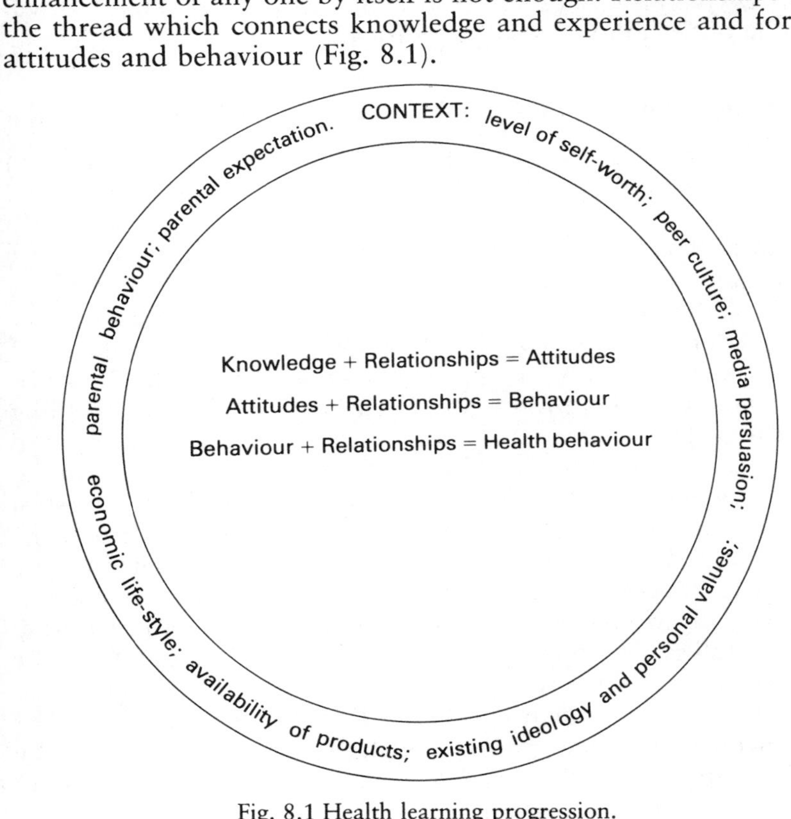

Fig. 8.1 Health learning progression.

Courses Available

Over the last decade, health education programmes have been built on these concepts. Pupil-discovery methods have developed the child's curiosity and initiative, leading to discrimination between what is valuable and valueless and to the exercise of the child's own judgement in decisions concerning his own health.

Prepared Programmes

Today there are various packaged programmes of health education based on these lines. Many sources of information are used in the courses. The school departments that can be drawn upon include biology, history, home economics, physical education, religious education, social and moral education, geography and literature. Some schools have designed their own schemes and others use or adapt the nationally publicised programmes prepared by the Schools Council, the Health Education Council, the Teachers' Advisory Council on Alcohol and Drug Education (TACADE) and more recently the Family Planning Association.

There remains some reluctance on the part of administrators—both teaching and nursing—to provide time and material for the preparation and presentation of health education. Nonetheless the argument is gaining strength that, with the prospect of increased non-employed time and retracted public provision of health services, the promotion of self-responsibility in personal care will be one of the most crucial issues for the future.

The Contribution of the School Nurse in School Health Education

The remainder of this section will concentrate on the ways in which the school nurse can be involved in health education.

Rationale

As the nurse is the representative of health in the education setting, school children cannot avoid learning from her. Her work is among children who watch and listen; she is inevitably a source of information and she continually presents a certain pattern of attitudes and health behaviour. She is a practising health educator in all her responses to any health query; any advice concerning self-care, any explanation of doctor's examinations and immunisation programmes, and all health interviews contribute to the personal growth and development of the child. Once a trustful relationship with the other staff is built up, it is probable that she may be asked to extend her role out of the medical room. She may start with a talk about menstruation and, as her inclination, abilities and willingness are recognised, she may be asked to give further talks. The opportunities that arise will depend on the idiosyncrasies of each school—its ethos, staffing and geographical position and the climate engendered by the head teacher. The school nurse possesses positive assets by her very position. The fact that she is not a teacher, but moves among teachers, gives her a potential that is not always recognised.

Positive Assets

Her role is lateral to the teachers, neither competing with it nor interchangeable with it. The notion that she is 'as good as' implies substitution, rather than that she has skills that are distinctive. Some of the results of her professional laterality are that:

- She is not connected with the awarding or withholding of test marks, with demanding homework or with administering school discipline. She is usually seen by the children as being *non-autocratic*.
- She can therefore more easily be thought of as *alongside*. In many homes today, the time available for chatting over the day's events is eaten into by television, computer games and videos. Many children find that nobody listens at home. Teachers often have too many children to be able to listen to any one child in depth. The nurse can tap a vast need among children for someone to pay attention to their own views. This need coincides with the recommended methods of handling health education.
- She is usually comfortable in a *group*. Various reports record that because teachers have the skill to control 30–40 rowdy teenagers from the front of the class—or indeed because they have to have this control—they frequently have difficulty coping with a small group of young people on equal terms.
- She has ready *access to information* from outside the school, in particular from hospital personnel and facilities, community workers and voluntary organisations.
- She encourages self-care, and in the exercise of this role she can *use touch* more easily than teachers.
- She is presumed to be *free from embarrassment* when discussing delicate topics.
- She does not need to feel constrained by any *risk of over-familiarity* with particular pupils, since the size of her case-load and the number of schools she attends counterbalance such risks.

In spite of the value of these assets, there are also some practical difficulties that face the nurse undertaking health education in schools:

- As yet not all school nurses have training in how to educate.
- Time must be made for the preparation of the subject, collection of the material, setting up of equipment, and packing and returning of any aids used. This time is seldom allowed for in a busy nurse's day.
- There are difficulties of accountability: to whom is she accountable for what she says or does in front of the children? The class teacher? The head teacher? The nursing officer? The health education officer? The health visitor? The school doctor?
- Practising nurses often emphasise that they went into nursing in order to nurture, not primarily to instruct.

These are real obstacles and, in the absence of adequate training and expertise, the school nurse should not be pressured to take part in educating. However, there are many examples of good practice where the school nurse is used to the full in the school health education programme. The subject areas in which the contribution of the school nurse has been found to be most vital are listed in Table 8.1. It is significant that these areas are not confined to physical conditions, but emphasise the total personal development of each child.

Table 8.1
Subject Areas where Nursing Experience is Valuable

Infants	Responsibility for cleanliness, especially: Washing hands after toilet, before meals Teeth cleaning and mouth care Blowing nose—use of handkerchiefs/tissues Dressing Infection—'Mr Filth'.
Juniors ↑ all subjects are applicable at varying depth ↓	Dental care How a baby is born First aid Role of the school nurse Safety Infection Accidents in the home Puberty Self-care: body odour, halitosis, 'the unseen bits' Grooming: hair, nails, skin Clothes: advantages of natural/synthetic cloth to health, shoes Misuse of the body: exercise injuries, obesity, anorexia, use of purgatives/laxatives Sleep and rest Use and abuse of alcohol, drugs, caffeine, solvents Smoking Nutrition Parentcraft Domestic pets and health hazards.
Seniors	Sexually transmitted diseases Pre-conceptual care Contraception Personal relationships and health Coping with stress (own and others), relaxation techniques Attitudes to elderly and disabled people Separation, loss, bereavement, death Provision of community services—who to contact, where, when and how Ecological changes and their effect on health.

Most of the subjects listed above require a combination of aids to learning, depending on the needs of the children, the nature of the subject and the abilities of the educator. All methods of educating, whether they are formal or informal, traditional or innovative, require a high degree of commitment, training and application. Decisions about which method is best for which subject and audience should be made with the class teacher, and this can be a satisfying interdisciplinary exercise.

Formal Educating

External sources can be tapped for material for a formal talk. Straightforward information may be insufficient on its own, unless it can be seen by the child to relate to his own experience. If he finds it difficult to make a connection between what he is being told and what he has already found in life he may become bored and apathetic. A useful way to counteract passivity is to encourage questions, and sometimes to allow for time during the packing up of equipment for children to 'help' and voice their queries quietly.

Informal Educating

Many school nurses prefer the informal approach. In their daily contact with children and parents, nurses become comfortable with informal communication. This relaxed attitude can be used when discussing sensitive subjects with small groups. However, if time is not to be wasted it is good to make it clear to the group that there is a definite goal to be reached and that the leader should retain control of the structure of the session. Informal groups cannot be used in school as therapy or encounter groups.

Discovery Educating

The discovery method of education involves each pupil in his own learning. He is shown a considerable amount of accurate information that could be appropriate to him, and then he is encouraged to work out which bits fit together, what is of significance to him in his situation, and what is less so. This method can be used with individuals or groups: with young children discussing their own dental care habits, for instance, or with a senior group looking at their attitudes to contraception or the care of the elderly. It has several advantages:

- The pupil's interest is harnessed to the idea that he has power in his own life and can effect results by his own behaviour.
- His awareness of his environment can home in on what he learns about himself and his own concerns and confusions.
- Different solutions offered by different people can be explored.
- Questions can be used as tin-openers—not knowing what is inside but prepared to experiment.
- Disorder can be tolerated for a while, until a new order is discovered.
- An informed commitment can eventually be made to a specific attitude or action.

- Supportive measures which may be offered by the school nurse are accepted because they are not seen as imposed.

Materials to support such discovery methods can usually be supplied from the local health education department, the school library, local community sources and the school nurse's own creativity. The children themselves often contribute the most significant subject from their own experience. When they are encouraged to air things that have happened to them not only does the subject become immediately real, but ideas that have gathered around the subject can be disentangled and straightened out.

The Use of Reward Systems

Systems of reward are basic to any educating, but in health education they can become better identified and actually negotiated with the individual child. Later on more specific goals can be chosen, and the steps needed to reach these goals can be broken down into easily reachable successes. These steps should be sufficiently difficult to pose a challenge, but sufficiently easy to ensure success. Many small successes confirm each other, whereas a large failure can demoralise the pupil to the extent that he gives up the effort. The pupil's trust in his ability to cope with his own problem has to be built up by deliberately avoiding opportunities for failure. Each success is a step nearer the desired goal. This progress is confirmed by a system of reward that has been agreed in the original negotiation. The hidden back-up reward is the growth of self-respect and the knowledge that others recognise it. The eventual optimum outcome of any reward system is dependent on three things from the beginning: agreement with the child; back-up of all concerned including the parents, the teacher, and the nurse; and thoroughly consistent management throughout. Parents should be consulted in the original design of the plan, as they will know what goals are best for a particular set of circumstances. Rewards may take the form of points or counters which, when a prearranged total has been collected can be exchanged for a new cassette, a ticket to the football match, or a pair of coveted earrings. The following are some of the satisfactions that can result from a reward system:

- The gaining of self-empowerment.
- Adding to a collection—books, stamps, records, sport.
- Confirmation of approval—teacher's, parents', peers'.
- Challenge met, obstacle overcome.
- Competition with peers in similar circumstances.
- Ambition to excel.
- Pleasure in giving pleasure.
- Choice of motivation proved to be effective.

Self-care

The school nurse may find that all or any of the above methods of educating are relevant in her promotion of self-care by children. She may be involved in the modification of behaviour of a group of smoking teenagers, or she may want to interest a young child in calipers in the care of his own skin. The general pattern is similar in each case: cooperation of the child or children concerned, the choosing of an attainable goal, and the agreed small steps in time and skill in order to succeed.

Future Developments

As health education becomes more established in the core curriculum of our schools, it may be that the school nurse will become increasingly turned to for education. Her contribution is particularly valid wherever the body and mind interrelate. For instance, her particular concerns may be the *worry syndrome* and the effect of stress; the *grief syndrome* and the effects of loss, separation and bereavement; and the *hostility syndrome* and the physical expression of anger and frustration in protest, truancy and vandalism. An informed listening ear at school could forestall a serious breakdown of physical or mental health. *Crisis* is a factor in all the above issues. Nurses are trained to cope with crisis without undue disturbance. Nurses also *know*, sometimes without articulating it, that temporarily unstable situations can in fact be growing points for change. A certain degree of tension, frustration and struggle is necessary before summoning the drive to take a new direction. In the same way, a sense of dissatisfaction with the present state of things is often a precursor of the 'teachable moment'. Stress and crisis are uncomfortable, but they can also be pivotal points in a change for the better. Nurses have experienced these things while caring for people and their knowledge and empathy can be a valuable resource. Teachers have different 'givens': their goal is *achievement* for their pupils. The nurse, in contrast, may have special insights into *non-achievement*—how to cope with illness, inadequacy, non-success and loss. We all succeed at something, but equally we all fail at something else. Learning to look at and to accept this fact is an important aspect of developing coping skills.

Loss is a wide subject. It can apply to the loss of a pet, the disillusionment of an ideal or a fantasy; the non-attainment of an ambition; the loss of a bodily function or ability or part; the loss of friends when moving home; the separation of parents, or the death of a relative. When a child becomes aware that a person he knows is dying, whether it is a favourite relative, a family friend, or a classmate with terminal illness, he will be full of puzzlements. He will be prone to alternative periods of fantasy and reality, misconceptions and understanding, detachment and concern. Our children should be given the opportunity to explore and verbalise how they feel about loss and death just as much as they are encouraged to articulate feelings of success. Through imaginary role exchange, they can come to terms with the fact that other people's lives are different and sometimes difficult, and that they will have to learn to cope in similar circumstances. In this way, children can develop a concern for others and other people's responses, as well as a better understanding of themselves.

Health education in the stress-related areas outlined above should always be accompanied by the following measures of support and back-up:

- A well-publicised time when the school nurse can be regularly available for a chat in private. If possible, this should be at a time when the child can obtain permission to be absent from class.
- Advice to classes, groups or individuals on relaxation techniques and where to find further opportunities to practise them.
- It is sometimes possible to set up peer counselling groups with the approval of the head teacher. Children are often surprisingly adept at listening to each other's problems, and quickly learn sensitivity in doing so without the presence of an adult. The aims of these schemes are to: verbalise feelings unchallenged; elicit support for new or threatening responses; practise experience-distancing; rehearse emotion expressivity tactics; and ventilate problem-solving suggestions.

How can the school nurse become more aware of learning opportunities?

The short answer is by being constantly ready to learn herself. At present, the ability to recognise such opportunities may depend upon her own skills of observation. Furthermore, the more school nurses clamour for more training in these areas, the more likely it is that training will be forthcoming. Health education departments advise not only on direct instruction methods, but they also have libraries containing more information on the subjects discussed here. The school nurse who wants to be creative will find the resources and cooperation she needs with a little perseverance, determination and diplomacy. A commitment to personal responsibility for health will provide a service to the school, satisfaction for her and, above all, lifelong values for the child. One of the greatest rewards she will receive will be to hear students make statements like the following:

> I think my ideas have changed to be quite strong because:
> I feel I know them better.
> I am lovable.
> I am important (i.e. have worth).
> I am not on my own.

9 Special Needs

All children are full of needs. However, 'special' needs are those that are over and above the claims which can be dealt with by an ordinary family in the ordinary community. Special needs are those that we all have—only rather more so. The needs that we all share are:

- to be aware of our surroundings.
- to communicate with those who surround us.
- to control our own body and its activity.
- to care for our own body's functions so that they are socially acceptable.
- to be approved of and accepted as individuals, and to be able to hold on to a sense of worth, hope and fun.
- to exercise our curiosity; to be able to learn to stretch within our world and improve it.

These basic wants only become special when we cannot manage them without outside help. Special needs are a heightening of our own needs, they are not strange or of a different order; there is no 'we' and 'them' with regard to needs. It is only a matter of the degree of extra attention that is required by different people in different circumstances.

Basic Considerations

The threads which go into the make-up of each person are interwoven, but they can be traced to body image, the attitudes of self to self and others to self, mental reaction to these, and the moral and spiritual network which reinforces the whole. The effect of any contortion of body, mind or spirit can be spread into previously unaffected areas, including family and social concerns. This *spreading effect* from an original source can lead to devaluation of the whole of life or of revaluation. It is often the responsibility of the outside carer to help a disabled child convert a negative attitude towards himself into a positive one. The following comments are relevant to the professional worker in such a situation.

The sense of personal devaluation felt by a child with a disorder that is not immediately observable can be as great—or greater—than the devaluation felt by a child whose disorder is visibly severe. Therefore, the degree of care that may be required cannot be measured against the observable degree of disability. The child with fluctuating deafness, for instance, can be burdened with as much embarrassment and anxiety as a child in a wheelchair—perhaps even more so since the expectations put upon him are higher and the leeway offered to him to compensate for his disability is less.

Overt pity can undermine a child's confidence in himself and confirm in him a feeling of not being worth much. A balanced mix of 'poor you' and 'let's get on with it' usually comes with practice.

If it is allowed to get out of hand, a child can use the perception that he is 'special' to his own detriment. 'You have to help me' and 'poor little me' can become powerful weapons in games of manipulation, whether they are used consciously or not. If the child finds that he can control people, he becomes confused at the lack of omnipotency of his carers or parents, and this increases his social bewilderment. It will bring him more self-assurance to be allowed—or enabled—to pick up his own clothes, turn his own page, wash his own face, explain his own actions and make amends for his own unkindnesses, than having these 'ordinary' things done for him.

Following on from the above, carers may need to resist their natural desire to compensate for their own able-bodiedness by working out their feelings of compassion on the children.

Many of the areas that require special care can be seen as phases of ordinary care that have simply been delayed. There is a 'normal' time for a child to learn to walk, to talk and to use the potty, and all his surrounding circumstances lead him towards the urgent acquisition of each particular skill. The child who has had to postpone such learning because of hospitalisation, lack of stimulation or sensory/motor deficit, must tackle it in isolation for all the accruing incentives and influences and motives have been lost. In addition, the sensitivities within the child appropriate to that critical phase are reduced, and his ability to adapt to the relevant reflexes and responses has to be re-educated.

The needs of the child with special difficulties will always be uneven and overlapping. There will be times when his need of extra attention is great, and others when he is independent. One consequence of learning delays is that the retention of a newly acquired skill is often unreliable. The skill taught or the explanation received a short while ago may have to be repeated. Performance, comprehension and memory recall may all be liable to fluctuate.

Attitudes to Disability

There are many attitudes to disability on the part of the professionals, parents and peers. These range from the passively fatalistic, in which the individual believes he has little control over what happens to him, to the assumption of full self-responsibility. If the latter is accepted to its absolute extent, the disability becomes the 'fault' of the sufferer. Perhaps the idea of marginality is the most practical—that needs are marginal, we all share them, and whereas we are all better than others at some things, equally we are all worse than others at different things.

The professional carer should encourage:

- *Optimism*: but this has to be measured to fit the likelihood of attainment. Over-optimism may lead to disillusionment and frustration.
- *Goal-setting*: but this must be carefully designed to confirm success and not failure—as one disabled adolescent remarked 'I'd rather succeed in doing what I can, than fail at doing what I can't'.
- *Integration*: but if this is attempted without meticulous preparation, the isolation of the disabled child can lead to greater ultimate segregation than if the identity given him by his special need had been maintained.
- *Individual planning* for each child in educational and nursing terms: but these plans have to be continually reassessed; if they are followed too strictly, new opportunities may not be recognised and new needs remain neglected.

The Role of the School Nurse

The specific role of the school nurse in attending to the needs of children with special difficulties involves assessment, management, support, ensuring safety and liaising with community resources. These services are available to all children in ordinary schools—they are simply concentrated and crystallised in the needs of the disabled child. A child has limited experience, therefore it is up to the school nurse to pick up clues and follow them through. She may develop a particular sensitivity to the minutiae of changing needs and in the re-patterning of developmental programmes. When non-trained ancillaries and teachers and not the nurse are the people who see the child daily, she can see whether improvement has taken place over a period of time or whether the *status quo* needs to be interrupted and new ideas introduced. It may be that the immediate attendant needs to know that what she is doing is right, and then she can be taken on to a new goal. In this non-static approach the nurse can bring in many advisers; she will not be dependent on her own resources nor will she need to be an expert herself in all fields. Figure 9.1 is an example of how one school nurse interacted with other disciplines in the case of one particular child.

There are a number of practical considerations which will be within the responsibility of the school nurse.

- *Pressure areas* of the child with walking aids or in a wheelchair. The child can be taught to care for these himself, examining parts at risk each evening and rubbing them gently with spirit when he undresses. It is advisable for him to adopt the habit of lifting the weight of his body off the chair seat with his arms and shaking himself. This short exercise should be remembered every two hours or so throughout his waking hours.
- *Cleanliness* can be easily neglected by a young person with mobility difficulties. Washing and special care with drying have to be taught deliberately and patiently, as do self-management of dental care and body odour.
- *Clothing* is often chosen and bought by another person if the child cannot get about easily, but he should be encouraged to voice his needs and preferences. The use of cotton directly next to the skin is particularly important for children who sit in hot and clammy plastic wheelchairs or wear heavy surgical boots. Many mothers think nylon is preferable because it is easier to buy, cheaper, easy to wash and 'makes him sweat more so it must be warmer'. However, the close combination of plastic, nylon and sweat will cause sore skin and considerable discomfort.
- *Insensate limbs* need particular care. It is often difficult for people to fully grasp the implications of the fact that a child has no feeling in a part of his body. If his feet are allowed to dangle

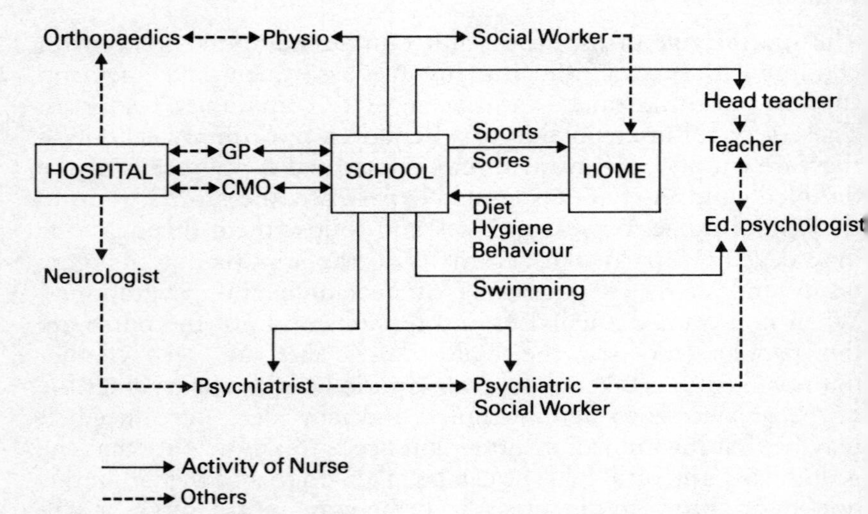

Fig. 9.1 Interdisciplinary liaison by a school nurse (concerning one child only).

off the foot-rest of the chair, he may sustain a spontaneous fracture; if he is encouraged to sit too near a radiator he may receive a burn that takes weeks to heal; if he sits carelessly in his chair, his buttocks or genitals may become pinched and haematose; if his urinary drainage becomes blocked underneath him, he may have back pressure to his kidneys—these are all real dangers disproportionate to the small degree of negligence that might cause them. Teachers and ancillaries who take care of a child with insensate areas in his feet should be reminded that a boot put on without due care may result in a bent toe which turns gangrenous. Athlete's foot, ingrowing toenails, pressure on heels and/or toes are all signs to look for as they will not be felt. When feet are inadequately covered, the child may get frostbite or carpet burns (if he has been allowed to crawl).

- *Walking aid maintenance* is the responsibility of the technician. However, if the nurse notices brakes that are weak or faulty, arms that are difficult to move or replace, screws on calipers or chairs that project and need padding, creases in cushions that mark the skin, or leg extensions that give inadequate support, she should make sure that these faults are rectified. For example, she can encourage mothers to cover plastic seats with attractive cotton towelling and she can give advice about suitable clothing for children in calipers or with urinary appliances. The guiding principles for these clothes will be ease of changing, access to areas that may require attention during the day, and disguise of disability.
- *Nursing procedures* in addition to the above may be required if the nurse works in a special school for physically handicapped children. These procedures may include sterile dressings post-operatively or for severe pressure sores, catheterisation, bladder washouts, rectal examinations and irrigations of various types. All these procedures will be undertaken on the advice of the medical specialists in charge of the child, and it is always helpful for the school nurse to keep in close touch with the hospital clinic.

Lifting

It is important for the school nurse to be able to advise all school staff handling disabled children on the skills of *lifting*, and to be able to instruct the children themselves how to make the best use of their limbs. The strain of weight and movement should always be taken by the most efficient muscles—for example, the legs rather than the back, but conversely the least efficient muscles of the paraplegic or hemiplegic child should not be allowed to atrophy unnecessarily. Physiotherapists will advise on gentle or passive exercising. Similarly, transference from wheelchair to school chair, wheelchair to car seat, wheelchair or sticks to floor and back up again, wheelchair to bath or toilet, can be demonstrated by paramedics to the school nurse as a resource for others within the school. Wherever possible, sufficient time must be allowed for the child to do these things for himself—he will gain independence and the helper will preserve her back.

Pivotal Needs

To be Aware of Environment

The growth and development of an ordinary child includes the gradual absorption of experience of the world about him through his mouth, his ears, his eyes, his touch and his activity. If any of these paths of assimilation are obstructed, his experience of his surroundings will be deficient and the people who care for the child become mediators between him and his world. The way he accepts himself may largely depend on the way he is accepted by his carers; anxiety over his condition and protectiveness over his experience will inhibit his curiosity and natural sense of adventure. The adults involved may have to take risks so that the blind child can feel and learn, so that the epileptic child can gain confidence in spite of his seizures, and so that the asthmatic child can understand what predisposes him to his attacks.

Experience leads to learning; without it not only will understanding of the environment be less, but a lack of early experience can compound later difficulties. For instance, if the child has little experience of play on account of early hospitalisation or over-protection, he is deprived not only of enjoyment and stimulation of toys, water, sand and games, but at the critical learning stage, he does not acquire knowledge of space and volume, or of the relationships between things and people. This deficiency may lead to a lack of *basic perceptual concepts* as well as underdeveloped social awareness. Perceptual concepts have to do with the grasping of comparisons such as big and bigger, positions such as together or apart, and spaces such as above and below. A simple but telling example of how difficulty in these areas can affect a child's apprehension of the world about him and the acquisition of reading, writing and number skills is shown in Fig. 9.2.

Remedial work for children with these difficulties is time-consuming and specialised. Some authorities consider that over

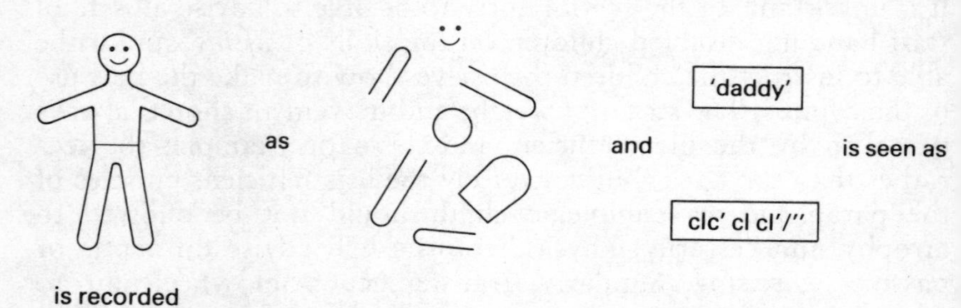

Fig. 9.2 A child's drawing and writing which exhibits difficulty with perceiving concepts.

the age of eight or nine it has a limited effect. The child with limitations should therefore be encouraged at the earliest age practicable to use whatever faculties he has. He must discover as much of the world as it is possible for him to reach or the spreading effect of disability may be more inhibiting than the disability itself.

Another significant aspect of the secondary effects of handicap is less recognised. Most children in ordinary circumstances can watch themselves in mirrors whenever they want to. As they grow older they can examine their bodies, their appearance and their facial behaviour in a mirror and in privacy. Often they observe the normal bodies of their siblings and their parents as they are bathing and dressing, and they grow up with ordinary expectations of how an ordinary body appears and functions. The child with physical limitation is inadvertently 'protected' from all this natural learning. If he is toileted, washed, bathed and dressed with his mother, his attention will be on her and not on his own mirror reflection. His carer may even 'protect' him from seeing what she thinks is not quite 'normal'. He is physically unable to casually bump into others who are changing. The corollary to these circumstances is that:

- he seldom examines his own body.
- he cannot fully apprehend the image he presents to the world.
- he cannot recognise 'normal' body make-up or behaviour.

A child cared for in this way may feel that his body is something that other people look after for him and he may disassociate himself from it. Yet body image is an important base of self-concept. The school medical room can provide some positive experience in the constructing of his body image, especially if the child can watch himself in a three-sided mirror while he is being attended to and can assess for himself the image he projects to others.

Some of the inappropriate social behaviour common among children with physical disabilities is due to these causes. Their acceptance of infantilisation, their disaffection for their own bodies and their comparative immunity to social feedback, can add to the segregation from their peers that is evident in many schools.

To be Mobile and Control Activity

We all need to be in contact with other people. When the effort of reaching them is great, when we cannot be easy and casual in our contact, it is up to those around us to make good the gaps. There are many degrees of activity control. The child with a minor degree of spasticity may merely be seen as 'clumsy', but he will feel that his deficiency in physical prowess is a keen failure and, like the child with a coronary defect, he may find compensation in becoming 'bookish'. The children who are more severely curtailed and can only get about with calipers, sticks, crutches or a wheelchair are being increasingly seen in the ordinary school.

The following guidelines may not apply to every case, but ideas can be adapted from them to fit the child in mind.

Any difficulty with balance will produce physical insecurity. This is often matched by a feeling of *social insecurity*. For instance, a child who is relying on sticks for equilibrium cannot hold out his hand to another; an athetoid spastic may have to forego close contact with another because it distracts from the concentration he needs to control his own movements; the mechanics of hugging a child in a wheelchair can be so obstructive that the child has to get by without being hugged; where an ordinary child might receive approval by a hand on the shoulder, the child in a wheelchair receives such gestures on the *handles of the chair*; indeed those who wish to be friendly with him tend to push the chair and talk to him from behind unseen by the child.

The attitude of such children to their calipers, sticks and wheelchairs is an ambivalent love/hate. The aids become an *extension of their bodies*. Although walking in calipers enables a child with spina bifida to stand tall(er), to relieve some pressure areas, to exercise flaccid limbs, to stimulate his lower limb circulation and to increase the efficiency of his elimination systems, the child himself may see the wheelchair as being more comfortable, as requiring less effort and, best of all, as enabling him to get around faster than with walking aids. If he succumbs to the last considerations too easily, he will find adult life more difficult. He will be unable to use public transport, find only limited access to shops and places of entertainment and need specially widened doors, lifts and adapted toilets in his prospective place of work. Table-top levels, basin or sink tops, door handles and electric switches may all need adjusting for a person in a wheelchair.

Adolescents and Activity

Some adolescents with mobility difficulties can use this fact as a scapegoat. If they have been overprotected, they may lean towards apathy and a lack of initiative and they may hesitate from experimenting. On the other hand, some with severe physical limitation may excel at chess or computer operations. As the child grows older, he will increasingly become aware of the ways by which his peers prove themselves. They can be competitive in sport, aggressive in fighting and self-assertive in running out and slamming the door. These normal expressions of development are denied to him. Sometimes there are other avenues open, such as wheelchair badminton, archery, table tennis, netball, swimming, canoeing, horse-riding, pony-carting, wheelchair dancing and boxing. Some paralytic young people compete with radio-controlled cars and aeroplane models. Special sensitivity is needed on the part of the health worker when an adolescent with limited mobility becomes sexually aware. There is little opportunity for either privacy or experimentation when he has to take a wheelchair wherever he goes. The worker will have to explain to teachers that he needs extra latitude when he is trying out new behaviours to do with the opposite sex in school; he probably does not socialise anywhere else.

Where physical dependence is still strong, the school nurse may have to encourage an adolescent to question the way things are done, to stretch himself and try out new methods that he could manage on his own, and to sort things out for himself. He may build myths about the possible changes which could happen in the future. Fantasy can keep hope alive, but he may need help in seeing his condition realistically and in learning to cope with the frustrations that are inevitable.

In all work with children with limited mobility, the prime consideration is the promotion of an idea of self which is the most positive possible in the particular circumstances. Care for the actual mechanics of the defect, and encouragement of any gifts and leanings that the child may have, will mean the child can make the most of what he has without too much focus on what he has not.

Management of Body Functions

Special needs in keeping socially and medically clean include daily hygiene of the body; choice and care of clothes; skin care; and incontinence of the bowel and/or of the bladder—which may have a neurological, mechanical or psychological cause and may be temporary or permanent, congenital or acquired. Each of these is a large subject on its own, but for the health worker at school there are several main principles to bear in mind.

- If the child is allowed to become *malodorous* at school, for whatever reason, his peers will keep away from him. Visits to the home to discuss daily hygiene management and laundry facilities may help. When it is difficult to get the child in and out of the bath, the occupational therapist may be able to give good advice and the social worker may be able to provide aids. If clean clothes are a problem, the health visitor may suggest sources of outside help for obtaining laundry equipment. If the class teacher cooperates in allowing extra time, the school nurse may be able to build on the child's interest in grooming and sense of proper pride and encourage him in self-care in school.

Recent research (Parker, 1983) has shown up a lack of simple practical help suitable for mothers and older children in the management of hemiplegia. Often very basic advice is needed:

- Advice on the care of skin folds and creases as sweat can collect where poor hand control is combined with a lack of feeling. Adequate washing, rinsing and drying of creases in the axilla, midriff, abdomen and groin will prevent soreness. Loose cotton underclothing can separate skin folds.

- The need for moderate use of talcum powder may have to be explained as immoderate use will lead to damp caking and consequent soreness.
- The importance of the proper use of deodorants.
- The fact that poor circulation may result in dryness of the skin, making it more friable. A small amount of baby oil added to the bath can counteract this tendency.
- Sometimes mothers appreciate advice about how best to disguise wasted limbs, and how to make it easier to dress inert limbs. There is no need to risk upsetting any solution that the mother and child have worked out satisfactorily for themselves. 'Velcro' can be a useful fastening, but the stiff corners of the tape should be made round.
- Ideas about the timing and positioning of defaecation are generally welcomed. For instance, the traditional time in the morning before school may be fraught with anxiety and haste—relaxation may be easier in the afternoon after school when the child has unburdened his news over a hot drink and can then sit on the toilet with a radio and a book or comic. An added help will be a small stool or upturned bucket to raise the child's legs to a proper angle whereby gravity can be an advantage.
- Temporary enuresis or encopresis can be referred to the local

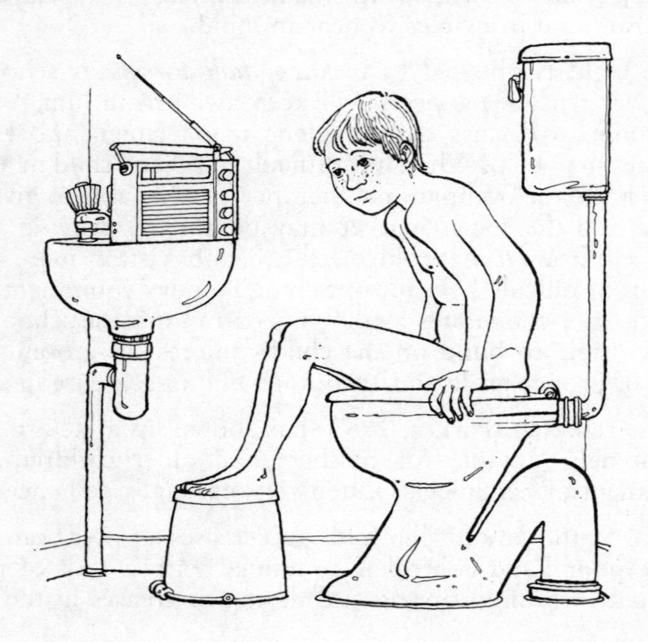

enuretic clinic or the health visitor via the school doctor or through the mother to the family practitioner. The school nurse will have to decide whether it is appropriate to tell the class teacher so that she is aware of the extra anxiety of the child or whether this information might label him in the eyes of the school. Confidentiality and understanding are of utmost importance.

- All treatments ordered from medical sources must be scrupulously carried out. This may involve supporting the child in regular toileting and the formation of good habits, in bladder expression; or in helping him to learn to change his own padding, empty his own urinary bag, apply his own continence device or carry out self-catheterisation at school. If any of these procedures are unfamiliar to the school nurse, she can make an appointment with the hospital or the peripatetic stoma therapist to refresh her technique.
- In some situations, it may be the nurse's responsibility to be aware of the possibility of urine infections. She may be asked to collect samples for testing and to alert the mother or the hospital, if she observes a raised temperature, raised irritability, or raised complaints of feeling unwell on the part of the child.

It cannot be over-emphasised that wherever possible the developing child should be encouraged to take charge of his own body management. It can be difficult to persuade an apathetic child of this and sometimes even more difficult to persuade the parents who can do it quicker and more efficiently themselves. But if physical dependence is not weaned away by deliberate small steps as early as possible, a time will come when disengagement will be traumatic. The ordinary mechanisms with which a teenager asserts his independence are seldom available to the child with special needs: life 'outside' is too precarious for him.

To be Approved and to Socialise

The universal need for approval and acceptance as an individual is as important to the special child as it is to other people; it may be even more difficult for the special child to hold onto a sense of worth, hope and fun. Usual cues may be distorted due to social inexperience, and this inexpertise may itself put off the normal responses of ordinary children. The resulting social inhibition can be counterbalanced by the school nurse who attends to his physical needs. As he teaches him self-care, her whole approach, touch and technique can convey respect for the other. She can make sure he enjoys coming to the medical room. In the secondary school, in particular, reality is bound to encroach upon the childhood fantasies which upheld him in early years. Most adults will humour the five year old boy who boasts 'I'm going to be a racing driver when I grow up'. But when the same boy reaches his mid-teens and suddenly realises that the only transport available to him is a car adapted to his disability, all his expectations have to be recast. Pathological depression is not uncommon.

Suspicion of others and their motives can prevent him from accepting help when it is offered. He may display gauche or ambiguous behaviour which misfires with his contemporaries. This is due to social maladroitness rather than deliberate intention. The lack of an accepted role may be difficult for his peers to tolerate, especially in sexual situations. Sometimes the school nurse can broach these matters naturally to him, but if she feels discomfort or has doubts about her ability to cope with the psychosocial position she finds, she should refer him for outside help through the school doctor or head teacher. It may be helpful to discuss with the parent the ways in which the child's experience of life can be widened. This may take the form of joining in board games with his siblings, helping with the drying up or taking part in club activities outside the home. It is worth investigating any means of drawing out the approval and the acceptance that he must have in order to function positively. Sometimes a mother's sense of loss as her dependent child increases his independence can be compensated for by an enrichment of her own life—she can join pottery classes while he goes swimming, for instance. Work experience for the young person about to leave school may pose a great threat to his mother if she has been his main support; to counter this, she may be able to branch out into a part-time job too. It may be the nurse can suggest ways of retiming her essential management of the child in order to take on a job.

Many mothers of children with special needs feel devalued about their part in society. Both mothers and children need reassurance that their experience has, in fact, increased the contribution they can make, rather than lessened it. Some people find confirmation in taking part in self-help groups and others prefer the company of people with different interests—either way, as long as their experience of value is deepened, their ability to cope with their difficulties will improve. The siblings of a handicapped child have been found to be emotionally and socially deprived also; their needs for attention may be demoted in favour of the disabled member of the family and they will need social boosting at school.

To Exercise Curiosity and to Learn

Every child needs tools with which to experiment in how to improve his own world. The child with learning delay or sensory deficit lacks some of these tools, and those around him need to identify how to provide him with substitutes. The educational psychologist uses tests through which he can interpret the level of each child's learning ability, so that teaching plans can be designed to meet his exact need. The most usual of such tests are known as the WISC (Wechsler Intelligence Scale for Children), the Stanford-Binet scale and the Goodenough Draw-a-Man tests.

Revisions and replacements for these tests are constantly being devised.

It must be understood that such tests measure and compare verbal performance and motor performance only; they do not measure social adaptation, cultural expectancy or emotional equilibrium. The effective exercise of intelligence is found in all of these factors, so it is important that a high rating in one area is not taken to mean there is a high rating in all areas or the converse. A gifted child with an abnormally high IQ may have a low emotional ability; a spina bifida child with a high verbal performance may have a very low learning performance; an epileptic child who has adapted well socially may be held back by the culturally low expectation surrounding him. Results such as these illustrate the value of treating tests as useful pointers, but they can be misleading unless the results are used with caution. Once a problem has been accurately identified, a solution can be designed to get around it or adapt to it. Realistic observation may avoid goals that are set too high. As Brechin and Liddiard state (1981), 'It is generally acknowledged that learning occurs through action, and that simply telling someone how to do something has little impact'. So the nurse who understands and accepts a difficulty and encourages the child and other staff to look at it together will strengthen the foundation for his further learning.

Part of facing reality may be helping the child understand what is different about him. Many adolescents have been found to know very little about their own disability and how it will affect their future. Often they do not want to ask their parents about their disability 'in case it hurts them' and there is little time to ask teachers; the privacy of the medical room may be the most secure place to discuss such matters. When the school nurse finds herself explaining the cause and effects of a particular condition, it is a good opportunity to also suggest sources of further help. Community services, youth organisations, and self-help groups may be especially useful (see references and addresses for each specific condition in Chapters 10 and 11).

Finally, we should look at ourselves. What do we, the 'helpers' expect of independence and integration? Are our feet on the ground or are our heads in the sky? Do we try to see the world by standing in the child's footprints—our feet will not fit them but how near can we get? What does the child with special needs want himself? Are we as nurses any good at helping him to get it? Can we trust him to do it right and can we risk him doing it wrong? Can we see to it that he is not on the receiving end only, but also on the doing end and the giving end? Can we accept an uneven performance? Organic disorder involves congenital, biological, physiological, psychological, emotional, social and mental difficulties in differing degrees. Can we hold them all in mind? No single factor can be dealt with in isolation; the effects of one affect all the others. And when we finally construct a nursing plan, do we mistake the map for the territory itself? A defined plan can be dangerous if there is too much confidence in it; can we still feel the need to review the situation constantly, think again and never allow ourselves the luxury of having it all under control?

10 Specific Physical Disorders

This chapter presents short descriptions of the major disorders found in our schools today. It must be emphasised that none of the following passages contain in themselves sufficient information for the total nurture of any disabled child. The information presented is designed to be a reminder only; the nurse who is not already familiar with the condition should inform herself further, using the recommended references provided. Most managers, libraries or bookshops should be able to obtain these books without difficulty.

Nursing Concerns Shared

The school nurse who carries responsibility for several schools can obviously not take care of every child needing care every day. Therefore there will be several cases in her work-load where special needs—including nursing care—are supplied by non-trained ancillary staff employed by the LEA. The relationship between these workers and the school nurse is crucial in developing a programme that advances the health status of each child. The other staff involved should be encouraged to see that the health care of disabled children in school is not a matter of plugging gaps, but rather of furthering self-care. The mutual exchange of messages and information between the school nurse nd the school secretary is vital. A good and creative working relationship will bring about an improvement of the general awareness of all health concerns within the school. It may be that the school secretary will have to practise first aid and cope with emergencies in the absence of the school nurse. Trust and confidence that have been fostered on less eventful days will underpin the care required in crises.

The transport of a child who is ill or hurt is the responsibility of the head teacher and *not* of the school nurse. If this duty is undertaken by the school nurse out of goodwill, it must be remembered that there may be no insurance cover for such practice and often no escort.

Parents should be contacted as soon as possible and arrangements made that:

1. the parents collect their child themselves; or
2. if they are not contactable or have no transport, that a member of staff with an escort takes the child and delivers him into someone else's care; or
3. an ambulance is called to the school.

The following section deals with the school management and expanded nursing role of specific physical disorders that may be encountered in the ordinary school. Where a special diet or medication routine is prescribed, it will form part of the school nurse's role to ensure that these directions are carried out smoothly. Physical disorders whose management does not impinge on school over and above the general nurture already discussed in this book have not been included here. Although conditions have to be identified by names, great care has to be taken to avoid 'labelling' a child. The personality and development of the child is always more important than his condition. Also his condition may change and his 'typing' become inaccurate and stigmatising. It should be remembered that some children are multi-handicapped, and the diagnosis of one condition cannot be allowed to blind carers to the needs that may emerge due to another.

Allergy

This term has recently become emotive and it should be used with caution. Asthma, hay fever and chronic rhinitis have long been recognised as allergic reactions to pollen, house-dust and animal fur. Similarly, skin rashes, mucous membrane inflammation and some pyrexias have also been seen as the allergic reaction of some children to medication and treatment, particularly penicillin and adhesive plaster. However, there is now such a wide range of claims made for symptoms that are physical, behavioural and psychiatric that a tendency is developing to identify almost any chronic ailment as an allergy. Some of the allergens that have been implicated in allergic reactions are listed below (p. 193).

Clinical ecologists maintain that if the offending allergen could be identified by the use of a rotating diet and eliminated thereafter from the diet, all disturbing symptoms would cease. Dramatic experiences of cures from long-standing illnesses have been described in the literature, but there is, as yet, little collected hard data from sufficiently large numbers of allergy sufferers trying this treatment.

Allergens		*Resulting Conditions*
pollen house dust fur and feather food additives (preservatives, colourings, sweeteners) sugar milk cheese eggs chocolate potatoes wheat, corn tea coffee beer synthetic clothing manufactured drugs oranges strawberries	have been claimed to be responsible for	asthma catarrh conjunctivitis hay fever rhinitis migraine lethargy nausea, vomiting abdominal pain colitis skin rashes local eczema high blood pressure chronic constipation multiple sclerosis cancer hyperactivity in childhood depression schizophrenia emotional maladjustment criminal behaviour learning disability memory and concentration deficit

Management at School

Special clothing and special diets requested, or sent into school by the child's mother must be respected. It is wisest for the school nurse to do nothing to inflame the situation, which may be causing considerable anxiety to the child. Shared discussion and exchange of information with the class teacher is always useful. It may be advisable sometimes to emphasise to the teacher that certain dietary precautions have been prescribed by the doctor and are not childish fads. Some deficiency diseases require strict control of food intake, and these must not be confused with limitations that are recommended rather than prescribed.

Self-help organisation: Action Against Allergy, 43 The Downs, London SW20 8HG. A stamped self-addressed envelope (SAE) is requested if information is required.

Further reading
There are many articles in journals in the USA. The chief literature in this country comes from Dr Richard Mackarness, published by

Pan Books Ltd., Cavaye Place, London SW10 9PG. Titles include *Eating Dangerously*, *Not All in the Mind* and *Chemical Victims*.

Asthma

It is commonly estimated that asthma and 'bronchial wheezing' account for over one-third of all chronic illness in childhood. It is a condition with a wide range of predisposing factors; it presents attacks of breathlessness that range from mild to life-threatening; and its control may range from simple prophylaxis to an extended spectrum of treatment. The school nurse has the difficult task of allaying anxiety in the child, his parents and the school staff—chiefly because relaxation is one of the most potent factors in avoiding attacks—while bearing in mind that an attack never can be treated lightly and that the annual death rate for asthmatic children is still unacceptably high.

Causation

Genetic, allergic, bacterial and psychosomatic factors can all contribute to the aetiology of asthma, but in no case can all these factors be presumed. Asthmatic children are not necessarily over-anxious or over-emotional, and they cannot deliberately 'bring on an attack'. Exercise may predispose to breathlessness, but if it is managed properly and positively, exercise can strengthen resistance to attack. Some athletes who have won gold medals at the Olympic Games have been asthmatic.

Clinical Presentation at School

A child may complain at school of tightness in the chest, wheeziness, night coughing or acute breathlessness. Some experts urge that all such symptoms should be investigated for asthma, particularly if the child belongs to an 'atopic' family—that is, one with a common history of repeated respiratory inflammation, eczema, allergies, hay fever or disturbed sleep. Early diagnosis followed by treatment with prophylactic inhalants can arrest further development of the disease. Once this 'mild' stage has become more severe, the resulting over-protection, school absence and inevitable introspection may lead to spiralling effects.

Management at School

Many diagnosed young asthmatics will be advised by their doctor to take pocket inhalers to school and use them 2–4 times a day. This small mechanism delivers a substance directly into the bronchioles by inhalation; the drug, in powder form, inhibits histamine sensitivity and prevents the over-production of mucus which is the cause of bronchial spasm. Some of these inhalers are *not* suitable for the treatment of an actual attack. Where it is prescribed, the use of the inhaler must be regular, whether attacks occur or not.

If a child becomes wheezy and breathless at school, he should be taken to a place of calm and seated with his elbows over the back of a cushioned chair placed in front of him to allow the fullest expansion of his rib cage. He should be spoken to quietly by the nurse seated close to him, and encouraged to breathe slowly and deeply and deliberately. Smaller children may find that resting their arms on a table is more comfortable. Sometimes inspiring and expiring in common with the nurse can help. The distraction of a story or a book being read aloud will often calm the child.

Any bronchodilator which has been brought to school should be administered as prescribed. More sophisticated drugs, such as corticosteroids and nebulisers, are usually left at home. Antibiotics may be brought to school. When it becomes obvious that these simple measures are not working, the patient must be taken to hospital without further delay for treatment by injection and oxygen. His parents should be contacted immediately.

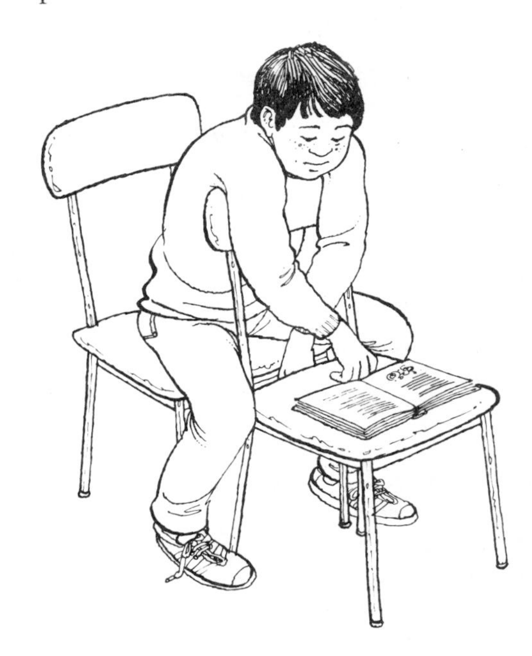

The Role of the School Nurse

Her role is primarily to encourage self-care, to help the child to learn to live with his disability, to explain the extent of his capabilities to PE teachers, to link parents with school staff, and to give continual support to the child. She may be asked by the doctor to record a pattern of the asthmatic attacks, and to make use of a peak flowmeter at school to measure the child's air capacity at different times and with varying activities.

The school nurse will play an important part in helping staff and children at school to accept the inconvenience of the child's asthmatic attacks and to accept the child as a person. The child with asthma will need continual reassurance in practical ways that he is not 'ill' and that his way of life is 'normal'. The more he can be encouraged to be extrovert at school, the more he will respond physically and belie the folklore that asthmatics are necessarily sheltered and delicate.

Self-help organisations: The Asthma Society and Friends of the Asthma Research Council, St Thomas' Hospital, Lambeth Palace Road, London SE1 7EH. These organisations will supply information, the *Asthma News* and addresses of local branches.

Further reading

Leaflets from the above society include titles such as *Asthma at School, Coming to Terms with Asthma, Exercise Asthma* and *I Have Asthma* (a booklet for children). Also useful is *Breathing Instruction for Children* from the Chest, Heart and Stroke Assoc., Tavistock House North, Tavistock Square, London WC1H 9SR. Also:

Godfrey S. (1975). *Your Child with Asthma*. London: Heinemann Health Books.

Knight A. (1982). *Asthma and Hay Fever*. London: Martin Dunitz.

Lane D. J., Storr, A. (1979). *Asthma: the Facts*. Oxford: Oxford University Press.

Rackman K. *et al.* (1976). *The Child with Asthma*. London: Invalid Children's Aid Association.

Autism

Most of the 3000 children of school age in England and Wales who have autism will be in special schools; one-half of these children are further handicapped by spasticity, epilepsy or mental retardation. However, there is a larger number of children who have autistic-like tendencies. Their diagnosis is obscure, but they can be encouraged to socialise in an ordinary school with the extra attention of an ancillary worker. Where this is the case, the chief contribution of the school nurse will be that of a 'listening ear'—to receive the puzzled queries of teachers, carers and parents alike—and to help the child's classmates appreciate his positive qualities.

Autism is still not fully understood. Research is continually disproving the assumption that an autistic child comes from parents who are middle class, intelligent and either over-solicitous or emotionally cold. This group of parents is perhaps less tolerant of strange behaviour and more vocal when finding it, but in fact autistic children are spread throughout the socioeconomic range of families.

The chief feature of autism is negative development rather than physical abnormality. The distinguishing marks of early autism are a lack of ability to respond or relate, a lack of curiosity and a lack of imagination. The children appear to be unable to make connections or patterns of stimuli that they receive. This means that although they can see, hear, taste, smell and feel with normal accuracy, the ability to link together the sensory data and make meaning out of it appears to be lacking. For instance, when they have learnt a few words, they will use them in inappropriate orders. They may draw or complete puzzles or enjoy constructional toys, but often these will be upside down and unrelated to their immediate context.

The consequence is that access to the firm foundation of loving relationships, which support the 'normal' child, is denied to the autistic child. He must find his security elsewhere. Often he finds it in repetitive, stylised and socially meaningless routines. This obsessiveness can attach to actions that are monotonously simple and any slight change in a recognised pattern may produce prolonged screaming. His reaction to anything unfamiliar is erratic and unpredictable; loud noises may leave him indifferent, whereas a whisper can produce real distress. The bewilderment of the child with autistic tendencies is even greater than the bewilderment of those who care for him.

Many people can tolerate a well-behaved child with a visible handicap better than a visibly pleasing child who has distorted and uncontrollable behaviour. Parents put so much into the care of these children and often become so worn down by the unresponsive nature of their condition, that they find it difficult to see the situation objectively. The school nurse has a positive part to play in getting to know them. Sometimes she can suggest a means of respite care for the child so that the family can take a short holiday or enjoy a good night's sleep; sometimes a surrogate family will look after the child for short breaks; or she may be able to put them in touch with the DHSS which has a list of holiday places with financial help for handicapped people.

Management at School

There is as yet no specific *medical* treatment.

Psychotherapy has, so far, produced only disappointing results, largely due to the limited possibilities of word exchange.

Educational success will largely depend on the degree of aphasia present and the level of effective communication. Sometimes non-verbal language is as confusing to the autistic child as verbal, so exchanges should be simplified as far as possible and directed on one level only. Many otherwise puzzling children have displayed strengths in unexpected areas—usually those which are not reliant on many words, such as music, mathematics and construction. These gifts should be developed.

Socialising in school is important. Autistic children are seldom able to sustain close friendships. The autistic child has been described as the 'child apart' or the 'involuntary stranger'. This description is apt, but the child's social isolation should not be accepted by the school nurse as inevitable. The presence of other children around him should be encouraged, even if they are puzzled by his behaviour and even if he cannot take part in their activities. Eventually many children with autistic tendencies do grow into young adults who can cope in general society, although usually in a limited fashion.

The Role of the School Nurse

Nursing involvement may include the promotion of toilet training and encouragement of hygiene. School nurses in this situation should be familiar with the techniques of behaviour modification and operant conditioning (see references below). The child who has autistic tendencies often enjoys physical contact. The nurse is in a good position to reinforce self-care skills by using her hands to teach and to show approval; this may be more successful and satisfactory than words.

Self-help organisation: The National Autistic Society, 276 Willesden Lane, London NW2.

Further reading

From the above society—*The Handicaps of Autistic Children*; *Children Apart*; *Information for Parents*; *Body Awareness and the Development of Basic Skills in Physical Education*; *What is Operant Conditioning?—Successes and Limitations*. Also:

Copeland J. (1973). *For the love of Ann*. London: Arrow Books Ltd.

Deich R., Hodges P. M. (1977). *Language without Speech*. London: Souvenir Press Ltd.

Everard P. (1980). *Involuntary Strangers*. London: John Clare Books Ltd.

Lovell A. (1978). *Simple Simon*. Herts: Lion Publishing.

Wing L. (1976). *Early Childhood Autism: clinical, educational and social aspects*. Oxford: Pergamon Press.

Wing L. (1980). *Autistic Children—A Guide for Parents*. London: Constable & Co. Ltd.

Cerebral Palsy

Cerebral palsy is an umbrella term; about one baby in 500 is born with some damage to some brain cells. The damage may be mild—for example, the child's right arm may have reduced power and reduced coordination—or it may be extensive and cause a child to be confined to a wheelchair, without speech or hearing. The degree of severity is variable, whatever the site of brain damage.

The classifications of spasticity, athetosis and ataxia originate from the part of the brain affected—whether it is outer cortex, basal ganglia or cerebellum respectively. In practice, however, these effects overlap one another and the difference between them is not important in nursing terms. The definition of cerebral palsy as a disorder of posture and movement resulting from a permanent, non-progressive defect of the immature brain is, on the other hand, useful for understanding the condition and planning care. The disordered movements and posture can affect one limb (*monoplegia*), two limbs (upper or lower, but usually lower only—*paraplegia*) or one side of body (*hemiplegia*), three limbs (spastic *triplegia*, which is rare) or all four limbs (*double hemiplegia*, *quadraplegia*). Some children with cerebral palsy have the added disadvantage of epilepsy and are prone to seizures.

There have been rare cases where a child who is quadraplegic has been mentally unaffected and has been able to obtain a university degree. Unfortunately, there are a larger number at the opposite end of the scale who live in institutions all their lives, particularly those whose speech and hearing centres in the brain have also been damaged. The great majority, however, fall in between these extremes and they are likely to go to ordinary schools.

Early diagnosis and early provision for identified needs can greatly improve the outlook for most children with cerebral palsy. If the early years, with their sensitive learning periods, are not made the most of, the spreading effects of the handicap can be more disabling than the original brain damage. Cerebral palsy itself is not degenerative. Once a child reaches school, teamwork and continual assessment are of the utmost importance. Those involved in overall care along with the teacher and the nurse will be:

- *the physiotherapist* (peripatetic, community clinic or hospital-based)—whose role is to design active and passive exercises to strengthen working muscles, stimulate weak ones and stretch spastic ones, and thus minimise muscle atrophy.
- *the occupational therapist*—whose role is to provide aids both at home and at school for writing, eating, drinking, dressing, and toileting and washing.
- *the orthopaedic surgeon*—whose role is to diagnose and

prescribe treatment for the next goal, whether calipers, walking aids or surgery for the relief of contractures.

- *the speech therapist*—whose role is to develop available speech and language potential.
- *the audiologist*—whose role is to provide hearing aids where necessary. Athetoid children are particularly prone to high-tone deafness and this range may include the teacher's voice. Any implication from a teacher that their CP child is dull or inattentive should be referred for hearing tests.
- *the optician*—whose role is to diagnose and prescribe treatment for squint, myopia, or less often nystagmus.
- *the educational psychologist*—whose role is to advise concerning remedial special education.
- *the educational welfare officer*—whose role is to investigate and make allowances for school absences.
- *the social worker*—whose role is to be involved with possible problems at home.

Management at School

The child with cerebral palsy has many of the special needs that have already been discussed. With adequate oversight and provision for these needs, he can contribute as much to 'normal' children in the school—by showing 'how to make the most of what you've got'—as 'normal' children can offer to him in friendship and support. School management will be different for each child, and detailed care will vary from episode to episode.

The Role of the School Nurse

Nursing skills as such may not feature prominently in the care of the cerebral palsy child in ordinary school, but her continual nurturing role will give him support. Her main concern will be to provide warmth, acceptance and liaison with other sources of help. The school nurse should take the initiative in finding out the individual daily and long-term plans for the child from his consultant, his teacher and his parent, and then decide how best she can reinforce them.

Self-help organisations: The Spastics Society, 12 Park Crescent, London W1N 4EQ, and AFASIC (Association for all Speech Impaired Children) 347 Central Markets, Smithfield, London EC1.

Further reading

Finnie N. (1974). *Handling Your Cerebral Palsied Child at Home*. London: Heinemann Medical.

Howe B. (1969). *Crossed Wires*. London: The Spastics Society.

Mitchell R. G. (1961). *Cerebral Palsy in Childhood and Adolescence.* (Henderson J. L., ed.) Edinburgh: Livingstone.
Morgan M., Kendall S. (1979). *Them and Us: Working Together.* London: The Spastics Society.

Childhood Cancer

Malignancy takes various forms in children: leukaemia accounts for about half of the total, with sarcomas, neuroblastomas, brain tumours, lymphomas (including Hodgkin's disease), retinoblastomas and cancer of the kidney (Wilms' tumour) making up the remainder. Cancer is at present the commonest disease-related cause of death in children of school age; nonetheless modern treatment is extending both the survival rate and the degree of remission. In these circumstances, it is of paramount importance that a child with diagnosed malignant disease comes to school as much and as often as possible. The more 'normalcy' that can be retained in his life, the more can be relieved of his stress and the more effective his treatment will be.

Management at School

The child with cancer will probably be undergoing surgery, chemotherapy or radiotherapy or a combination of these treatments, and he will be experiencing the side-effects that go with them. Order, acceptance of whatever happens and calmness will be pillars of security for him.

At home, the emotions of both child and family will be fluctuating—constantly readjusting to the changing circumstances. In hospital, the child's experiences may be alarming or reassuring, but they will certainly be out of the ordinary. At school, life goes on as steadily as always and the child often finds it an enormous relief to be allowed to be 'ordinary'. The child will sometimes tire easily. A rest may be needed before the child can return to class activities. Alternatively, arrangements may be made for a shortened day or regular half-day attendance.

It is important to emphasise that if the child with cancer can be enabled to attend school, he will feel that he is living in a positive and constructive way and his feelings of inadequacy, failure and threat will be minimised. If he can be convinced that his company is still enjoyable in spite of everything and that it is sought by others, his morale and self-esteem will remain high.

Nonetheless tensions will exist. If the school nurse can help teachers, other staff and perhaps even pupils to understand some of the feelings of the child with cancer, they will be able to offer greater support on his 'low' days. Sensitivity will be needed to decide whether a particular child *wants* to discuss an issue and needs help with opening it up, or whether these feelings are sufficiently aired at home and school is the place where he has relief from facing up to them. If he asks questions at school, his answers should be truthful at the level at which they are asked; if he trusts the answer, he will feel free to ask further, but he should not be pressed to dig any deeper than he wants to. The staff should be aware of the areas he might decide to expose.

Table 10.1 illustrates the various stages of emotions that shocked or grieving people are likely to pass through. A child who knows that he has a serious or life-threatening condition will indeed be grieving. Those around him may need to go through anticipatory mourning too. If some of these emotions are shared, they can in time become stepping stones to reconstruction.

Table 10.1 does not describe definite stages; not all will be experienced by everyone and some will overlap with others. The child may not be able to verbalise such things, but nevertheless his emotions will fluctuate in a way that alarms him. Regular school attendance can be an enormously steadying influence.

The Role of the School Nurse

The role of the nurse is to support the child; to support other staff; to support 'watching' classmates, who may identify personally with the child and feel very threatened themselves; and to maintain close links with all disciplines concerned with the child's treatment.

Quite early in the situation, the nurse may have to decide where she will take her own distress. She may decide to go to a colleague outside the school or she may point out the need for a carer of carers to her nursing manager. If the school nurse is to retain her sensitivity as well as provide a secure support for others in situations that are difficult for everyone, she should not batten down the hatches of her own emotions. For the sake of the help she gives others, she must make sure she can 'let it all out' somewhere and then refill her own resources.

Side-effects of treatment that may be met at school include fatigue, lassitude, depression, pallor and loss of hair. It is seldom that a school nurse will be required to undertake medical treatment at school, although she will carry out palliative measures. She must maintain close contact concerning these with the child's doctor, whether he is home-based or hospital-based. Teaching staff may need explanations concerning the dulling of learning abilities associated with radiation therapy or aggressive chemotherapy.

School staff may also need help to understand the reactions of parents. Two particular issues may arise:

- an apparent reluctance on the part of the child to attend school may, in fact, be a reflection of the parents' separation complex,

Table 10.1
Phases of Mourning for the Loss of Health (can be experienced by parents and/or child)

Term	*Behavioural Reaction*	*Verbal Expression*
Limbo (during time of diagnostic testing)	Hyperactive behaviour. Indecision can be terrifying. Hide it.	'Be bright and brittle, pretend you don't care.'
Numb disbelief/ excruciating stress (on hearing confirmation of serious diagnosis)	A first 'death'. Hopelessness.	'Why strive further?'
Shock/denial	Apathy. Verbal difficulties. Thought processes slowed.	'It's not true, this is only a bad dream. This isn't real reality.'
Rage	Sullenness; periodic irrational outbursts towards carers, close relatives, medical staff. Need to fix blame.	'It's not fair.' 'It's all the fault of . . .'
Guilt	Vagueness, withdrawal, stammering.	'What have I done to make this happen? Where did I go wrong?'
Idealisation of child	Aggressive advocacy, sentimentality.	'Of course he can have whatever he wants.'
Somatic sympathy	Physical pains felt by nearest and dearest—even to the point of feeling they are dying.	'If I hurt too, yours might be less' or 'I can take yours on.'
Bargaining, with fate, God or self	Usually internalised. Unrealistic demands made on self.	'If I behave perfectly, then . . . won't happen. If only I can . . .'
Fear/panic	Future appears out of control. Competency skills go absent.	'I'm going mad.' 'I can't cope.'
Depression	Inward venting of helplessness, non-verbalization, detachment from sufferer. Suicidal fantasies.	'Nothing I can do will change things. It would be better if I wasn't here.'
Resignation	Fatalism, passivity. No point in anything.	'No use trying.'
Given time, support and continued nurturance, such grief work can grow into:		
Acceptance	Constructive peace of mind. Growth of maturity.	'The world isn't going to end. Ultimately all shall be well in spite of the scars.'
Re-establishment of emotional attachment, trust, hope, conviction. Construction of meaning to life, incorporating loss.		

rather than a school-phobia. It may be possible to persuade such parents that it is in the child's interests to continue to attend school as often as possible, even if this entails 'sacrifice' on the parents' part.

- parents' reactions to remission can sometimes be hard to justify. Mixed with relief and joy will be anger—fierce anger—at the pointlessness of all the grieving they have been through. They think to themselves 'after all that it's all going to be all right'. Reasoning is unlikely to help; receptivity and tolerance will help to speed the passing of these negative emotions.

Self-help organisations: National Society for Cancer Relief, Michael Sobell House, 30 Dorset Square, London NW1 6QL. Leukaemia Society, 28 Eastern Road, London N2.

Further reading

Burton L. (1974). *Care of the Child Facing Death*. London: Routledge & Kegan Paul.

Gynlay J. (1978). *The Dying Child*. Maidenhead: McGraw-Hill Inc.

Stedeford A. (1984). *Facing Death: Patients, Families and Professionals*. London: Heinemann Medical.

Cystic Fibrosis

Until recently, the child who was born with cystic fibrosis had a very poor outlook. Research into the causation, medication and treatment of this disease has intensified only over the last two decades; therefore, the number of young adults at college and in the community is still small and the level of general knowledge concerning the condition is low. The children who now survive the risks of infancy are not impaired in their intellectual or communication skills and their mobility is normal. A large majority can attend ordinary school, given some extra provision for their physical treatment. The prognosis of these children depends largely on the degree to which respiratory infections can be avoided and lung damage controlled (Table 10.2).

The name cystic fibrosis does not describe the cause of the condition, but rather one of its effects. The cause is a genetic abnormality, carried by both sexes, and as many as 1 in 20 adults in NW Europe may be a carrier. When two carriers marry, there is a one in four chance that they will produce a baby who has the extra gene—this means that about 1 in 2000 babies are born with this disease. It cannot be detected as yet before conception nor in the newborn child.

The single abnormal gene affects one enzyme's activity in the body's chemistry. The effect is to make normal secretions extra viscid. The symptoms of this develop with the child.

Table 10.2
Cystic Fibrosis

	Medical Condition	*Parents*	*Child*
Stage 1	Neonates and infancy High risk of morbidity and mortality	Parents often exhausted, anxious, totally involved.	100% dependent on others.
Stage 2	Early childhood Infancy survived, outlook improved.	Parents sometimes reluctant to pass care to others. Hesitant to expand child's experience for fear of infection.	Intellect, curiosity and mobility are 'normal'. Child desires increasing independence. Strength of body, character and immunity may develop.
Stage 3	Teenage to adulthood The older, the better the prognosis. May train, hold a job, marry.	Over-protection may provoke rebelliousness and non-compliance. Parents should be encouraged to widen their own interests.	Responsibility for self-care, diet and exercise needs should be promoted. Medical oversight maintained. Genetic counselling may be advised.

1. At birth, the meconium may be so thick and difficult to discharge that an obstruction is caused in the ileum, sometimes requiring surgery. During childhood, faeces may continue to be bulky, pale and offensive.
2. Thickened secretions block the ducts of the pancreas. Cysts form, which then fibrose—hence the name of cystic fibrosis. The flow of the digestive enzyme pancreatin is inhibited, normal digestion of fats cannot take place, and the body becomes under-nourished. This means that:
   (a) the new-born child may be severely underweight.
   (b) a special diet must be followed throughout life, with the addition at each meal of pancreatin.
3. Secretions in the lungs of normal mucus are thickened. Bronchioles can become blocked and this has three effects:
   (a) the risk of respiratory infection is high.
   (b) coughing becomes persistent.
   (c) breathlessness can result from sudden exercise.
   (d) there is an ever-present risk of lung collapse or lobal atrophy if treatment is neglected.

To alleviate this third condition, special breathing exercises have to be undertaken at least twice a day and sometimes two hourly.

Physiotherapists will be responsible for designing this regime from infancy, and they will instruct parents to take over as proves practicable. When the child grows older, he can be encouraged to understand why and how he needs this treatment. An increasing number of 10–12 year olds' are performing their own programmes. Many affirm that they themselves know exactly when and where to percuss, and how to compress and shake and then expire with a 'huff' and cough. Postural drainage enables each lobe of the lung to be cleared individually. To facilitate this at school, the nurse may have to help with arrangements for floor mattresses or a couch with an appropriate tilting mechanism, together with pillows or foam wedges, to be available at school. In some cases bronchodilator inhalants are prescribed for use before postural drainage. Antibiotics may be inhaled after the lungs are cleared.

In children with cystic fibrosis, excretion of sweat has an abnormally high salt content. Cleanliness of the skin is particularly important and older children may need help in controlling body odour.

Management at School

The pattern of the disease should be borne in mind when considering the management of cystic fibrosis at school. When the child first comes to school, it is likely that he will be provided by the LEA with personal ancillary help. A peripatetic physiotherapist is likely to visit the school to oversee the programme of exercises and relaxation periods. It may be that the school nurse is not directly involved in these, but there will nonetheless be a distinct role for her to play as resource person in other areas.

The Role of the School Nurse

In her role of back-up support for the child, his parents and other services, there are some practical pointers.

- The child with cystic fibrosis should be included in all the usual *immunisation* and *screening* procedures. It may be advised that the child and his close contacts have an annual dose of influenza vaccine in addition.
- Exercise should be encouraged to the extent that the child himself can tolerate. If *breathlessness* should occur, he should be helped into a position where he can breathe diaphragmatically in a relaxed way; he may find it helps to rest his arms on a table nearby and lean over them, or sit leaning forward, or lie on his side but supported upwards—any position where the weight of his shoulders and upper thorax is taken off his diaphragm.

Over-breathing should be avoided: the aim is to make quiet, normal air-exchange easier.

- *School meals* can be adjusted for his diet. He should have a high calorie intake in the form of protein, vegetables and sugar with minimal fat and low starch. He will bring his enzyme and vitamin additives from home—the school nurse may be responsible for negotiating storage and administration arrangements.
- Extra care with *dental hygiene* will be necessary on account of his high sugar intake.
- The teenager must realise that *smoking* cannot be tolerated.
- A close liaison with the *medical social worker* from the child's hospital team should be maintained throughout his school life.
- The nurse should make sure the following points are clear to the *class teacher*: CF coughing is not infectious itself, but the CF child is very prone *to* infection. Therefore, absences from school may be frequent, and transport in public buses and trains may have to be avoided. Frequent absences may contribute to academic backwardness, but intellectual function is unaffected by CF.
- *Parental attitudes* of protection may need caring modification. The school nurse can do much to boost their confidence in the school's care of their child if she acts as a link agent.

Self-help organisation: Cystic Fibrosis Research Trust, Alexandra House, 5 Blyth Road, Bromley, Kent BR1 3RS. The free information leaflets from this organisation are particularly useful.

Further reading

Anderson M., Goodchild M. C. (1976). *Cystic Fibrosis: a manual of diagnosis and management*. Oxford: Blackwell Scientific Publications.

Gaskelly D., Webber B. (1982). *The Physical Treatment of Cystic Fibrosis*, from above address.

Lawson D. (1984). *Cystic Fibrosis*, from above address.

Eczema

Eczema is seldom called a disability or a special need, but among children it can cause considerable distress, embarrassment and peer segregation. It is an umbrella term, which can be used to describe skin conditions that are:

1. congenital or acquired as allergies.
2. either wet and oozing or dry and scaly.
3. either due to infection or atopic (without reference to a cause).
4. either disturbingly itchy or barely noticeable to the observer.

Some types are hereditary, some are considered psychosomatic and appear only when the patient is upset emotionally—such as before exams—and some are seen in conjunction with asthma and/or hay fever. Eczema can also be the response to a particular substance being in contact with the skin.

In any of these conditions, whatever the cause, the affected child is apt to feel 'marked'. Lessening tension and attention around the child will help him to see that having eczema should be of no significance in school. It usually disappears during the early teenage years, although it may be superseded by acne. The basic practical management of most eczematous conditions is similar. The child should be advised to:

- wear cotton clothing next to the skin where possible. Some children may be advised to avoid wool or nylon altogether. Change underclothing daily.
- wash gently with a non-irritating soap. Avoid crude or perfumed soaps. Pat affected skin dry with paper tissues. Avoid talcum powder.
- use soap powder for laundry, particularly keep away from enzyme washing preparations. Always rinse clothes very thoroughly.
- keep fingernails as short as possible, but try not to become anxious over scratching. Rubbing is preferable.
- try to work out what makes it worse. Touching anything particular? Eating a certain food? Getting too hot or too cold? Feeling frightened or worried or excited?

Management at School

Teachers, peers and the mothers of peers will probably need reassuring that eczema is not catching; holding the hand of a child whose fingers are affected will do much for his sense of acceptance and no harm whatever to the other person. It may also seem puzzling to the non-medical person that one day the child will have such a bad eruption that he cannot concentrate, his skin is too tight and dry to allow him to hold a pencil, and he feels too low and lethargic to play football; yet within a couple of days he can be as lively and active as any in the class. Explanation may also be needed about the sleepiness and learning difficulties that sometimes accompany steroid treatments or wakeful, itchy nights. School nurses should also note factors that tend to exacerbate the eczema, such as overheated rooms, chlorine in the swimming pool, ropes in the gymnasium or the attention of dinner ladies who mistake a young child's diet for fussiness. Tactile playthings such as clay, sand and modelling media may also irritate his skin.

If a bout of scratching occurs in class, the following practical hints may be useful:

- allow the child to leave the room, to cool down physically and emotionally.

- encourage him to splash cold water on the itching area or to use a cool flannel for relief.
- let him apply his own anti-irritant cream—he knows best where it is itching, and the self-control and distraction will both be useful.
- he can ask for his own antihistamine medication from the appropriate person.

The Role of the School Nurse

Close contact should be maintained with the mother. Sometimes the child, mother and nurse can construct patterns together of behaviour and reaction, as suggested above.

The child should be encouraged to take care of his skin and to have a sense of humour rather than self-pity about the state of his skin. Group discussions with peers can be initiated as a way of meeting real relationship difficulties if these occur.

Sometimes sore areas will need to be re-dressed at school, and the school nurse will need to instruct a permanent member of staff about the best means of managing this with the least embarrassment to the child.

The immunisation programme need not be modified, although smallpox vaccination is usually contraindicated.

Self-help organisation: The National Eczema Society, Tavistock House North, Tavistock Square, London WC1H 9SR. This organisation prints the following excellent titles.

Eczema—Some Hints and Facts
Coping with School
What is Eczema?
Let's Talk About You—a booklet for children

Further reading

Atherton D. J. (1984). *Your Child with Eczema*. London: Heinemann Medical.
Mackie R. (1983). *Eczema and Dermatitis*. London: Martin Dunitz. Positive Health Guides.
Orton C. (1981). *Learning to Live with Skin Disorders*. London: Souvenir Press.

Diabetes

Diabetes is a complex of disorders, a syndrome rather than a single disease; the basic defect common to all diabetics is a failure to produce adequate insulin. Suggested causes include virus infection, inherited factors, and the presence of autoimmunity antibodies which destroy or damage the insulin-producing cells. Although extensive research is being carried out, there is not as yet a cure.

It is likely that 1 in 12 000 children attending ordinary school will be diabetic. Considerable apprehension has been shown to exist among school staff about diabetes, but the care of the child with this disorder is straightforward once the basic principles of management have been fully understood. He can be treated quite normally and can withstand the usual demands of discipline, sport, outings and school journeys once the fundamental theory has been recognised by all who attend him.

The *normal conversion* of carbohydrate into energy has five clear stages:

1. Sugar and starch are taken in as food.
2. This carbohydrate is digested and converted into glucose.
3. The glucose is carried by the bloodstream to every part of the body.
4. The pancreas normally excretes insulin into the bloodstream.
5. In the presence of sufficient insulin, glucose is released into functioning energy wherever it is needed; it may be in the muscles, the brain, the eyes or the skin.

The normal pattern is disturbed where the insulin secreted by the pancreas is insufficient. The position then is described as *mal-adapted functioning*. Where there is insufficient insulin, glucose cannot be converted, and it builds up in the bloodstream to a level that is toxic. At the same time, energy is at a low level, and none of the specific areas mentioned can function normally. This stage is known as incipient diabetes, and if undetected may reach a state of *hyperglycaemia* (too much sugar in the blood). Its effects are: fatigue, weakness, loss of weight (due to unexercised muscles), headache, dizziness, vomiting (lack of energy in the brain), frequent micturition (in an effort to excrete toxic levels of glucose), and high levels of thirst (due to frequent micturition). At this stage, diagnosis is made and treatment is immediately effective. If it should remain untreated, however, coma will ensue.

Treatment is two-fold. Insulin will be administered to the child to correct the balance of energy production, while a diet is designed that will control his carbohydrate intake. When properly adhered to, this combined treatment will mean the child can lead a totally normal life, with all the usual demands made upon ordinary children. However, human beings are not robots, and changes in the pattern of daily living do occur. If the balance between the supply of insulin in the blood, the intake of carbohydrate and the need for instant energy is disturbed, then unfavourable symptoms may reappear. Where there is too great a demand for energy and too small a supply of insulin or convertable glucose, there will be a state of *hypoglycaemia* (too little sugar in the blood). Its effects are: unusual vagueness, wandering attention, obstinacy, a glazed, drunken appearance, irritability that can be mistaken for naughtiness, shakiness, sweating, pallor, changes in vision, speech and fluency of reading.

Treatment: GIVE GLUCOSE—or any food or drink with a high sugar content. Dextrasol tablets, sugar lumps, sweets or sweet biscuits may be carried by diabetic children in their pockets. In the absence of these, the child should be given a drink with plenty of sugar stirred into it. Most children recover quickly from hypoglycaemic episodes, and usually they can be trusted to judge for themselves when they need a snack and also when they feel fit to resume normal school activities.

NB: IF THE CHILD SHOULD BECOME UNCONSCIOUS DO NOT GIVE ANYTHING BY MOUTH

If medical aid is not available within a few minutes he should be taken to hospital.

The situations which can cause hypoglycaemia can often be foreseen and steps can, therefore, be taken to avoid them. Some of these causes are:

An extra demand for energy, such as arises from sports.
An unexpected delay in eating a meal.
A bout of high fever.
An unusual excitement.
An accident in the administration of the insulin—either too large a dose given or an injection directly into the bloodstream.

Extra food or sugary snacks should be taken in all these instances.

Management at School

When diabetes is confirmed in a child of school age, its onset brings a sense of affront to both child and family alike. While the implications for the future are being grasped, the uncertainty and confusion will require constant and repeated reassurance from those advising the family. In many areas, a specialist diabetic community nurse or health visitor is available to counsel the child and his parents. In non-specific terms, however, the following points may be useful:

- Adaptation to diabetes involves a total reassessment of life-style and goals by the patient. In the case of a young child, much of this will be done for him; as he grows older, it is of the greatest importance that he is able gradually to take over some of the choices and decisions concerning his life. An attitude can be fostered at school that avoids over-protection, disassociation or alienation, and which raises the level of his own shared responsibility.

- The adaptation undertaken by the child will include:
  1. the necessity of a controlled diet.
  2. the daily administration of insulin by injection.
  3. knowledge of self-injection techniques.
  4. a readjustment of his own self-concept and body image.
  5. the questions which concern others' attitude to him and expectations of him.
  6. a consequent diffidence about his approach to others.

  These are hard tasks for a young child to have thrust upon him. He may react with resentment and anger, or with over-compensation, or he may withdraw socially. All this demands empathetic understanding.
- This adaptation is not completed in a short span of time. As his body grows and his energy output changes, so his treatment, diet and attitude will all have to readjust. This will be a lengthy and on-going process, and will require the adults around him to be tolerant and relaxed, while keeping a watchful eye unobtrusively open.
- In making this adaptation as smooth as possible, it has been found possible to create a small group in a school where peers can air their difficulties to each other and share their own insights. Sometimes just offering them a chance to blow off steam, or express real fears, or explain antagonisms can be of mutual help—especially if it is 'allowed' by an adult, though not manipulated by her. This type of offering and receiving can help restore a sense of equilibrium to a child, and help him tolerate reality rather than retreat into fantasy or denial.

The Role of the School Nurse

The treatment, administration of insulin and dietary advice for diabetes are currently topics of considerable research, and it will be necessary for the school nurse to update constantly her understanding of the subject. Not only will she be turned to for information and advice by other staff, but if both nurse and teachers can feel comfortable and confident in the care they provide, this confidence will be reflected in the child's attitude also. Uncertainty in the carers will increase the anxiety of the child, which may dangerously add to his non-compliance. Individual management varies from child to child and area to area, so it will be essential for the school nurse to establish direct contact with the doctor in charge of a specific case and familiarise herself with its details. In addition to her part in the forming of attitudes at school, and being a resource to the other members of staff, the special responsibility of the school nurse with a diabetic child at her school will be:

- To remember that the primary aim is to equate calorie intake and energy outlay throughout the day. Small meals, with snacks or drinks or sweets taken in between, are better than large meals. Teachers will have to make allowances for the child who carries a biscuit or sugar lump to take when he feels he needs it. Most children who attend ordinary school have been previously encouraged to experience and recognise the onset of a hypoglycaemic episode, and they should be trusted to exercise their own judgement concerning the need for instant glucose.

- Her advice may be sought regarding the diabetic child's access to the school tuck shop or ice cream van. Some form of an agreement or contract could be made between the child and school staff. On the whole, offering him self-responsibility will be the way through. Similarly, there may be discussions with the child's parents, dinner ladies and providers of school lunches, in which the school nurse will have a part. High fibre, unprocessed foods are preferable to low fibre, refined foods; they may be similar in calorie *intake*, but the former is slower in absorption *uptake* and thereby a level of blood glucose that is steady can be maintained. 'Highs' and 'lows' of energy intake should be avoided.
- The school nurse will need to make sure that the standards of hygiene and cleanliness of the diabetic child are high; where the peripheral blood circulation is affected, there is increased risk of skin infection.
- She may have to reinforce the specialist nurse's guidance on self-care, the rotation of injection sites and urine testing.
- She will have to bear in mind the long-term risks of obesity, vascular disease and blindness.
- Routine inoculations and dental treatment can be undertaken as normally, and 'flu immunisation is often recommended in the late autumn. The child's doctor should be consulted if a general anaesthetic becomes necessary.

Throughout her care, the key values will be tolerance, responsibility and, where appropriate, a sense of humour.

Self-help organisation: British Diabetic Association, 10 Queen Anne Street, London W1M 0BD. This organisation has an active Youth Department, which arranges holidays and weekends for young diabetics with or without their parents. It also publishes many pamphlets including such titles as: *An Introduction to Diabetes*, *The Diabetic at School*, *Childhood and Adolescence* and *Exercise and Sport*.

Further reading

Craig, O. (1982). *Childhood Diabetes: the Facts*. Oxford: Oxford Medical Publications.

Farquhar J. W. (1982). *(a) The Diabetic Child, (b) Diabetes in Your Teens*. Edinburgh: Churchill Livingstone.

Tattersall R. (1982). *Diabetes: A Practical Guide for Patients on Insulin*. Edinburgh: Churchill Livingstone.

Down's Syndrome

Down's syndrome is the most common congenital defect me today. The children who inherit it make up over a third of those who, until recently, were categorised as mentally retarded. Because their condition is so immediately recognisable at birth, in the past they were labelled early and sentenced as educationally unrewarding. During the last 20 years, however, the situation has changed dramatically. It is now recognised that most Down's syndrome children are *slow* to develop and not *unable* to develop. Once they have survived the immediate physical risks with which some are born (heart defect, oesophageal atresia, anal obstruction and susceptibility to respiratory infection), they can be exposed to early developmental learning programmes such as the Portage Scheme. It has been proved that with such specialist training, most can learn the basic social skills eventually and many can enter normal school.

Children with Down's syndrome will seldom be more than below average academically. As if to compensate for this and for some physical and behavioural clumsiness, they are very often amenable, affectionate and happy. They can form close attachments to others, although their immediate peers may not find it easy.

Management at School

The Down's child may need the attention of an adult to help speed up toileting times and to be with him at meals. On the whole, ordinary school will advance his chance of gaining general independence, given sufficient time. Teachers may concentrate on special learning techniques and behaviour modification may prove useful in varying degrees. These children are the subject of teasing in school, but often they are not made unduly unhappy by it and it seldom reaches the point of physical molestation. Sporting activities may have to be geared to their limitations, but again if managed with good humour, they do not necessarily become sensitive to being 'different'.

The Role of the School Nurse

If it is known beforehand that a child with Down's syndrome is coming into the school, the school nurse may explain about Down's syndrome to his class before he arrives. Role play by puppets has been found to be a useful way of voicing apprehensions or uncomfortable antipathies through a third arty; with a little imagination, it is possible to convey a onsiderable amount of information and demonstrate appropriate ttitudes through the mouths of puppets. The nurse may want to nvolve the parents in talking to the child's teacher about his ondition, his abilities and special needs.

Nursing skills will apply to the care of the child's eyes, his vision nd, in particular, to his ears and his hearing; children with own's syndrome are prone to upper respiratory tract infections. here will be an increased risk of hearing loss that is partial and ntermittent, due to catarrhal conditions, and this needs continual nonitoring. Middle ear infections may cause permanent scarring f the ear drums or damage to the inner ear, and this will lead to oor speech.

His immunisation programme will be as normal. Obesity is a trong tendency among Down's children, and it should be ountered as far as comfortably possible. Sometimes, in discusion, parents may display feelings of guilt at having produced an nomaly that is known to be inherited—particularly if they are lder parents. It may help if the nurse assures them that a Down's aby can be born to parents of any age, race and social ackground, and that the abnormal chromosome may have come rom either the father or the mother. But, where possible, young arents should be advised to ask for genetic counselling before mbarking upon another pregnancy.

Self-help organisation: Down's Children's Association, 4 xford Street, London W1.

urther reading

arr J. (1980). *Helping Your Handicapped Child.* Harmondsworth: Penguin Books.

rawfurd M. d'A. (1980). *The Genetics of Down's Syndrome.* London: Down's Children's Association.

unton M. (1979). *Medical Help for Children with Down's Syndrome.* London: Mark & Moody Ltd.

ugh G. (1981). *Parents as Partners.* London: National Children's Bureau.

pilepsy

he child who may have some form of epileptic seizure at school is ot uncommon—there may be 100 000 of them in the United ingdom today. These seizures are demonstrations of temporary eurological disorganisation in the brain. Many children experince convulsions in infancy as the result of a fever, and many dults experience a similar fit as the result of a shock or trauma. he term 'epilepsy' is reserved for those conditions where seizures, onvulsions or fits recur—perhaps once a year or several times a ay—and where medication is usually required for their control.

The neurological disturbance can be localised in a single part o
the brain or it can be more complex and involve large and differen
parts of the brain. Epilepsy may be a condition experienced i
isolation or it may be a symptom in the syndrome of othe
disabilities such as cerebral palsy or mental retardation. Of itsel
it need not affect the physical or mental development of the chilc
But where over-protection or stigmatisation is strong and th
growth of self-esteem is stunted, then the child's personalit
development may be jeopardised. Large doses of anticonvulsan
drugs may slow down learning ability and shorten the attentio
span, but children needing this degree of control are less likely t
be in ordinary school.

There is a great deal of fear and misunderstanding about th
nature and consequences of an epileptic attack. Nurses may b
familiar with the following, but a large part of her role will be t
explain these facts to school staff and pupils because she may no
be present to deal with the attack herself. It can be beneficial t
actually enact a seizure for a group of people most likely to be i
contact with a new entrant who is a diagnosed epileptic. This ca
allay their apprehension and open up the way for questions whicl
otherwise might be embarrassing.

A partial, non-convulsive, minor fit—sometimes known as peti
mal—is much more common than is generally realised.
temporary absence of attention, flicking of eyelids, slurring o
speech or twitching of one limb will often pass unnoticed in th
classroom but may be recorded on an EEG as a neurologica
disturbance. There are children who look 'normal', but fail t
respond to the teacher's questions or appear vacant for a fev
minutes at a time; they too may be diagnosed as epileptic. Sucl
children should not be penalised for their temporary 'absence
Repeated 'absences' over a period of time can accumulate
cognitive deficit, even though they are categorised as 'mild
Seizures vary in every degree from this end of the scale to the mor
easily recognised 'classic' epileptic seizure described below.

Generalised, convulsive, tonic-clonic major fit: The child may
but not necessarily, have an aura—a sensory warning that a fit i
about to occur. He may have time to get to a place of safety or h
may fall where he stands. Any of the following can occur, but no
always all of them.

An aura
A cry
Falling, either rigid or flaccid
Loss of consciousness
Jerking of all limbs
Saliva flow or vomit from the mouth
Incontinence of urine
Clenched teeth
Apnoea and sometimes some cyanosis

'his active stage may last a few seconds or up to several minutes. : is followed by a period of flaccidity. The child may recover onsciousness and be drowsy and confused or he may appear to be .eeping. Sometimes he becomes argumentative and tries to resume is normal activities while still disorientated. In all cases he should e encouraged to rest until he has really recovered his own control.)rdinarily he can then resume his life where it was interrupted, ut sometimes the child will need to go home for the remainder of ie day. Further medical help should be sought if:

The fit is repeated.
The fit lasts more than 15 minutes.
The child does not appear to regain consciousness after 20–25 minutes.

'he Role of the Attendant

'he attendant's role is to maintain calm and prevent crowding. he should not attempt to restrain thrashing limbs, but should emove obstacles that could harm the child. As soon as practic-ble, the child should be laid on his left side in the recovery osition, his mouth and airway sloping towards the ground. The dult should not attempt to force open his teeth to gag his tongue nd she should not offer him a drink until fully recovered. She hould reassure the child verbally as soon as he can hear. The child hould *never* be left on his own.

'he Role of the School Nurse

.s soon as she knows that a child diagnosed as epileptic is coming ıto her care, the school nurse should see the parent to make erself familiar with the usual pattern and frequency of seizures, he medication regime and the accepted method of obtaining urther help (through GP, by ambulance to casualty department, y car with parent to medical centre). Thereafter her role will be ne of explanation and reassurance to all concerned.

There will be a major contribution from the school nurse as oon as the child is old enough to undertake his self-care. Some arents may feel that epilepsy is shameful and should be hidden nd they may discourage their child from discussing it. The school urse should try to persuade them that the child's self-esteem will ncrease when he can accept the condition and be in control of it as nuch as possible; in other words, when he is given the esponsibility of taking his own medicines and avoiding the factors hat might trigger an attack. She may also undertake group iscussions with the epileptic child's classmates and practise with hem the appropriate first aid they might need. Unfortunately, it is till common to find children—and adults—who think that epilepsy is 'catching'. As a result of this fear, their reaction is to stigmatise or avoid the person known to suffer from fits. If peers can be supportive and not deride or label the child, everybody will take a positive step in their own development.

The school nurse should report to the school doctor any change in the general behaviour of an epileptic child—increased drowsiness, overactivity and the frequency of fitting. She should also make herself responsible for passing on advice concerning sport—especially swimming, head-contact and climbing—and the advisability of the child participating in activities with loud noises and flashing lights, such as discos, stage lighting or television. Some children may have to avoid such stimulation. Every opportunity should be taken to maintain friendly contact with the child's mother—both school and home should be aware of the pattern of fits in each environment. A spare set of clothing kept at school may be advisable for the child who becomes incontinent during a fit.

Self-help organisation: The National Society for Epilepsy, Chalfont St Peter, Gerrards Cross, Bucks, SL9 0RJ.

Further reading
A comprehensive teaching pack has been devised by the above Society for the use of nurses and teachers.

Heart Disease

The children with heart defects who go to ordinary school are there because they have already proved the efficiency of their adaptation techniques. The 'weakly' child whose heart was damaged by infections such as rheumatic fever or acute nephritis is now seldom seen due to the effectiveness of modern antibiotics. The child who is born with a severe congenital cardiac defect is unlikely to survive the first year of life; those who do are liable to experience cyanosis, stunted growth, clubbed fingers and breathlessness, and these children will need the restricted activity and extra supervision of a special school. Children whose condition is amenable to early surgery, such as the correction of the position of the blood vessels, coarctation of the aorta, stenosis of a coronary valve or closure of a defect, may thrive thereafter and reach ordinary school. Those children born with a smaller ventricular septal defect may be encouraged to take full part in school life while retaining close medical monitoring. Spontaneous closure of such defects is not unknown, and compensatory development of smaller vessels of the heart to take over the functions of larger vessels can sometimes be expected. Children with pacemakers are also occasionally to be met in ordinary school.

The corollary of this brief outline is that most children who get to the ordinary school with some degree of heart disease are aware of their condition and their limits. In general, they can be relied upon to be self-pacing, given proper support. The child himself will know what makes him uncomfortably breathless and when to stop for rest. Since his disability is not obvious, he will be keen to keep up with his classmates and to be treated as 'normal'; he is less likely to develop the demanding or introverted attitudes of some children with more obvious handicaps. Sometimes a direct phone call to the child's physician will enable the school nurse to understand the situation and what can be expected of the child more clearly.

The Role of the School Nurse

The school nurse is a resource for school staff, parents and the child; she should be able to explain the child's condition and the management it entails. As the child grows older, his level of understanding of the mechanism of his heart may lag behind because adults 'forget' to go over the details with him. The nurse is in a good position to fill out his knowledge of terms, tests and expectations. Drawings and models from the local health education department can be of great help in this area.

One of the nurse's main functions is to be a listening ear for the child's confusions and frustrations. She should encourage him to participate to the greatest degree possible in all school activities and help him to come to terms with his limitations.

The nurse should ensure that any medication to be taken at school is stored, delivered and taken correctly.

Self-help organisation: Association for Children with Heart Disorders, 11 Milthorn Avenue, Clitheroe, Lancashire.

Muscular Dystrophy

Chidren with muscular dystrophy are often among the most cooperative, most spirited and most insightful people to be met in school. Their goodwill and good humour is remarked upon by staff and visitors alike. But it should not be counted upon. The children who know that they have the disease—and their parents—are living against a backcloth of prolonged mourning. It may be a relief from intense personal emotions to come to school, which is a place where the child can act as if all was normal for a large part of the time. Yet the staff must be ready to catch and hold him—both physically and emotionally—should he feel like falling.

Muscular dystrophy is a hereditary condition, usually transmitted by females. The term covers several rare conditions of gradually deteriorating muscle-power. The most common is the Duchenne type, which most usually affects boys. Sometimes the early symptoms of stumbling and difficulty with stairs will be apparent before the child enters school; but there are cases where the first observation of undue falling has been made when the young boy is playing football. Deterioration takes place over several years and is irreversible; the age at which a wheelchair may become necessary varies from 6 to 15 years. Children with muscular dystrophy tend to remain at school for the earlier stages especially. During this period, the effects of their increasing weakness and all its implications will grow upon them.

Diagnosis is ascertained by a small muscle biopsy. Often there is a family history of dystrophy, but as accurate medical recording is a comparatively recent phenomenon, this evidence may not be available. When diagnosis is confirmed, the mother may feel deeply guilty and may reject her child temporarily. Full realisation only comes gradually. Contact with other families who have gone through the same experience may be helpful.

Disease career: At first the child will be able to pick himself up when he falls, often by the classic technique of walking with his hands up his own straightened legs. At this stage he will feel humiliated if he is 'helped'. When the muscles of his pectoral girdle start to fail, he will be unable to raise his arms above shoulder level; teachers must understand that they should not ask him to draw on the blackboard or reach for a book. He will develop a typically 'waddling' gait, with feet spaced apart, as his pelvic girdle muscles weaken.

There are different types of treatment at this stage: he may be recommended to wear light calipers or night splints, or he may be put in plaster casts for a limited period. Physiotherapy to avoid contractures and stimulate remaining muscle power will be important. The hospital will provide spinal bracing or a spinal jacket to minimise lordosis and eventually to provide support while sitting. Assessment for all treatment and all equipment may be undertaken at one of the special units in the country over a period of several days of close observation and testing. At this stage the muscle fibres will have been replaced—either by connective tissue, leaving the child wasted and thin, or by a deposition of fat, making mobility more difficult on account of the extra weight. Diet appears to have little effect; moderate avoidance of high calorie intake is acceptable, but sometimes it may seem pointless to further restrict the child's range of choice. Foods of high fibre content should be encouraged nevertheless.

When breathing or coughing becomes difficult, it is unlikely that the ordinary school will be the best place for the child. He may be changed to a special school before it is strictly necessary so that he can settle into a new environment while he is fit. Or he may be left among his friends until home tuition seems advisable. In either case, whenever he is away, continued contact with his classmates by letter or by visit is of the greatest importance, both for the patient and for his peers. Eventually respiratory infection or myocardial failure will bring an early death. Many bereaved parents have found support and strength in being welcomed back to visit the school, and they like to hear members of staff reminisce about the 'good' times.

Management at School

A principle of the management of muscular dystrophy at school is to prepare the way for the next stage ahead of time. The effect of this is twofold.

- It relieves feelings of pending insecurity. Unvoiced anxieties about how to cope with the next stage in debilitation are made superfluous.
- Both child and parents will be relieved that provision has already been made and that needs can be met when they arise, without the further frustration of proving that they need services and waiting for them.

Examples of this principle are:

- Making sure there is provision for postural drainage in school (possibly a plastic foam wedge) before the child needs it.
- Positioning of rails in the toilet or obtaining supplies of disposable urinary bottles before they are necessary.
- Allowing a wheelchair/electric wheelchair to be in school, unused but occasionally tried out, before it is relied upon totally.

Such preparations need not be made morbidly, nor need the sympathy be laid on too thickly, but the whole school will gain confidence from the fact that they will not 'be taken unaware'—just as the family may move to a bungalow to get used to it before facing the trauma of actually having to move.

Similarly, it is good to build up interests in the child which can be pursued and not stopped when he becomes less active. Examples are listening to music, reading, collecting stamps or football stickers, playing computer games or racing radio-controlled cars. There may be several years ahead when his mind will be active and his interest keen, although his body is weak; resources for this period must be laid up beforehand. Personal relationships and friendships which will sustain him through this period are of enormous importance and these too must be fostered during his active days.

The Role of the School Nurse

The school nurse will be a link agent between parents and school, hospital and school, physiotherapist and teachers, social worker and parents, doctor and ancillary worker; she will be of great importance to the total nurture of the child. In her own field, the school nurse will have to make sure that the child's toileting arrangements are satisfactory, that his meal time care is adequate, that his skin-care and hygiene have proper supervision, and that others understand how to lift him. Support under his axillas is insufficient once his shoulder muscles weaken and his whole body can slip through such a hold. The trunk of one carrier should support his back, using her arms to cross his chest and grasp his raised wrists, while another carrier lifts his legs at the knees.

In later stages, the child will need total nursing care, and in some cases the school nurse can prepare his mother for this by teaching the principle of mouth care, bed-bathing and other procedures. As his peripheral circulation is poor, it may be advisable to demonstrate to his mother a simple massage technique of exposed limbs and areas which are at risk of pressure. The school nurse may be asked to explain medical terms and advice, such as genetic counselling and the importance of testing for carrier indications in the girls of the family.

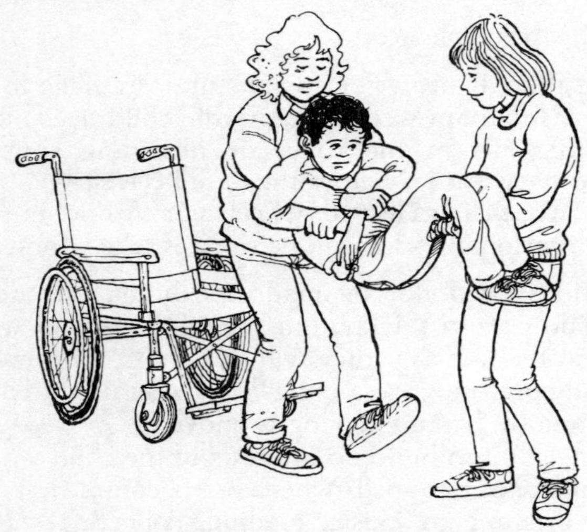

At all times the school nurse will be aware of teamwork and being alongside the family, whatever problems they have to meet.

Self-help organisation: Muscular Dystrophy Group, Nattrass House, 35 Macaulay Road, London SW4 0QP.

Further reading
Leaflets available from the above address are:
Children with Neuromuscular Disease, *Passive Stretching*, *Postural Correction*, *Breathing Exercises*, and *Exercises*.

Migraine

It is becoming increasingly acknowledged that children suffer from migraine. This condition has many factors attached to it, and there is still uncertainty about its exact cause and definition. Because many children are not skilled at localising physical symptoms and because experts themselves find definition difficult, there has been hesitation in diagnosing childhood migraine. However, if this periodic syndrome becomes established untreated, it can lead to years of misery in adult life. Early diagnosis and management can avoid such an outcome.

Young children may complain of a 'tummy-ache' and forget to mention that they cannot see very well or that the brilliant sunshine coming through the window is adding to their discomfort. Alternatively, they may complain of feeling sick, and while the adult associates it with overeating chocolate the day before, the child does not have a sense of how much he ate and will not add that his head hurts. If the school nurse has cause to believe there are repeated episodes involving nausea, vomiting, dizziness, disturbed vision, headache, slurred speech, travel sickness or anxiety—or any combination of these symptoms—she should consider suggesting investigations for migraine.

If the child tends to be a perfectionist, the trigger situation may be over-striving at school or worries concerning home life. The trigger may be one of the classical food provokers such as chocolate, cheese, or citrus fruit; or the attack may come when the child is hungry, having come to school without breakfast. Known allergies and sudden weather changes can also contribute to the situation.

The Role of the School Nurse

If the nurse can relate such episodes from her records into a pattern, she may like to ask the parents if they know of any precipitating factors with which it might coincide. Such evidence can be offered to the school doctor, who may decide to refer the child for further investigations.

A calm and accepting attitude among all staff at school will decrease the tension which underlies the 'headache'. Approved analgesics may be allowed at school; if an episode can be anticipated, a rest in the medical room might be appropriate. With suitable management, childhood migraine is frequently outgrown by young adulthood, and there is the added satisfaction that a lifelong disorder has been pre-empted.

Self-help organisation: The Migraine Trust, 45 Great Ormond Street, London WC1N 3HD.

Further reading

Understanding Migraine is available from above address.
Clifford R. E., Gawel M. (1979). *Migraine: the Facts*, Oxford: Oxford University Press.

Osteogenesis Imperfecta (Brittle Bone Disease)

This hereditary disease is rare; about 1 in 20 000 people are affected by it. However, since mental and social development are normal, children who have it are generally in ordinary school. In these cases it is the nurse who will be looked to for advice concerning the activity and management of the child.

In the past there has been some diffidence on the part of people who care for children with brittle bones as there have been unfortunate cases where children with unexplained fractures have been taken from their parents and put into the care of the local authority on the grounds of suspected non-accidental injury. General understanding of the condition is growing, however, and staff can be reassured that today no one is ever imputed with 'blame' for the fracture(s) incurred by these children. Spontaneous breakage may be the result of a quick turn or even a surprise tensing of muscles. Some children have years free from fracture and then have several within a few months, without apparent added cause. The basic congenital defect is in the collagen—the binding protein of the bones—and not in the laying down of calcium or the formation of marrow or blood.

Management at School

The child with brittle bones may be seen by his peers to be disabled more than he is. He may be small and used to considerable protection by adults. He is, in fact, 'normal' in intellect and personality, and the more he can mix in ordinary activities, the less 'sheltered' he will appear. Deliberate muscular exercise, such as swimming, will strengthen the skeletal protection of his bones, although sports which require sudden jerking or head bumping should not be encouraged. He may tire easily, and due to the laxness of his joints—including fingers—he may take longer to write than his classmates and may require more time to finish an exercise or a test paper. His desk top may need to be adjusted to his height and a tilting writing surface may help him reach to the top of the paper, but his actual performance should be expected to match that of his peers. A young girl's friends may have to be warned not to hug her too tightly, as hugging may fracture her ribs, and both girls and boys may have to be warned of the risk of skull fracture, but too much special adaptation of behaviour is inappropriate.

It is often advisable to take the inclinations of the child himself seriously—he will often know instinctively what situations are unwise for him to tackle. Similarly, the parents will have learnt through experience how much he can safely undertake in the form of exercise.

The Role of the School Nurse

The nurse may have to absorb a certain amount of anxiety from staff when the child first enters school. If he complains of pain, or if there is the least 'new' deformity in a limb, he must go to hospital for investigation. Some fractures occur without trauma—the tissues are not bruised and capillaries are not broken, so there is little of the swelling, heat or redness commonly associated with bone breakage. If there is any doubt, the limb must be relieved of weight bearing, so the nurse should have slings, a wheelchair with leg extensions, and possibly inflatable splints, in the medical room in case they should be needed. There is no specific medical treatment and the condition is not curable as yet, although as the child grows older and his muscles grow stronger and larger, he should incur fewer fractures.

Orthopaedic treatment will include the immobilisation of broken limbs, the resetting of distorted weight-bearing limbs and sometimes the insertion of intramedullary metal rods in particularly fragile bones. Dental care is particularly necessary for the child whose teeth are affected and have only a thin layer of enamel. The audiologist may detect hearing loss if the ossicles of the middle ear are damaged. The child's eyes sometimes have a bluish tinge due to thin sclerae, but vision is normal. Immunisation programmes should also be administered as normal. The school nurse can ensure that the child's diet contains sufficient vitamin D and fluoride, although added calcium is unnecessary. Extra body weight must be avoided.

Many parents have difficulty with the guilt they feel on two counts: the fact that one of them may already suffer from the disease and have passed it on to the child, and the fact that whatever their care, they cannot totally avoid bone breakages. If possible, the nurse should avoid discussions about 'how it happened'—this can only add to their feelings of ineffectiveness. Support will always be necessary. Advice on genetic counselling for the older child and his siblings may be appropriate.

Self-help organisation: Brittle Bone Society, 112 City Road, Dundee DD2 2PW.

Further reading
Leaflets from above organisation, including: *Education for Children with Brittle Bones* by J. Alston. Another useful reference is the article 'Brittle bones—a plea for sensitive handling' by G. R. Paterson in the *Journal of Community Nursing*, May 1979.

Sensory Deficits

This group of physical disorders includes a vast range of defects that require an equally wide range of special provision. However, while the specific diagnosis and treatment of each variant will be dealt with outside the school, there are general principles which are common to all these conditions and which apply to the nurse in school.

Sensory deficits include:

Visual Deficits These range from the child who needs reminding and support about his need to wear glasses in school, to the child who has just sufficient vestigial sight to enable him to remain in ordinary school. There may also be some totally blind children in an ordinary school.

Auditory Deficits These range from the young child with fluctuating catarrhal deafness or the child who has deafness only in a limited tone range, to the profoundly deaf pupil who relies on phonic-ear aids.

Tactile Deficits Insensate skin areas are usually restricted to children with paraplegia or neoplasms and these problems have been dealt with previously. Scarred areas from burns will also be without surface feeling.

Multi-Deficits Multi-deficits may follow rubella in a pregnant mother. Deaf-blind children may also have aphasia. They are usually late with social skills and they may also have some mental retardation. These unfortunate children generally have several needs that are best provided for by special schools.

Management at School

Many of the children affected by sensory defects who are in the ordinary school will be visited regularly by a peripatetic education specialist. Some may also be attached to special units or need teaching in remedial classes. Many may have the care of an ancillary worker to help with daily living skills at certain times of the day. These staff members will need steady encouragement, particularly when it becomes necessary for them to withhold their care, so that the child can learn to cope for himself. They will be giving the child a greater benefit if they allow him to develop confidence and calm in dealing with obstacles, as inevitably he will meet them throughout his life. The child will need to be given scope to discover how to ask for help, when necessary, without minding, as well as how to receive or reject the offers of help that come to him unasked. He will need to develop a particular indifference to jibes or condescension from others, while keeping his self-esteem intact. This 'socialising' can only be learnt at school.

Priorities in the management of all children with sensory defects are:

1. self-help.
2. the ability to move freely around school.
3. communication with his immediate carers, his peers and teachers.
4. knowledge of the outside world.

The world of the child with sensory defects can become very narrow and isolating: the wider world is unseen, unheard or untouched. Deliberate efforts should be made to introduce experience that expands his understanding.

The Role of the School Nurse

The school nurse will naturally be involved with screening these children, although their detailed testing will be undertaken by others. She may be asked to describe their daily coping skills at multidisciplinary assessment meetings. If she is not invited to these meetings, but has comments that she feels would be useful, she can put them in writing and offer them to the team through their nursing representative.

Her major role among children with sensory defects will be explanation. She will need to explain the effects of his condition to the child himself—underlining whatever the consultant has already told him that he did not understand or cannot recall. She will need to explain the same material as well as the meaning of unfamiliar medical terms to his parents and teachers. She can point out to all these people that apparent indifference, apathy, rudeness or disobedience on the part of the child may simply be because he does not understand why he does not understand. Information concerning the precise nature of his deficits—what pitch he cannot hear, what area or size of print he cannot see, what makes him clumsy, why he tends to 'flare up' unexpectedly—is of particular use. If she does not know herself, the school nurse is in a better position to find out from the specialist exact details of the condition, and its relevance to learning ability and school life than anyone else in school.

The child will be puzzled at his lack of interaction with his peers. His unaffected senses will tell him something is going on around him, but he will be unable to assess it for himself. The nurse's welcoming greeting and acceptance of him as he is may do much to explain the world to him, and his place in it. She may be the best person to help him understand *why* he has to wear glasses and what he should do with them when they are not on his face, so that they are kept undamaged. Many children are inexpert at cleaning their lenses, especially when they cannot see well, and a regular check should be made to make sure spectacles are clean.

Similarly, the nurse can check periodically that heavy wax is not occluding a child's hearing unnecessarily.

Advice to Teachers Concerning Those with Disadvantaged Sight

The proper source of light is of primary importance:

- it should be sufficient; normal daylight is best, therefore curtains or plants hanging in windows should be removed.
- it should not be glaring; therefore highly polished or glossy surfaces should be avoided. Speakers should not stand against a window nor the child's chair face the source of light. Glare and reflection can be as trying to those with poor sight as insufficient light.
- it should be properly directed; daylight which falls onto the child's work, without casting shadows, is the optimum.

The position of the child and also that of his equipment is important:

- the child with tunnel vision or restricted visual field from other causes must have consideration when classroom layout is designed.
- the child himself will find the most comfortable angle and level to hold his reading material—this should not be disturbed unless directions come from the specialist.
- crowded walls and blackboards are confusing and fatiguing—single clear pictures or charts will convey more meaning.
- felt-tip pens can be easier for a partially sighted child to see than pencil or pen, and dull yellow on dark green or matt black makes signs easier to distinguish.

Advice to Teachers Concerning Those with Disadvantaged Hearing

The source of sound is of primary importance:

- speech must come directly in front of the child so he can simultaneously see non-verbal indications of meaning and also learn to lip-read; music or non-articulated sound should be directed at the phonic aid or the better ear.
- confused or background noise should be avoided.

Hints Applying to Both Partially Blind and Partially Hearing Children

- Concentration with the use of the defective sense is tiring, therefore 'seeing' or 'hearing' work should be alternated with times of activity.

- Sources of light and sound should be aptly placed to avoid shadows and echoes.
- Concentration span is short, and the handicap makes the child distractable, so use the limited spans effectively.
- Group work is difficult, and group looking or hearing nearly impossible. Time should be allowed for the child with this special need to attend to the subject on his own, after the group.
- Continual feedback from the child is necessary, to make sure he has understood the matter in hand.
- Accuracy, rather than speed, should be encouraged in work.
- Method, order, regularity and consistency in all areas will increase the child's confidence in the reliability of his environment. His work, his movements, his timetable should all reflect this, so that valuable energy does not have to be spent on sorting out confusion. Any change in the classroom furniture will mean a rearrangement of his mental picture of shadows and echoes, and may take a considerable time for him to become used to.
- Adults must always remember that non-verbal communication such as hand gestures, pointing, facial expression, nuances of voice (for deaf children) or eyes (for blind children) will be lost. Instructions have to be clear and simple, often repeated, and approval/disapproval has to be conveyed directly, not merely implied.
- The child will be unable to take in environmental information without deliberate help. He will have to be taken to store-cupboards, shown the way to the toilets, helped to find the banister to the stairs (so he can stay securely out of the way of hurrying children). Sensitivity and imagination will be needed to discover those things he cannot find out for himself, while leaving him room to experiment safely.

Information from the Teacher

School nurses should encourage class teachers to report to them whenever the following difficulties are observed in the classroom. She can then give such children individual vision and hearing tests, followed by a confirmatory test two weeks later, and refer her findings to the school doctor.

- Any child who appears fatigued or bored by long periods of listening, reading aloud or writing work.
- Any child who responds badly to a request to hurry his work.
- Any child who constantly loses his place on the page or misunderstands what he is told to do.
- Any child who has difficulty copying from the blackboard—because he has not heard or cannot see properly.
- Any child who appears clumsy or awkward playing in a group; those who stumble or bump or trip often.

- Any child who complains of headaches, dizziness, nausea after close work, or who covers his eye(s) or ear(s) unusually often.
- Any child with discharging eyes or ears.

The above illustrates the close cooperation that is advisable between nurse, teacher and ancillary worker. Integration of many children who have sensory deficits is not only possible but highly satisfactory if all those who care for them interrelate well, so the children can themselves learn about the world around them to the very best of their abilities. They will teach those children who do not have the same obstacles how to make the most of what they have got.

Self-help organisations: The National Deaf Children's Society, 45 Hereford Road, London W2 5AH.
The Association for the Education and Welfare of the Visually Handicapped, Church Road, Gorleston-on-Sea, Great Yarmouth, Norfolk.
Royal National Institute for the Blind, 224 Great Portland Street, London W1N 6AA.
The National Association for Deaf-Blind and Rubella Handicapped, 311 Gray's Inn Road, London WC1X 8PT.

Further reading

Fraiberg S. (1977). *Insights from the Blind*. London: Souvenir Press.
Nolan M., Tucker I. (1981). *The Hearing-Impaired Child and the Family*. London: Souvenir Press.
Woolley M. (1984). *Being Deaf*. London: Souvenir Press.

Spina Bifida

This is a condition which has a wide range of severity. On one end of the scale is spina bifida occulta, in which part of two or three vertebrae are malformed and the dura of the spinal cord bulges through. This relatively common malformation is covered by normal fascia and skin, presents no immediate problems and may remain undiagnosed throughout life.

On the other end of the scale is severe myelomeningocele, in which the openings of the vertebrae allow both the dura and the meninges of the spinal cord to protrude and break through the exterior skin. In this multifactorial condition, few systems of the body remain unaffected.

There are many more children with spina bifida in ordinary schools than is generally recognised. In order to be able to attend, they will already have achieved an adequate level of independence. Nonetheless, the school nurse must remain aware of the potential difficulties that might arise from the child's congenital defects.

The history, aetiology, selection for treatment, continued

treatment and management of spina bifida is a lengthy discussion. Therefore, the school nurse who is involved with children who have spina bifida is urged to consult the references given below.

The school nurse should consider the following in the care of children suffering from this multifaceted condition.

- Encouragement of *self-care* of the body and *independence* is essential before the early teens. Young children with spina bifida tend to be attractive with their 'cocktail-chatter' syndrome; they are appealing in their young helplessness, and they tend to be willing to have things done for them. But as the young child grows older, it becomes more obvious that the cocktail chatter is imitative and repetitive and that it disguises a usually low IQ: his 'helplessness' becomes intolerably weighty to manage both physically and emotionally; and his acceptance can turn into passivity, apathy, low self-esteem and teenage depression. For his own sake, therefore, as well as for the sake of his parents, training for self-responsibility must start young.
- The *family dynamics* are often such that the child with spina bifida can hold power over his mother and his siblings. Research and experience have demonstrated that a father is more likely to be able to detach himself and may indeed leave the household if the power of the affected child is not brought into proper perspective. Siblings may become emotionally deprived or damaged if the handicapped child is allowed to monopolise attention and interest. Social workers do much in this area, but sometimes the school nurse can catch early hints of the direction things are going, and offer suggestions that might deflect the dangers before they develop.
- When the child spends *periods away from home*, it often highlights how emotionally involved the parents are with their handicapped child. However, such excursions bring great benefit to all concerned and with hindsight are recognised as milestones in the personality of the child. Holidays geared especially to the needs of disabled children, residential independence courses, respite care at a family unit, school journeys, and further education at residential holidays are all means of expanding the child's experience and increasing his self-confidence. Sporting events arranged for those with disabilities include athletics for the Disabled Olympics, canoeing, archery, wheelchair dancing and pony cart driving; these events usually include residential facilities.
- The controversy surrounding clumsy calipers and sticks or dependence on wheelchairs is difficult and involves physiological, psychological and social issues (Table 10.3).

These considerations are all difficult to quantify. The ultimate decision will be a compromise and it will depend on individual

Table 10.4
Spina Bifida

BODY SYSTEM	*as AFFECTED IN SPINA BIFIDA*	*MEDICAL/SURGICAL TREATMENT*
BRAIN	Can range from no effect to gross hydrocephalus; may have associated epilepsy.	Insertion of catheter drainage with valve control, e.g. Spitz Holter; CSF directed into right atrium of heart or into peritoneum.
CENTRAL NERVOUS SYSTEM: SPINE	Can range from spina bifida occulta to myelomeningocele, some lordosis, contracture of limbs and paralysis.	If other factors are favourable, surgical closure of spinal lesion in postnatal period.
EYES	Some visual field defect. Squint.	Correction of squint.
EARS	—	—
TOUCH	Can range from patches of insensate skin to total anaesthesia of lower limbs. Erratic and unreliable interpretation of peripheral stimuli	—
MUSCULAR/ SKELETAL SUPPORT	Lordosis, scoliosis, kyphosis. Hip dislocation, deformity of feet. Often strong pectoral girdle, broad shoulders, but weak pelvic girdle, requires external support. Various degrees of lower limb paralysis, requiring calipers or wheelchair.	Spinal supports of many designs. Milwaukee brace. Surgical fusion of vertebrae; insertion of steel rod. Surgical correction of distortion of hips, knees, ankles, feet, by redistribution of muscle attachment. Permanent boney prominences are to be avoided.
RESPIRATION	Becomes difficult if lordosis is severe.	As above.
DIGESTION	Slow passage of food through alimentary tract results in high rate of absorption and tendency to obesity. Flaccid bowel results in chronic constipation, see below.	Low fat, high fibre diet.

Table 10.4
Spina Bifida

NURSING MANAGEMENT in SCHOOL	*TEACHING INVOLVEMENT*
Watch for intracranial pressure: headache, vomiting, blurred vision. Watch for blockage of valve drainage system: as above, plus drowsiness, nausea, swelling near scar of lesion, reduced concentration in class.	Learning/perceptual difficulties: blunting of all responses; limited memory recall; poor hand–eye co-ordination; restricted concentration span; usually below average IQ.
—	Ensure access to all relevant areas: ramps, rails, lifts, widened doors as appropriate. Individual attendant for personal needs. Allow time out for physiotherapy etc.
Test vision annually and following complaints by child or teacher.	Provision of correct lighting. Ensure spectacles/occlusive patches are worn as prescribed.
Routine screening for hearing defects, and care of paediatric infections as for ordinary children.	Provision as necessary.
Watch for pressure erythema, sores, bruises, burns, scalds; meticulous skin hygiene. Guard against frostbite, sunburn. Oversight of feet—watch for athlete's foot, ill-fitting boots, distortion or overlapping of toes, in-growing toe nails, carpet-burns, maladjusted foot rests.	Avoid contact with warm radiators. Protect extremities and exposed areas when outdoors.
Skin-care under braces and plasters. Postoperative rehabilitative care. Nursing care of pressure areas. Watch for spontaneous fracture due to osteoporosis from lack of use.	Counteract low body image. Increase spatial perception.
Skin care of folds under rib cage.	—
Mastication of raw fruit and vegetables is sometimes uncomfortable for those with a post-aural catheter—encourage chewing for control of obesity and for balanced diet.	Avoid sweet treats or rewards, for instance on school outings or parties.

Table 10.4
Spina Bifida

BODY SYSTEM	*as AFFECTED in SPINA BIFIDA*	*MEDICAL/SURGICAL TREATMENT*
BLADDER	Sometimes congenital kidney damage Effects of neurogenic bladder include: inadequate storage→frequency of urinating inadequate emptying→ stagnation of residual inadequate sensation of distension→constant dribbling inadequate sphincter closure→constant dribbling inadequate sphincter opening→back pressure to kidneys inadequate voluntary control of sphincter→incontinence	Options available: Urinary infection can be treated long-term or episodically. Surgical urinary diversion performed via ileal loop to stoma opening on abdominal wall. Penile collecting bags. Regular catheterization.
BOWEL	Lower intestine may be inert and yet residual reflex action may remain. Anal sphincter may be patulous without sensation or control. Reduced gut motility. Descending colon/rectum may be straightened.	Medical management is usually preferred. Possible formation of colostomy.
SKIN	Heavy perspiration. Child is often unaware of temperature. Soreness or stickiness of insensate areas of skin.	Preventive measures.
REPRODUCTIVE SYSTEM	Girls: early menarche—from 8 yrs onwards; can conceive easily, due to prolapse of fornix; fertility usually unaffected Boys: reflex erection, but difficulty with ejaculation; semen may be infertile.	Counselling. Genetic advice.
HEART AND CIRCULATION	Hypertension present sometimes. Peripheral circulation of lower limbs poor. Slow healing. Anaemia due to menorrhagia.	As appropriate.

Table 10.4
Spina Bifida

NURSING MANAGEMENT in SCHOOL	*TEACHING INVOLVEMENT*
Encourage fluids to prevent infections. Meticulous skin care. Education for self-care. Regularity training, with charting/ rewards. Incontinence control.	Time to be allowed out of class for toilet training; application of own urine collecting bags; provision of privacy.
Bowel training, taking advantage of residual reflex action. Timing is crucial. Control of diet, fluids, laxatives, positioning and education concerning these. Teaching of self-administration of suppositories, enemas and cleanliness.	Time to be allowed out of class for self-care training.
Hygiene, care of clothing, effects of different washing powders, use of natural and synthetic materials. Control of body odour.	Grooming education.
Extensive counselling. Use of menstrual protection: internal tampons can be more comfortable for those in a wheelchair. Explanation of physiology of reproduction. Introduction of community youth advisory centres.	Health education, including sex education and personal relationships. Social experimentation should be tolerated in view of limited social opportunity and experience.
Healing of sores is very slow. Extremities can become too cold; legs become blue and should be raised to facilitate venous return.	There may be absences from school due to infections, hospitalisation, treatment, etc.; liaison with home and school; home tutor can correlate pupil's work. Letters and visits between class and absent child should be always encouraged.

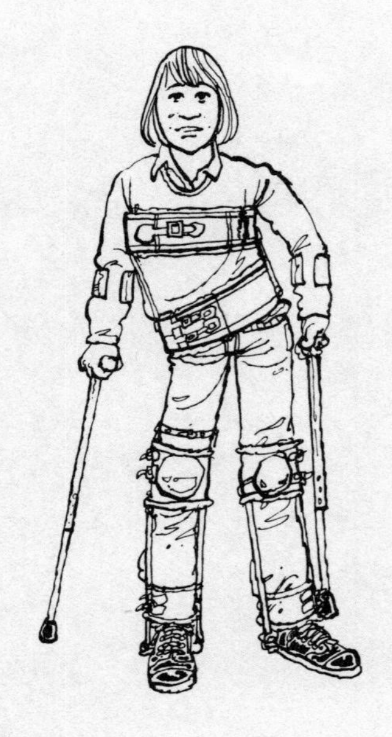

Table 10.3
Advantages and Disadvantages of Calipers and Sticks, and Wheelchairs

Calipers and Sticks	
Advantages	*Disadvantages*
'Walk tall'	Slow and clumsy
Raised eye level	Limited distance
Exercise	Public embarrassment
Easier access through all doorways	
Improved circulation	
Improved renal drainage	
Improved respiration	
Inhibits osteoporosis due to disuse	
Wheelchairs	
Advantages	*Disadvantages*
Increased speed	Lowered eye level among standing people
Self-powered mobility	Restricted public access
Increased distance	Restricted toilet access
Immediate public sympathy	Restricted employment opportunities
	Restricted physiological functions (cramped breathing, drainage, lack of stimulation to circulation and musculoskeletal system)

circumstance, including the particular child's motivation, desires and job prospects.

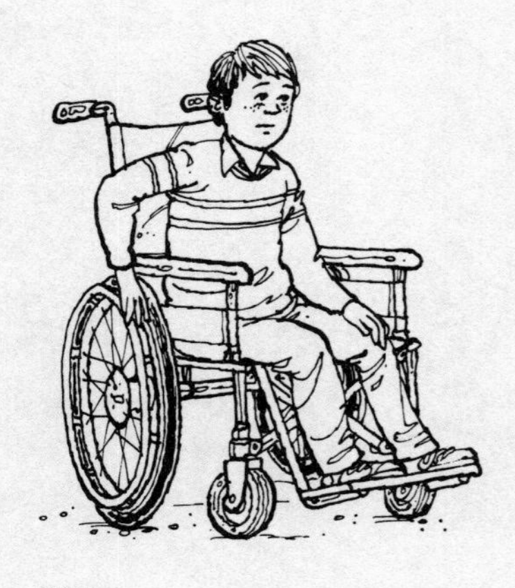

Management in School

This will involve team-work and case discussions that include everyone concerned with the child, both inside and outside school.

The Role of the School Nurse

The primary function of the school nurse in the care of the child with spina bifida is to keep everyone who is involved with the case well informed of what the others are doing (Table 10.4). She is a link agent between professionals, and she will give crucial support to parents and ancillaries. Her supervision of clinical procedures can weld the self-care education of the child at school with the parallel management of the child at home. With such a multifactorial condition, no regime can be allowed to become static. There must be continual reassessment and awareness of new opportunities or new difficulties; often it will be the school nurse—who only intermittently sees the child—who notices these changes.

In addition to general care, she will be responsible for making herself familiar with the signs of raised intracranial pressure, suspected blockage of the CSF drainage valve and of spontaneous fracture—all of which require direct transport of the child to hospital. When such episodes occur, it will be up to the school nurse to keep the atmosphere in the school calm and balanced, while time is allowed for a proper assessment. Meanwhile the child should be kept no lower than semi-prone—gravity should be taken advantage of to drain pressure from the head as much as possible.

The nurse will only obtain the confidence to reassure and advise parents, staff and child when she understands the details of the situation as far as possible. The references below should help in her self-tuition.

Self-help organisation: Association for Spina Bifida and Hydrocephalus, Tavistock House North, Tavistock Square, London WC1H 9HJ.

Further reading

Many leaflets produced by the above association; details are available upon writing. There is a large bibliography. The following are selected recommendations:

Dorner S. (1976). 'Adolescents with Spina Bifida—How They See Their Situation'; *Archives of Diseases in Childhood*. **51**:439–44.

Dorner S. (1977). 'Sexual Interest and Activity in Adolescents with Spina Bifida'; *Journal of Child Psychology and Psychiatry*. **18**:229–37.

George S. H., Hart B. (1983). *Physical Education for Handicapped Children*. London: Souvenir Press.

Reid R. (1977). *My Children, My Children*. London: BBC.

Stark G. D. (1977). *Spina Bifida: Problems and Management*. Oxford: Blackwell Scientific Publications.

Incontinence

Incontinence is only a symptom. The inability to control the emptying of the bladder or the bowel is due to a number of different causes or a combination of these. The following pages present a summary of the points that need considering when childhood incontinence is met at school. Both nurses and teachers may need reminding of the complexity of the situation. However, it is the parents who face the full brunt of the problem. A mother who is already fraught as a result of disturbed nights and

Table 10.5
The Causes, Effects and Management of Incontinence

Causes	Effects: *On Bladder*	Effects: *On Bowel*	Management
Environmental sources			
i. Lack of provision at home or at school of privacy, time, cleanliness. Some children will avoid using toilet because of absence of paper, soap, or fear of cold or of bullying.	Retention and overflow of either bladder or bowel, resulting in 'accidental' excretion, particularly with young children.		Ensure toilet arrangements are adequate. Position on toilet is important for small, young or disabled children. Provide necessary support for feet and handrails for security.
ii. Inappropriate diet, resulting in too loose stools or constipation with overflow (liquid contents of higher gut bypass obstruction—can be mistaken for diarrhoea).		Soiling of underclothes—encopresis	Nutritional advice to both child and mother. Health education in class?
iii. Difficulties with clothing: insufficient fine motor skills to cope with awkward buttons and zips, shoulder fastenings etc.	Cannot hold on long enough—wets clothing		Advise mother on more manageable clothing. Arrange for child to practise dressing and undressing.
iv. Too much to drink before bedtime.	Bed-wetting		Suck an orange in place of a night-time drink.
v. Hurried morning routine: too little time to relax and evacuate properly.		Accumulated faecal obstruction with overflow.	Suggest rearrangement of routine. Is it easier to relax on toilet after school? or following a hot drink and hot bath in evening? Child can take book or radio with him to help relaxation.
Emotional sources			
i. Reversion to baby habits and rejection/denial of own responsibility on account of: *anxiety*—concerning arrival of new baby, teacher's expectations, bullying by peers, parental discord, or bereavement. *fear*—e.g. of dark, or stairs, or toilet bowl—'I may fall down the hole.' *insecurity or jealousy*—needing extra attention from mother or father. *anger*—'getting back' at mother, thwarting her directions, damaging her mothering.	Bed-wetting at night—enuresis	Nervous 'hurried' bowel syndrome increases gut motility. May produce wind; fluid, loose stools with encopresis, e.g. before exams or times of extra tension. Constipation resulting in retention with overflow and encopresis.	Listening to, and reassurance of, both child and mother. Interruption and modification of behaviour patterns which may re-establish confidence. Teacher to be tolerant and understanding. Use of buzzer unit may restore acceptable habits of dryness. Reward small successes. Counselling of child, practise new habits regularly at school—more objective atmosphere.
ii. Over-eager or coercive toilet training may lead to phobias.	ditto	ditto	Child guidance if necessary
iii. Inability to 'open-up', usually of 'tight' personality.		ditto	ditto
iv. Sudden over-stimulation when bladder is full; nervous giggling which tightens bladder wall, reducing its elasticity, simultaneously increasing abdominal pressure. Sphincter gives way.	Stress-incontinence.		Relaxation. Pelvic floor exercises. Practise social skills.

Physical sources			
i. Infection—enteritis or cystitis.	Dribbling	Loose stools	Consult GP about medication and investigation.
ii. Overdose of laxative: over-zealous parent or efforts of 'slimmers'.		Loose stools	Advise parents; beware of anorexia.
iii. Dyschezia—habitual over-distension of large bowel desensitises the urge to evacuate. Faeces are held, become dehydrated and are hard and painful to expel.		Retention of faeces with overflow.	
iv. Spinal injury, e.g. road traffic accident, neurological impairment: motor messages to lower organs and sensory messages from lower organs are inhibited. Limit to voluntary control of sphincters. Limit to conscious sensation of fullness.	Bladder may dribble continuously due to collapse of muscle wall, extended bladder retaining urine with overflow or bladder may empty unexpectedly.	Involuntary peristaltic reflexes may remain or bowel may empty without warning or sensation.	Even insensate rectum can be 'trained' to empty regularly and appropriately. Intervention procedures, in progressive order, include: For bladder: charting of pattern, volume, timing, stream, consistency or urine. —Regular toileting at predetermined intervals. —Manual expression from fundus. —Intermittent catheterization. —Self-retaining catheterization. —Ileal loop diversion and urinary stoma. For bowel: charting of pattern of evacuation. —digital peri-anal stimulation —laxatives, enemas, wash-outs —manual evacuation. Provision of protective padding and clothing.
v. Congenital malformation of bladder or rectum: imperforate anus, sphincters too tight or too lose, fistulas or obstructed passages.	Obstruction	Obstruction	
Mental sources			
i. Delayed habit formation due to: mental retardation, inconsistency of instruction and physical arrangements, unclear directions.	Intermittent or continual wetness.	Occasional or regular defaecating into clothing.	Physical arrangements should be matched to mental comprehension. 'Reminding' should be continual if there is little memory recall. Facilities must be immediately on hand if 'holding' is difficult.
ii. Lack of comprehension of what is required.	ditto	ditto	Habits can usually be established if directions are exact, regular and reliable. Acceptable behaviour is to be rewarded; non-acceptable behaviour is to be ignored.
iii. Dysfunctions of reflex patterning.	ditto	ditto	Padding and protective pants can be provided when necessary.

burdensome laundry will also have the bother of strict training schedules; she will be sensitive about opening her home to visitors; and she will often feel unhappy about her own mothering ability.

Nonetheless, when child, parents and staff are cooperating together, the outlook can be optimistic. It may take a little while to establish, but enabling a child to gain control over his own functions and take responsibility for his own body-care is worth all the patience and sensitivity that it takes. With increased self-confidence the child's work, behaviour, and value of himself will all expand.

Nurses may have to explain sometimes that whereas some children use frequency and apparent urgency as excuses for getting out of class, and are penalised for it, those with incontinence should never be included in this category. Young children want to conform to basic social expectations, and the inability to do so is seen by them as something demeaning which needs to be hidden or denied. This is a heavy secret for them to bear.

Management at School

The child who has the problem of being wet or dirty at school has attitudes to contend with as well as practicalities. He may feel that he is a 'soiled' personality; that others feel it is all his fault and that he could help it if he tried hard enough; if his clothes smell, his peers will avoid him and thus reinforce his feelings of isolation. The child may only be able to cope with the situation by convincing himself that it is preferable to be a loner anyway, or by covering his bewilderment with an armour of unconcern. Sometimes the armour may be hardened and difficult to lift, but small changes in practical arrangements can show him there is someone on the way with him. Allowing him time in the toilet before the rush at the end of class, making sure clean underwear is unobtrusively available, or seeing that soap and towel are easy to come by, are some suggestions.

Any degree of censure towards either the mother or the child is totally inappropriate.

Role of the School Nurse

To acknowledge the problem, and make some headway towards identifying its cause.

To back up medical directions where disorders are already diagnosed. To act as link agent between school and home.

To be a confidante and health adviser for the child.

To act as link agent to further expert help where necessary.

To be a source of information to teachers, child and parents on cause of condition, likely outcome, explanation of investigations, and management.

1. Where incontinence has not been previously diagnosed, the nurse may be the first health worker to detect it or to be alerted to it by the teacher. It is a fairly common occurrence for the school nurse to be asked to deal with a child who smells. In these cases she must initially find out for herself that the complaints are soundly based and not built on prejudice. She can gain the child's confidence by being straightforward ('let's admit there's a bit of difficulty and work at it together') and it will probably be advisable for her to visit his home. Some authorities prefer home visits to be undertaken by health visitors. The child's teacher will have to be told of practical difficulties there may be at home, and help for extra clothing or washing facilities usually comes through the social services. The child himself should be encouraged to take his responsibility for his own hygiene seriously and, where necessary, he can be taught to wash his own underwear overnight.
2. Already established medical directions may include any of the measures included in Table 10.5. If the LEA has provided a special helper for the child in school, it may be up to the school nurse to support her efforts and to initiate a developmental programme for the child. Small steps in the progress towards self-care can be made practical in the school setting, even when hospital advice seems remote, and an untrained aide does not have the relevant knowledge to make suggestions. It will be up to the school nurse to familiarise herself with the possibilities and take the initiative to make them workable.
3. The school nurse is in a good position to remain alongside both child and mother.
4. The school nurse can offer privacy and clinical detachment where these are not possible in the classroom. Wherever possible, self-administration of any management programme should be encouraged, even where this involves the use of stoma appliances, catheters, enemas or emptying bags.
5. Further help is available primarily from the doctor. It will be up to the child's parents to choose between school doctor, GP, health centre or enuresis clinic. Some cases may benefit from child guidance. Some authorities advise direct links between school nurses and the staff of clinics. The school nurse may also be asked about the supply of protective pads and pants: the design and availability of these is being constantly updated, and details of the latest developments can be obtained from the Disabled Living Foundation (see below) or the local stoma therapist.
6. It will be the responsibility of the school nurse to forearm herself with as much relevant information as possible. The use of laxatives, for instance, can be for stimulating peristalsis, adding bulk, lubricating the passage of faeces, or drawing water into them—each action affects timing and administration and

should be explained to the parent/child. The difference between the static picture seen as the result of an intravenous pyelogram and the dynamic process revealed by a micturating cystogram requires explanation, as do rectal procedures and different types of equipment. It is often helpful for an individual school nurse to visit the hospital and ask to be present at some of these investigations.

If the effects of the Education Act 1981 are to progress in accordance with the recommendations of the Warnock Report (1978), many children with incontinence problems will be seen in our ordinary schools. Development of the skills required to control their own bodies, rather than to constantly submit to the attentions of 'being done to', will be greatly facilitated by the skill and patience of a committed school nurse.

Self-help organisation: The Disabled Living Foundation, 380/384 Harrow Road, London W9 2HU.

Further reading

Mandelstam D. A. (1978). *Notes on Incontinence.* London. Disabled Living Foundation.

Morgan R. (1981). *Childhood Incontinence.* London: Heinemann Medical Books Ltd.

11 Socially Related Syndromes

The word 'syndrome' is used to describe a cluster of symptoms that occur at the same time. Together they suggest that something might be wrong. The school nurse is a generalist; but she is special in that she recognises signs that are not general, and she is expert in knowing when and how to refer these to the relevant specialist. This chapter looks at several childhood conditions that may eventually need specialist attention in psychosocial therapy. They have been grouped in such a way that the school nurse can exercise her generalist skills with them.

Understanding, warmth and acceptance may be all that is necessary to lessen the worries of a disturbed child. Empathy with him and his family at this first contact will make it easier to disentangle the situation. The provisions that are then made will hopefully be more effective. Having gained the cooperation of the child and his parents, the school nurse can act as link agent—should this prove necessary—together with the school doctor. Between them, the most appropriate source of further help can be decided upon and contacted and requests can be made for specialist therapy.

By now the reader will be familiar with the overall emphasis of this book—to view the whole child within his total circumstances and to highlight principles rather than detailed aetiology and treatment of physical effects. This chapter follows this emphasis, making connections between several conditions in order to draw out the general attitude that is most helpful to the child in school. The organisation is as follows:

Group A—Misuse of a normal body function,
including obesity, anorexia nervosa and bulimia.

Group B—Abuse of child's body by others,
including non-accidental injury, sexual molestation and abuse.

Group C—Exceptional learning and its social relevance, including highly gifted and erratically gifted children

Group D—Personal dependence on external substances, including alcohol, solvents, drugs.

Group E—Personal deprivation due to external circumstances, including ethnic minorities, separation and bereavement.

Group F—The use and misuse of stress—to drive or overdrive?

Group A. Misuse of a Normal Bodily Function

Obesity is the most common disease of childhood today. If it remains uncontrolled, it becomes adult obesity with allied risks of heart disease, lung disease and diabetes and consequent adverse discrimination by insurers and employers. The cost of treatment to the nation and loss of working days through morbidity from obesity is incalculable.

Obesity is commonly described as a self-induced behavioural disorder of affluence, and as such is recognised as a socially related physical condition. In spite of the media's emphasis on slimness—acres of newsprint in girls' and women's magazines are devoted to slimming—many growing adolescents remain unconvinced of their personal need to reduce their calorie intake. What chance has the individual school nurse of enabling them to change?

It could be that calorie-counting has become counterproductive; perhaps the continual threat of nuclear catastrophe is confirming a lifestyle of instant gratification; or perhaps the incidence of anorexia nervosa and bulimia has been over-publicised. But whatever the cause or the reality, a deep dissatisfaction with life is driving some of our youngsters to overeat and be (too) full.

In school, the nurse meets with young boys and girls who are outside of their homes, who can meet together as a group, who are keen to develop self-responsibility, and who want to demonstrate that they can control their own lives. This would seem to present an optimum and objective environment for creating eating habits which can be tailored to fit each individual.

Food is Power

Food has the power to activate our lives, to fuel our physical needs and to satisfy our hunger. The rejection of food has power—power to hurt or annoy those who prepare and offer it, power to show our rejection of ourselves (as in anorexia), and power to protest against parental and adult control.

We learn very early in our lives that food has the power to satiate our craving. It does this so easily and so immediately that we often use this 'instant comforting' to compensate for other hungers. But sometimes it is simpler than this. Some people actually enjoy being fat and they are comfortable with it. And some families have a genuine ignorance about the moderate amount of food that it is necessary to eat in order to maintain good health. (Some children can function best on a diet regulated to as little as 800–1000 calories a day).

However, there are deep psychosocial factors that can result in child obesity; and it is because of them that it is often more effective to teach weight care at school rather than at home. A mother who is generous with her love may show it by being generous in her helpings; and the family may accept uncritically what she gives. A mother may feel that she ought to make up for the bits of life her disabled child misses by filling him up with extra chocolates. Some parents may say by their behaviour with food: 'if you're fat you needn't be clever or beautiful or athletic—just as we're not'.

Some of the significance food carries is shown in this poem:

The giving and the taking
the receiving or rejecting
the enticing or denying . . .
The offering and accepting
the preparing and responding
the creating and the serving
the sharing and consuming . . .
The filling or the fooling
the richness or the meanness
the joining or the spoiling
the nurture or the nuisance . . .
The loving and the breaking—
(The loving *or* the breaking??)—
What is it, this Food?

The emphasis here is on *weight-control*. In many cases, a growing child only needs to maintain his weight at the same level, while his height lengthens, to regain proper proportions. Thus the aim is long-term re-education of eating habits. Short intensive spurts of self-denial and observable weight loss are of questionable value in a developing child, and it is possible to do more emotional damage than physical good. The best short advice is often—eat what you eat already, but less of it—and priority here is given to group work as a mutual distraction, rather than the relay of detailed dietary advice.

The Nurse and Management at School

The school nurse interested in helping young people to control their weight must first obtain approval from the school doctor, the head teacher and the mothers. Agreement will also have to be sought for anyone already under the care of another professional, such as a dietician, child psychologist or hospital consultant. The nurse needs to consider:

1. how to make the programme attractive to those for whom it is intended.
2. how to identify and stimulate each individual's motivation.

3. how to ensure long-term commitment using neither coercion nor penalty.
4. how to avoid inducing anxiety in the children (or adolescents).
5. the dangers of eating psychoses.

Making the programme attractive: With the cooperation of the head teacher and class teachers, a time might be arranged in the lunch-break when a film from the health education department can be shown. Young people may attend voluntarily or as a follow-through from their regular health check-ups. Alternatively, a group of youngsters could be invited who have been selected by the subscapular skin-fold test (thus avoiding the problem of youngsters who look 'fat' being invited). Discussion after the film may lead to a plan to form a club of mutual interest within the school. Attendance must be self-elective, or the chances of success will be greatly reduced. A congenial time, place, programme and the provision of scales will have to be worked out together.

Stimulate individual motivation: This should be an early step in the formation of the self-help group. With some general discussion, each child can be helped to look at what he wants most out of life: to be in the football team, to have the latest pop album, to learn how to make a pretty face. These desires can be made into a special reward system unique to each child. 'I can have a new football shirt/the new album/a make-up set in 6 weeks when I've lost ... lbs. Each time I lose ... ounces, I will be given a counter and when I have ... counters my mother has agreed to exchange them for the money to buy the reward. *Or* every time I *don't* buy a snack, I can put my saved pocket money in a tin kept by .... and spend the total when I have lost ... pounds. (The total number of pounds to be lost will not be great by adult standards. Sometimes not putting weight on while a growth spurt is taking place is as effective as actual weight loss.)

If each child is responsible for writing out his own aims and rewards, he will feel further committed to the plan. The sheets of paper can be stored collectively in a club file and referred to as appropriate—on the understanding that they are totally confidential and can never be used against the child.

There is a hidden reward that reinforces all the more obvious material rewards: it is increased self-worth, enhanced well-being and the knowledge of being in control of one's own body. It is the reward that is of greatest value to child and nurse alike.

Ensuring a Long-term Commitment

There are two major ingredients to this:

1. *Goal-setting*: This is done using an agreed length of time, perhaps half a term, and is connected with an agreed lack of weight gain, and an agreed reward. The emphasis must always be on offering opportunities for small successes, rather than opportu-

nities for large failures. Sometimes in the initial enthusiasm, goals are set that prove to be unattainable in practice. This must be avoided as it confirms the feelings of 'I told you I'm no good; I knew I couldn't do it' which are often responsible for the obesity in the first place.

2. *Group loyalty*: There is a double advantage if the cohesion of the group is built up. Shared interests can put weight in its proper place as one of several strands of interest; and members will stick to the group for the sake of the common activity. In addition to the regular weighing and comments on diet, the leader of the group can instigate projects or activities undertaken together. For instance, if facilities are available, Five-a-Side and swimming are always popular. Team spirit and competition can be stimulated by relay-running or on-the-spot counting games such as step-jumping or push-ups. Exercise is essential for the building up of muscle tone and increasing blood circulation, but too much emphasis can be laid on the effectiveness of exercise in weight-loss. The effects of exercise are to create thirst and hunger and, except in persons with very strong wills, the end result can be disappointing. A good guiding rule is to become short of breath due to exercise once a day.

Sponsored activities will encourage togetherness and friendly competitiveness. Well-motivated weight-losers could sponsor a local charity such as a nearby children's home. 'Save a choc-bar a day, give the proceeds away!'

Other group projects are also recommended: collecting snapshots of school activities and making an album; taking responsibility for a certain flower bed in the school grounds; growing vegetables; planning a convincing request to the school tuck shop to have on offer fresh fruit, tomatoes, ready washed celery sticks or yoghurt—instead of only sweets, crisps and fizzy pop.

Common activities will increase the individual child's loyalty to the group and its long-term goals. As they like each other more, they will like themselves more and the whole scheme can remain enjoyable and light-hearted.

Being Aware of the Dangers

Nonetheless, the nurse in charge must never lose sight of the danger of obsessional preoccupation with weight-loss. She should understand the emotions which predispose to *anorexia nervosa* and *bulimia*, as she is in the position to observe those children who may be prone to them. Boys, as well as girls, can suffer from this complaint, but often the sufferers are young girls who seem to positively reject friendliness in case they re-experience previous rejection. The school nurse should notify the school doctor if she comes across any of the following, particularly if the attitude appears to be persistent in young people:

- who are withdrawn and isolated.
- who appear to be unacceptable to themselves.
- who attempt to 'earn' approval by striving for the impossible
- who cannot allow themselves a let-up or an occasional treat.
- to whom failure is unbearable or disproportionate.
- who seem fearful of responsibility and the idea of growing-up
- who find it difficult to respond to good humour or light teasin and always treat life with great intensity.

Any hint of weekend bingeing, self-induced vomiting or sel administered purging should be reported immediately to th school doctor.

Cheerful optimism in the school nurse that long-term eatin habits *are* being reconstructed helps everybody. Coaxing an gentle persuasion are more positive than pressure and induce anxiety. Below is an example of a health education project i obesity control.

Trigger situation: 14 year old girl approaches school nurse with worry concerning her weight gain.

Action: Discuss long-term re-education of eating habit Should she join group? Or would she prefer t go-it-alone?

Goal: Mutually agreed: realistic first stage, to lose 3 lb in 6 weeks and to do it on her own. *Motive* i wanting to be more attractive at discos. *Rewar* is jeans of a smaller size. *Programme* is to los 8-10 ozs a week, by substituting peeled carrot brought from home to eat instead of between meal chocolate bars, and to resist second help ings of food. Is prepared to involve immediat peers in jokes about carrots. Hopes appetite wi shrink, so feeling of satisfaction will be mor easily attained with reduced intake. Mone saved from chocolate (30p a day = £2.10 week) will be collected in box at school. Tota after six weeks = £12.60; mother has agreed t top up with 50% of saved money = £6.30. Jean are therefore attainable.

Shaping Attitudes

There are healthy attitudes about food and body weight that ca be encouraged in the school child and the adolescent and in th adult.

Attitudes in the Child and the Adolescent

- Sweets aren't treats. Treats bring increased zest to life, sweet bring stickiness and toothache. Some people call sugar 'poison ous'.

I get more pleasure from my food because I eat it slowly and enjoy the feel of it. I don't just gobble it so fast that I can't even taste it.
I'm going to relax and chat to other people when I eat. Then I can enjoy the meal more and eat less.
Trash foods are overpriced, overhandled, overprocessed and overdone.
What would I like better to spend my money on? What will last longer and not be such a waste?
It's so inefficient to eat more than I need! And to spend money on something that lasts only a few seconds!
It feels good to be in control of my appetite.
Is there a better way than instant gratification? What do they mean by 'self-empowerment'?

am in charge of what I eat and not my mother—although she rovides the meals. I can ask her for smaller helpings or show that mean it by leaving some on my plate. When my friends or my ran offer me sweets, I'll just tell them why I don't want to eat nem. Then they won't pester me. *I'm* going to decide when I at—no one is going to force-feed me.

ttitudes in the Parents

t is very desirable that a child's mother should be part of his veight control programme. However, a large proportion of obese hildren come from families where obesity is a recognised pattern nd it may be too much to expect the parents to change their fe-style for the sake of the child. Nevertheless, if positive support annot be gained, at least active antagonism can be avoided.

If the school doctor agrees, the mother can be invited to school o discuss the situation. Alternatively, the school nurse can visit he child's home. The mother will be more understanding if she is old that her child's efficiency at converting food into energy is so ood that he can eat less. It can be suggested that it would be easier or him if she gave him smaller helpings. The nurse may find that he mother has been aware of the problems and needs only slight ncouragement to join a weight-watching group herself. She may e prepared to go to domestic science classes at school or to local vening classes to learn more about food values and about how to repare less fattening food. The school nurse may have to einforce the fact that 'none' can be bad if it becomes obsessional, hat 'some' is good, but that 'more' is not necessarily better.

Whatever protestations there might be about small consumpion, family tendencies or glandular causes, the fact is that if omeone is overweight there is more input of fuel than is necessary or the output of energy. One way of explaining this to the family s to say: in a car excess fuel will spill out; in the human body it is tored for 'emergency'. Stockpiling is anti-health and overstocking vith unused fuel has to be avoided. The only answer is to *eat less*.

Mothers may find useful the following practical hints on how to help a child to eat less:

- Talking together at a family meal is good distraction—it will also increase the child's sense of being valuable to the family.
- Start each meal with a drink of water or tea. This helps to fill the actual capacity of the stomach.
- Serve the child's meal onto a plate of similar design to everyone else's but smaller. A smaller helping will look proportionately the same.
- Increase the amount of vegetables in each meal and minimise the fat.
- A high fibre menu is beneficial in many ways—for bulk and for gut motility (see below)
- Refined foods are digested quicker and the calorie uptake is greater. Therefore try to avoid white bread, white flour, white rice and white sugar. Replace all these with brown equivalents.
- Don't leave half-empty serving dishes on the table, offering themselves for second helpings. The child should have sufficient in his first helping.
- Encourage the weight-watchers to eat slowly. The first to finish can do the washing up!
- Serve fresh fruit instead of pudding. Instead of sweets, sugarless chewing gum or diabetic jelly-tablets may be acceptable.
- If between-meal snacks are a well-established habit within the family, the nurse can suggest that 'crunchy' food is nicer to eat than sticky, chewy food. Finger-size sticks of any raw vegetable—carrots, swede, Chinese lettuce, celery, cauliflower, radishes or cabbage-stalk pith—can be kept available in the refrigerator to be eaten instead of snack bars or biscuits.
- If constipation is the result of reduced calorie intake, bulk will have to be increased or a laxative taken in the form of cellulose granules. Reduced gut motility can be a feature of obesity; it tends to be sluggish as part of the syndrome. Nervous, tense people generally have high gut mobility and are seldom overweight.
- Satisfactions that are alternatives to eating should be encouraged. Time spent on nibbling can be diverted into dressmaking, carpentry, caring for pets or an aquarium, collecting stamps, mending bikes or other hobbies.
- Balance between different food groups is essential. Most mothers these days know the basic facts about nutritional balance or have ready access to them. Their difficulties often lie in applying them.

Obesity and Physical Disorder

Obesity is not an illness: it is often associated with a lack of fulfilment and is a sign of ill-advised eating. However, some disorders such as Down's syndrome, muscular dystrophy, spinal bifida and diabetes involve an increased likelihood of obesity. Among the factors which predispose to obesity in these conditions are disorganisation of the hypothalamus and consequent erratic growth hormone release, the lack of exercise, the replacement of muscle tissue by adipose tissue and the irregular uptake of adrenalin. Such considerations are rare, however, and do not generally apply to the general population of obese people. For the majority, the only sensible direction is *eat well, but eat less*. If the school nurse can play her part in establishing healthy eating patterns for children, they are likely to remember her advice for life.

Self-help organisation: Association for the Study of Obesity, Psychiatric Unit, The German Hospital, Ritson Road, Dalston, London E8 1DF.

Further reading

The Health Education Department have a great variety of leaflets on balanced nutrition suitable for mothers and children. Calorie counting charts, if considered necessary, are distributed free by commercial manufacturers of margarine, for instance.

Royal College of Physicians Report (1983). 'Obesity' (leading article). *Journal of the Royal College of Physicians*. London.

Lennon D., Fieldhouse P. (1982). *Social Nutrition*. London: Forbes Publications Ltd.

Obesity

Craddock D. (1978). *Obesity and its Management*. Edinburgh: Churchill Livingstone.

Farrow J. S. (1981). *Treat Obesity Seriously*. Edinburgh: Churchill Livingstone.

Hayter J. (1981). 'Nutritional Science applied to Nursing'; *Nursing Science in Nursing Practice* (Smith J. P., ed.). pp. 152–69. London: Butterworths.

Hopson B., Scally M. (1981). *Life Skills Teaching*. Maidenhead: McGraw-Hill.

Anorexia Nervosa and Bulimia

Self-help organisation: Anorexic Aid, The Priory Centre, 11 Priory Road, High Wycombe, Bucks.

Crisp A. H. (1974). 'Primary Anorexia Nervosa or Adolescent Weight Phobia; *The Practitioner*; **212:** 525–35.

Crisp A. H. (1980). *Anorexia Nervosa—Let Me Be*. London: Academic Press.

Dally P., Gomez J., Isaacs A. J. (1979). *Anorexia Nervosa*. London: Heinemann Medical Books.

Lambley P. (1983). *How to Survive Anorexia. A Guide to Anorexia Nervosa and Bulimarexia*. London: Frederick Muller Ltd.

Group B. Abuse of Child's Body by Others

In the last decade there has been much discussion and research centred on non-accidental injury (NAI). Nowadays each authority has its own guidelines and procedure for its own staff, and every school nurse must make herself familiar with these and abide by them. Recommendations concerning observation and reporting are made later in this section.

The subjects of sex and death have, at last, become tolerable for discussion, but the trauma surrounding sexual abuse of children and incest is still kept hidden. By its very nature such a subject begets subjective responses; angers and urges are disturbed within the hearer herself, and this makes an objective appraisal extraordinarily difficult. These situations require a special calmness, combined with openness, and the school nurse dealing with such matters will have to reflect this in both her professional and her personal attitudes. She will simultaneously have to be warm with the people involved, and cool in her assessment of the situation. If she exposes a case of suspicion too early or too easily, the roll of events may be unstoppable. These can include the horrors of police prosecution, family separation, career and social termination, and may in fact be worse than the original situation. And yet, in the words of Mary de Young (1982, p. 163):

> ... child sexual assault, whether incestuous or non-incestuous, is prevalent, harmful and transmissible. To treat it as anything less than that is to deny sound scientific evidence and to discount the experiences of countless victims. And that in itself is its own form of child abuse.

It is crucial, therefore, that assessment should be well-timed and objective.

In terms of danger to the child, there is a continuum of degree in all types of child abuse. The risks of a downward continuation along this line without intervention have to be balanced against the possibility of over-dramatising and escalating a situation which might be self-limiting and self-healing if it is not disturbed (Table 11.1).

In dealing with cases of suspected child abuse, of whatever nature, there are three basic principles to bear in mind:

1. *Listen to the child.* Over and over again in the literature of child abuse, there are descriptions of adults turning away. The child may have got his facts wrong, he may be under some onus of 'secrecy', he may be overstating the situation, but he must be listened to. When someone who he has chosen to confide in and trust appears to disbelieve his story, his sense of betrayal and confusion is multiplied. Next time, instead of risking such denigration again, he will just keep quiet.

The overall behaviour and words of the child might be

Table 11.1

Range of Child Abuse Interaction

MINIMAL LONG-TERM EFFECT ← Continuum from Minimal⟷Gross Harm → GROSS EFFECT INVOLVING ENTIRE FAMILY

Non-Accidental Injury

'Accidental' fall downstairs: may frighten parent and child and bring about improvement in behaviour and care	Neglect, exposure, malnutrition, failure to thrive—may be due to ignorance. Teaching and counselling rectify the situation.	Repeated bruising and fractures, school absences, and hospitalisation. The child may be taken into care or there may be family counselling and the child may remain in the home, with social work support.	Skull fracture Abdominal rupture Starvation Fatality

← — →

Peer or sibling experimentation	Paternal 'interest and affection'. Isolated sexual incident.	Pederasty: organised circle of 'man/boy love', usually attached to 'reverence', not violence. Long-term adverse effects need not be marked. Boys may be heterosexual when adult.	Paedophilia: long-term or episodic molestation; may be violent, may be outburst by stranger, homosexual or heterosexual.	Repeated sexual interference with child, by parent, sibling or member of extended family. Secrecy enforced, tacit knowledge of spouse. Confusion of values and relationships compounded.	Established incest, violence, repressed rage in both molester and victim, total devaluation, introversion and psychic withdrawal

Sexual Abuse

contradictory; this is hardly surprising when his experience of th world teaches him that trusted adults say one thing but d another. His suppressed anger and bewilderment may make hir aggressive and want to pick a fight one minute, but withdrawn an stubborn the next. The person he elects to test his dilemma o must remain stable and trusting towards him, whatever sense c disbelief or outrage she may feel inwardly.

2. *Do not blame the parent.* If the nurse is to be in a positio where circumstances can be opened up and the adults involved ca become receptive to counselling, she must not be judgement towards them. In the vast majority of cases, their behaviour is repetition of the parenting that they experienced during their ow childhood. Research has demonstrated repeatedly that those wh mishandle their children—whether emotionally, physically c sexually—were mishandled themselves when young or witnesse their siblings' molestation. Those who victimise children con from all backgrounds and all social and intellectual levels an usually break only under considerable stress (Table 11.2). Mo mothers know from their own experience how little extra it woul take to make them enact the same drama.

3. *Beware of relying on your own opinion.* Where there is possibility of the situation repeating itself or deteriorating furthe the school nurse should share her concern with a senior colleagu Facts (but facts only and not guesses) should be recorded and kep in a confidential place, not necessarily at school. The head teache is usually informed of suspicious circumstances, but there shoul be vigilance against labelling a child without sufficient evidenc Nowadays each authority has its own guidelines and procedure for its staff in cases of abuse. Every school nurse must make herse familiar with these and abide by them. It is useful, however, fc her also to be familiar with the guidelines laid down by the DHS These are as follows:

First Action

When there is reasonable suspicion of injury the child should b admitted to hospital, preferably under the care of a paediatri cian. Each authority should have a planned procedure an should issue guidelines about obtaining a 'place of safety order' Parents should be encouraged to accompany the child and sta with him. In an emergency the child should be taken to a accident department. Where suspicions are not strong enoug to warrant removal to hospital the worker should discuss th case with the family doctor and at least one senior colleague i the same profession, or a colleague in a different profession; th risks should be weighed and a conference called.

Table 11.2

Social Factors, Commonly found in Child Abuse

Not all these factors apply to all cases. Where several separate items apply to one child, the health worker should be aware that *risk to that child is raised.*

Parenting	*Domestic Background*	*Child Behaviour*
History of own maltreatment as a child	Non-involvement in community	Ranges from playground aggression, initiating fights, to withdrawal, playground isolation and friendlessness.
Inadequate parent models	Socially isolated	Untrusting—untrustworthy
Low bonding with child	Far from extended family	Bragging and boastful or timid, defensive, low self-esteem.
Seldom 'enjoys' child	Mobile, has not stayed long in one place	Deliberate disobedience—anger reaction in adult is seen as preferable to indifference.
Seldom plays with child	May be unemployed	Lying, petty pilfering
Unrealistic expectations of child	Low job satisfaction	Fatigued, careless
Role reversal—'I'm not good, you're b... well going to be ...'	May be sole parent	Unkempt, poor hygiene
Blaming personality, punitive	Long-term stress	Attention seeking, clinging to adults
Low self-esteem	May be overcrowded, large family	Poor homework performance
Low daily coping skills.	May be alcohol problem	Low achiever—lacking parental support.
Parent often believes the following myths: that childhood is a happy, joyful time, that parenthood is easy, satisfying task that 'My children are mine to do as I please with'.	Marital disharmony	
The parent becomes angry when he finds out that these are just myths. He takes his anger out on the child—it must be the child's fault that life is different.	Role blurring in family	
Denial of the actual problem is perpetuated.	Absence or unavailability of sexual partner	

NB High incidence in total NAI figures of parental disruption; foster, adopted, step and illegitimate children; first and last births in family.

Managerial Duties

> Senior staff should ensure that workers likely to be in contact with the problem have adequate advice and support and precise written instructions. Staff should be aware of the procedure for obtaining a place of safety order and have adequate information about the use of the law to ensure the safety of the child when the parents do not cooperate. There should be a clear statement that major decisions should only be made by individuals in the case of an emergency. The long-term management of cases of child abuse should be kept under review and the course of action to be adopted should be the responsibility of a case conference. In spite of help given by supporting services, there will be times when the child should not be returned to his parents. In these cases, departments should be aware of the dangers of receiving a child into voluntary care without a court order or the assumption by the local authority of parental rights. Before the court makes an order the magistrates will need adequate medical and social evidence and it is the responsibility of all workers to keep accurate and careful records. It may be necessary to remind parents of the availability of legal aid.

School nurses and school authorities can adapt these guidelines to meet the needs of the School Health Service.

Students of the popular press will be aware that when tragedies have occurred and they have been the subject of a court case, usually there has been a failure of communication between the services, especially the social services and the medical services. The reason for this failure has often been the understandable desire to protect the client and avoid jeopardising the delicate relationship between the worker and the parent, for it is only trust that allows the worker to cross the threshold. The other reason for silence on the part of health or social workers is the fear of litigation if suspicions are passed on and not treated with sufficient caution. However, provided that the information is passed on in good faith to the person properly entitled to receive the information—for example the school doctor or the head teacher—it is unlikely that a case for breach of privilege would succeed. A balance has to be struck between preserving the trust of children and parents and the danger to life. If the scales have to be weighed the weight should be placed on the priority of need. When the need is urgent as when a child is in danger, the fullest information should be disclosed no matter what the risk to the client relationship. There may be occasions when the price of confidentiality is too high.

If a tragedy does occur and there is a court case, it must be remembered that no one involved is above the law, and if a school nurse is involved she would be well advised to get in touch with her professional organisation. However, in essence, evidence should be confined to strictly factual and accurate information and on no account should the school nurse be led to, or volunteer, giving an opinion. Opinions are the duty of the expert witness.

Sexual Abuse

This is not the place for a treatise on sexual abuse, but a few facts will show the reality (rather than the folklore). Statistics from the British Home Office state that in 1982 there were in all slightly over 2000 convicted cases of gross indecency, unlawful intercourse with children or incest; it is estimated that one in four of all adult women experienced some degree of sexual molestation as children. Molesters may be parents, relatives, siblings, babysitters, lodgers or regular visitors who happen to be left alone with children. Some molestation can be tolerated without permanent personality damage and accepted as 'interest' or 'affection'. But most cases of molestation cause value-confusion and when sexual advance is combined with violence, it is always damaging.

What to Do?

Children who are sexually abused feel exposed and unprotected, especially when their stories are not believed and are 'covered-up'. The elaborate webs of devious secrecy spun around them bewilder the children further and they become caught up against their will by guilt and stigma.

This 'trap' is one of the most destructive aspects of childhood sexual abuse. Once people are caught in it—whether abuser or abused—the spiral trap becomes self-perpetuating. To protect what security he has left, he involves the victim and witnesses (often siblings) and his wife (stunned herself by bewilderment and inadequacy) in a tacit, suppressed and fearful cover-up of the situation. At present, the only way out of the trap is for the behaviour to be 'found out' by a well-meaning professional, who must feel obliged to stick to the law. Illegal acts have to be prosecuted in court hearings, but the life of each member of the family may be irrevocably altered.

A continuing dilemma for parents or significant adults who maltreat children is where to turn for help when they recognise they need it. If what they have done is against the law, by the very act of exposing it to a professional, they run the risk of arrest and all the appalling consequences to their families which follow. In cases of this kind, there are telephone life-lines that can offer invaluable support and advice, reaching those who need such help actually in their own homes. School nurses may well feel it wise to recommend this help to parents who need someone to talk to who can understand their situation intimately. Telephone numbers and addresses are listed below.

Telephone Lifelines for Parents:

Resource Centre on Accidents to Children, 75 Portland Place, London W1N 3AL.

Parents Anonymous—many local branches, phone numbers are available from the Citizens' Advice Bureau.

Incest Crisis Line—for abusers who want help or children who need someone to turn to: Richard and Shirley Johnson, 01 422 5100 or 01 890 4732, at 32 Newbury Close, Northolt, Middlesex UB5 4JF.

Further reading

de Young, M. (1982). *The Sexual Victimization of Children*. London: McFarland & Co.

There is also a considerable amount of research and information available from the USA.

Group C. Exceptional Needs in Learning

Children who are exceptionally gifted, or who have specific learning difficulties or dyslexia, are grouped together in sharing common socially related issues for a special reason. It used to be suggested that many of the problems involved arose out of the child's social background; this idea is no longer considered adequate. However, identification of the children and their needs as well as their management do relate to social background. Parents who are less educationally aware are usually more tolerant of educational limitations, and therefore make fewer demands for special provision for their children. Conversely, those parents who are more educationally aware have greater expectations of their children; they notice any discrepancies more, and find them more difficult to tolerate. These are the parents who also have the abilities and the opportunities to be more articulate on their children's behalf; they are more demanding of the authorities, and hence this particular group of exceptional needs in learning has come to be associated with middle-class, aspiring, socially conscious families. In fact the needs are probably spread uniformly through the school population, but fewer children in the socioeconomic groups III–V are picked up.

In addition, it has been noted that the term 'dyslexia' may be more acceptable for parents of a particular social stratum than other labels that can be attached to low-achievement levels. Parents who are less academically demanding of their children seldom use the term in their domestic circle. The ground or matrix from which exceptional needs arise is therefore less significant than the outcomes, which can affect social relationships, life-style, higher education and employment prospects.

Having a child with 'unusual' learning needs in the family produces strains, whether the needs are due to exceptional gifts or learning difficulties. The signs the child presents are surprisingly similar. They range from levels of intelligence that are high through to those that are difficult to determine due to perceptual limitations. When an adult is confronted with such a child, it is simpler for the adult to assume he is spoilt, unmanageable or stupid than to penetrate more subtle origins of behaviour. This type of negative feedback from ordinary casual encounters with others confirms the child's retreat into frustration and non-conformity. Thus children at either polarity of exceptional learning may present as:

- rude, inattentive;
- bored, apathetic—either because they cannot understand or because the interest level of the interaction is too undemanding;
- frustrated, angry, and prone to temper tantrums;
- emotionally unstable—partly due to bewilderment and partly due to uneven development of mind and feelings. This can occur at either end of the IQ scale;
- hyperactivity—also sometimes called hyperkinesis or minimal brain dysfunction. An overactive child can be seriously disruptive in the classroom and an educational problem for teachers. The behaviour pattern may be associated with a minor neurological defect, but it is also seen in children whose exceptional learning needs are unrecognised. If the child is gifted, he will be hyperactive as a result of boredom; if the child is unhappy or of low IQ, he may be hyperactive because he is unable to relate to the material offered to him.
- tending to have few friends in same age group;
- poor sleepers and/or poor feeders, perhaps due to hyperactivity;
- limited in communication—either because they cannot coordinate the skills that are necessary, or because experience has taught them to be reticent about exposing their level of verbalisation. Adults and peers alike may react with disbelief at such unexpected speech skills, and 'cut-off' their attention.
- children whose parents are confused; some parents feel their child's unpredictability is their fault, and that they must somehow make up for that failure.

The remedial or special education of these children is the province of the teacher. Any adult who cares for children with exceptional learning needs to accept him at his own level and to occupy him at the reality which he himself knows, rather than at that at which 'he ought to be'. Adults' expectations can be too high or too low. The gifted child will require space to explore and to develop fields that are outside the general curriculum where he will not be in comparison with his peers. Such 'explorers' can use their intellect and energies in ways that are non-competitive, so they do not have to become conscious that they excel or are 'superior'; indeed they may remain unaware for a long time that their difference is relative. Children with special learning difficulties and perceptual problems will need spaces in their lives where their problems do not continually confront them; consultation with the teacher and the parent will help to define an area where freedom and play-experience go together.

Emotional Maturity

It has often been remarked by psychologists and carers alike that the emotional development of the gifted child may be well below his reading age, and perhaps well below his chronological age. Praise is relatively easy for him to gain, but his emotional control and understanding are weak when he is thwarted. Conversely, the child with specific learning needs has many difficulties with which he has to learn to be patient, and he can build emotional relationships more easily with give and take on both sides. Such relationships can absorb the stresses and frustrations of remedial work, for instance in reading.

Parents, in particular, need continual support in order that they can see they are not alone in their difficulties, nor in their feelings of 'failure'. Membership of the relevant self-help organisation can bring considerable reassurance. Often they feel embarrassed with other adults in a social setting at the unusualness of their children; they need help to see that their cooperation in an attitude of warmth and acceptance totally distinct from competitiveness plays an essential part in the unfolding of their child's full potential.

The nurse in school has a significant role to play as an informed observer of all these interactions. Since she is a non-participant in the child's academic progress, she may be in a position to influence the main actors in a positive direction. Listening with sensitivity and insight to the child, teacher and parent alike, may enable her to reinforce a sense of proportion in a situation that threatens to overbalance.

As a rough guideline, it is useful for the school nurse to be familiar with the following table. It must be emphasised, however, that the intelligence quotient is *only one* of the constituents in a child's learning abilities, situation and motivation can compensate for low IQ, and they can disguise high IQ levels, according to whether they are advantageous and positive or disadvantaged and negative. In addition, where there are problems of communication unrelated to IQ—such as with immigrant children; the testing itself raises difficulties and results can be unreliable.

General Levels of Intelligence Quotient

70% of all children come in the middle IQ range	85–115
2–3% of all children come in the higher IQ range	115–145
0.5% of all children come in the gifted IQ range	145–170+

The 'Gifts' of Parents and Teachers

These pages have outlined some of the difficulties of the child who has been identified as having unusual learning problems, but a plea must also be made for the ordinary child who is not recognised as being unusual. It can be both pleasant and reassuring to be the parent or teacher of a child whose general abilities lie within the 'ordinary' 70%. It is then all too easy to either become apathetically complacent, or to pressurise a child in a direction of the adult's choosing beyond his natural limitations. Yet the early budding of a talent that is within the child but still latent may wither for lack of nurture at the right moment. All adults who are significant in a child's life need to foster the gift of discrimination in themselves—to encourage the child to revel in discovery, so each natural gift can be given a proper chance to show itself, without becoming overshadowed by the adult's own preferred gifts. The truth of the matter lies in the understanding that all children are exceptional, and they look at us in an exceptional way. The nature of our response contributes towards the making or breaking of the child.

> 'Tis you, 'tis your estranged faces that miss the many-splendoured thing.
>
> Francis Thompson

Group D. Personal Dependence on External Substances (alcohol, solvents, drugs)

There is a great deal of material on the intake of damaging stimulants by young people: Why they take them, how it affects them, what they take and so on. But how is the individual school nurse to react in her daily round? The simplistic answer is that she should encourage her children to discover sources of developing strength within themselves, so that they do not resort to short-cuts which help them escape from their physical or mental uneasiness by giving them a 'high' which is artificial. How to put this answer into practice is more difficult.

A good starting point is with the child before he turns to the substance he thinks will change his life. As a result of many complex historical, philosophical and social trends, many adults today are reluctant to provide a model for young children to follow; the right to 'do your own thing' seems to be primary.

A common consequence is that children are left to make their own choices and to stand by their own decisions too early in life—before they have acquired the experience or wisdom to judge properly. Their self-esteem is weak, although it may be covered by a 'bold front'. The effect upon young children can be to leave them without an anchor to hold on to, and to deny them even a safe harbour within which to drift safely. Therefore, because so many of them have little guidance about where they should be heading:

- They have a sense of being left to fend for themselves.
- They feel underchallenged and become bored.

- They compare themselves with inflated public images (such as presented on TV) and feel inadequate.
- They have difficulty in moving from the viewpoint of the self which normally encompasses the very young child, to understand the point of view of others. The little boy kicking his way through the daffodils only sees that they are in his way. He learns to walk around them by hearing other people expressing their delight in them as he grows older.
- In addition, the child of today has more time and more money than his predecessors, with less supervision of either. He can 'please himself', and often does not have the experience of the pleasure he would get if others were pleased with him.

In these circumstances, many growing children turn for adventure and excitement to areas they know are interestingly illicit. Often experimentation with smoking cigarettes or cannabis, with sniffing solvents or with drinking alcohol begins as a group activity. A few boys and girls will egg each other on, giggling and secretive. Until recently, this type of behaviour was not viewed with any great alarm by experts. However, in the last two or three years, the development of the next stage—in which individuals find that the stimulus or the escape provided by the substance is irresistible and they increasingly practise it on their own—has assumed 'epidemic' proportions. It is becoming commonplace to see in the press that children have died while under the influence of stimulants. Furthermore, research findings are highlighting brain damage as well as kidney and liver damage, and some studies indicate the involvement of the heart and lungs as well.

Treatment for addicts of drugs, solvents or alcohol is expensive and traumatic; therefore, it is important to prevent addiction by understanding and anticipating the situations which produce the 'craving for out'. Prevention is particularly crucial now that the availability of tobacco, alcohol, cannabis, heroin and solvents of all types is so easy. The market for all these substances is at present so flooded that prices are within reach of most teenagers. This greatly increased availability is not only increasing the total volume consumed, it also allows for:

- earlier experimentation, at an even less mature age.
- longer-term usage.
- greater accumulated toxicity in any one individual.
- more widespread and overt practice which thereby becomes more acceptable amongst the peer group.

A transitory adventure, therefore, has all the back-up necessary to turn it into a full-scale addiction.

Disabled people depend on other people, but at least in those cases there is the possibility of give and take between persons. Children who are dependent upon inanimate external substances for support go through a depersonalising experience.

In her routine surveillance, the nurse can look out for those children whose attitude towards others seems to change over a period of time: the individual who unexpectedly becomes a loner—introverted and disinterested in what is going on around him—or who seems to be developing a sly, devious and secretive attitude to life, may be at risk of addiction. Physical signs and symptoms are difficult to isolate, since they are shared by many other childhood conditions. But those most common are: any gradual attitudinal change; becoming listless, sullen, non-cooperative; scabs around nose or mouth; puffy face; droopy eyes; rhinitis; conjunctivitis; sore lips; spots on arm from infecting needles; and coughing.

If the school nurse observes a combination of these symptoms in a child who is emotionally labile and irritable, she should make an opportunity to talk to him on his own. He may well insist that she should 'leave him be'; she may get the impression that he is solely caught up in his own problems, his own viewpoint, and that he is convinced that he has not 'got what it takes' to keep up with his peers' or his parents' expectations. She may feel she has got nowhere, but if this assessment is reinforced by his mother's complaints that she 'can't reach him', the nurse should think about referring him to the school doctor or youth advisory clinic.

If it seems that there is a risk of substance abuse, but there is no evidence, a programme of health education for the whole group may be useful. The local health education department can provide visual aids and information, but this should be backed up by discussion of values, human goals and particularly of why certain attitudes and behaviours are prized by society. The support of standards that have a binding effect and form a safety net for individual action may need to be verbalised and explained. Teenagers sometimes say that 'discussions at school are boring because they don't go deep enough'; the youngster who finds no satisfaction in ordinary living without external drug stimulation has not been helped 'to go deep enough'. His sense of self-worth may remain shallow until he finds that his environment is supportive and that he can safely give and receive trust and affection.

Once again, this is not an 'us' and 'them' situation. Most of us drink coffee and enjoy alcohol; we all need escape or excitement from time to time. Just because some of our adolescents have missed out the skill of moderation due to inadequate role modelling, they should not be penalised. They need to be helped then to learn how control brings self-respect and good feelings.

Group E. Personal Deprivation due to External Circumstances

Immigrant children	Children in care
Cultural disadvantage	Parental disruption

Living with life-threat in family | Bereaved children

At first sight this may seem a strange grouping. Why should immigrant children, for instance, be considered at the same time as children with divorced parents? All the children in the above list of circumstances have one thing in common; they have been parted from their familiar, traditional, nurturing situation and will all, to a lesser or greater extent, be affected by the syndrome known as *loss*. Children being cared for in other people's homes will have lost their family surroundings; children who have moved from other countries or other parts of the same country will have lost their familiar social culture; children of separated parents will have lost the constant presence of a familiar adult; other children may have lost a favourite grandparent or friend or beloved pet; and those with a life-threatening disease near them will have lost their security of the future. They will all be bewildered and feel they are not in any sort of control; they will not know where to turn.

Adults can objectify and rationalise; they can know that the next move is in a certain direction and that eventually their security will return. Children cannot identify how things will get better. Often behaviour such as clinging or giggling is an attempt to get attention and reassurance from adults who are supposed to be understanding and who, the children hope, will protect them from additional loss. Other children will put adults to the test, pretending that they do not care and that they are inviolate, in an effort to prove to themselves that they can manage on their own.

Such children are not asking for cosseting or soft treatment. From adults they need steady support, positive understanding and a readiness to listen if the opportunity arises. They are not 'naughty', although sometimes they may be confused about what is expected of them and how much society will tolerate. These children need consistency in the demonstration of what is acceptable behaviour and what is not, by those older people to whom they look for guidance.

The stages of loss or deprivation can include *anger and protest*—'it's not fair'; *guilt*—'it must have been my fault, I was too much for them'; *detachment*, when it hurts too much—'it's got nothing to do with me'; and eventually a *reorganisation of reality* as they see it. With adult support and maturity on the child's part, this reconstruction of his life may be more firmly based and embody a truer understanding of how things are than the stage at which change occurred. But without such help, he may end up with a greater degree of fantasy and shallower comprehension of life than before.

Education for Disadvantage, Vulnerability

Our society and our educational system are geared always towards achievement and success. The underlying philosophy is 'try hard and you'll get on'. But there are large areas of living that are not

oncerned with achievement. They usually involve disappoint-
nent, loss of opportunity or ability or health, and separation from hose things, events and people that had been relied upon for ecurity and meaning. Unemployment, home removal, disease, ereavement, change of any kind can require capacities that are arely hinted at in our present schools. The education for these najor components of life is still neglected in twentieth century ritain. In her contact with individual children going through such eriods of loss, the school nurse has considerable opportunities to elp children look at, accept and grow through such experience.

Positive Attitudes

What are the positive attitudes that the school nurse can endorse n her dealings with *children who are at a loss*? First, she will make ure the child understands that the demonstration of grief, anger, ewilderment and protest is allowable—that it is 'OK to let go'. Her support will remain constant; the child will be safe. Gradually she will encourage him

- to tolerate more uncertainty.
- to see that letting go of familiar, comfortable circumstances brings a chance to spread out and explore new solutions.
- to believe that coping with change increases confidence in the future, and can develop more understanding of how others feel.
- to know that if his value-system is broken open, he himself can be part of its reconstruction, and take part in the design of the new start.

Immigrant Children or Ethnic Minorities

Specific areas will have specific emphases. Many of these children will have to learn to live in a dual world: the family expectation may be that they retain their traditional language, clothes, diet, and life-style, while at school powerful figures will urge them to conform to the majority. Young children may have difficulty with the common verbal language, but even once this is mastered the adaptation to non-verbal cues and unfamiliar social expectations may take years. Physical problems should be noticed and referred for treatment: for example, rickets due to a traditional diet short in vitamin D and calcium; eye disorders and constipation due to circumstances that are different from those of the homeland; and lack of immunity to the British common cold. Home visits by the school nurse will help her understand the background from which the child attempts to cope with school. Insights can then be shared with other school staff and, in particular, with the head teacher and school doctor. The ethics of social and religious minorities should always be respected; fasting is part of the Hindu way of life, as travelling is part of the Romany way of life. Their effects should be taken into consideration.

Culturally Disadvantaged Children

How to react to unexpected responses, unrecognised cues and unacknowledged challenges will also be the problems of culturally disadvantaged children. Their disadvantage may be social, geographical or racial, but the effects may be similar. Sometimes less obvious discrimination can have more hurtful effects: for instance, the Welsh new boy does not have the visibly different family cell in which to retreat at the end of the day, unlike the Pakistani girl. Observation of behaviour and peer relationships is important in all these cases, and an attempt should be made to understand what it must be like to be where they are rather than where you think they should be.

Substitute Families

Children who are fostered or in care may not want it known among their schoolmates. They may sometimes feel they do not really belong anywhere, that adults are all playing an elaborate game of 'let's pretend' and that it is all bluff. Even happily adopted children will fantasise sometimes that the parents and background they do not know are so much better than that which they do know. Caring adults at all levels must help such children to develop trust and self-reliance; they will need special resources to manage the inevitable taunts with good humour.

Life-threatening Circumstances

Children who live among circumstances that are life-threatening to themselves or those they love will also be feeling insecure. The universal question 'why me?' has no easy answer. Other questions should, with the agreement of the parents, be dealt with honestly, but at the level at which they are asked. The truth, as it relates to the child's view of reality at that time, is always the best foundation for difficult answers—but not necessarily the whole truth and not necessarily the whole time. Sometimes there will be a need for 'normality' and a relaxation of intense emotions.

Further reading

Anthony S. (1973). *The Discovery of Death in Childhood and After*. Harmondsworth: Penguin Education.

Bowlby J. (1980). 'How Will Mummy Breathe and Who Will Feed Her?'; *New Society*; **51**(909):493–4.

Foster S. A. (1980). Death and Bereavement—What Shall We Tell the Children?; *Journal of the Institute of Health Education*; 18(2):41–4.

Gordon A. K., Klass D. (1979). *The Need to Know: How to Teach Children about Death*. Englewood Cliffs NJ: Prentice-Hall.

Varma V. P. ed. (1973). *Stresses in Children*. London: University of London Press.

White J. (1980). *Parents in Pain*. Leicester: Inter-Varsity Press.

Wolff S. (1973). *Children under Stress*. Harmondsworth: Penguin.

Group F. Stress—Drive or Overdrive?

Stress is part and parcel of healthy living. Its immediate effect is to produce energy—physical, mental, emotional or 'nervous'—to meet new and demanding situations. The creation of tension can be exciting and bring thrills and 'kicks' to life: the risk, speed, danger of fairground rides are highly pleasurable to many children and young people; the tension and power in organised sport and the stylised violence in spectator fights are enjoyable to vast numbers of the population. On the aesthetic level, it is the tension in the strings of a violin that make it possible for it to be played in tune. But when the strings of an instrument are overwound, they cannot harmonise and eventually they snap; when a car is overdriven, it burns out.

In keeping with the whole of this book, the intention in these last pages is to look generally at overstress. These general themes in fact reflect principles outlined at the beginning, and the holistic approach advocated throughout now appears to be drawing to a close in a full circle. Tension, risk and stress can develop abilities to cope with situations that are changing and challenging. They are parts of life that alert and motivate us to put more into life and to get more out of it. They are factors that need not necessarily be avoided; they can be put up with and they can be made use of. On the other hand, we can be overused, overstretched and overdriven (Fig. 11.1).

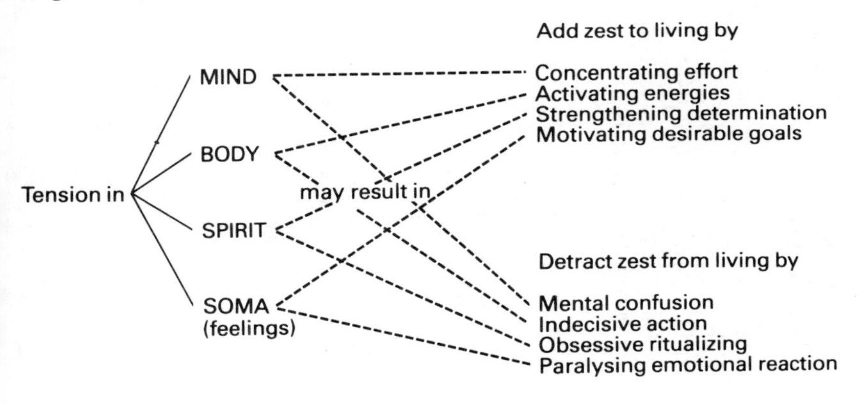

Fig. 11.1. The possibilities of stress.

Children are at risk of being overdriven because they have too little experience with which to judge how to proportion their energies. If anxious parents are driving them, ambitious teachers are urging them, and environmental factors are draining them, they have little to fall back upon when their personal resources of energy are depleted. There is an increasing recognition of the major importance school life holds in the emotional welfare of all children; it is during the school years that people can learn about

Table 11.3
Patterns of Increased Stress

Effects of tension to which individual may adapt positively ----------→	Effects of pressure to which individual may adapt negatively ----------→	Effects of anxiety to which individual may react with disturbed behaviour --→	Specific effects of overbalance into phobia or neuroses
Creativity Achievement Self-preservation Heroic acts to save others Perseverance Determination Ambition Extraverted anger channelled into drive	Introverted anger which becomes: Sullenness Withdrawal Fear Worry Shyness 'There's no point in trying' Depression Examination avoidance	Display of protest against ordinary societal limits/moral code, e.g. Lying Bullying Cheating Stealing Vandalism Truanting Fighting Disobedience Refusal to fit into family pattern	School phobia Separation complex Agoraphobia Obsessional rituals Irrational fears of e.g. trains knives germs dogs opposite sex
	MANAGEMENT	MANAGEMENT	MANAGEMENT
	Unconditional acceptance Non-judgemental listening Peer counselling Group work Social contacts allowing for gradual achievement and approval	Through counselling with social worker or child guidance clinic Through police and courts, child care and established penal system	By child psychiatrist and psychiatric social worker

hange and about how to exercise adequate adaptation skills to neet and even enjoy it.

Some stressors (stress-producing situations) are *in-built* to the uman situation and can cause anxiety from infancy. These are the nes that have to do with basic survival; gradually, as the child rows older he learns to control or not fear these fundamental hreats. Other stressors are *acquired* through experiences that are nitially painful. When these experiences are repeated later in life, hey confirm the pain, thereby increasing anxiety, rather than ringing control and reassurance and thereby diminishing anxiety. Yet other stressors may be *imposed* by the environment or confirmed by factors within it (Tables 11.3 and 11.4).

Table 11.4
Stressors—Sources of Anxiety

nborn	Acquired through personal experience	Imposed or confirmed by environmental factors
Abandonment	Separation	Anxious parent, especially mother
ight of blood	Situations of unsupported insecurity	Mobility of family
Darkness	Any sudden or prolonged pain	Chronic illness or disability
Pain	Emotional coldness in parents	Poor housing
Animal's teeth	Inconsistency of expectation from parents, teachers	Unemployment of parents
Crowds	Unattainable expectation of self	Marital disharmony at home
Strangers	Allegorical symbols—spiders, snakes, furry animals	Media influence—how 'things should be'
Heights	Strong, unreasonable disapproval	Constant change-over of teachers
Death	Bullying	Unrealistic expectations of parents, teachers
	Sexual confusion	Challenge which remains unresolved of siblings or peers

Most of the above stressors are met by most children at some time in their lives and adequately assimilated into their general experience. It is when a combination of pressures becomes too much that worry, anger or frustration can take a hold and anxiety sets in. Then the child is likely to feel that he is on his own, that no one understands and that he is so different he might be going mad. It is at this stage, when he is outwardly aggressive, emotionally inconsistent, behaviourably unreliable or just withdrawn and unreachable, that the school nurse should consult with her colleagues concerning further referral for specialist help.

The Role of the School Nurse

At the risk of repetition, it must be emphasised that the role of the school nurse in all these conditions remains that of the generalist. She will need to identify the child and his needs, listen to him, refer him when necessary and offer him support. She will continue to act as link agent between all the people involved with the child; it will be important for her to see the teaching staff and the parents' view of the child's behaviour and to keep them adequately and fittingly informed.

The techniques of counselling, desensitisation, saturation or aversion therapy, operant conditioning, family therapy or psychoanalysis are for the specialists. The nurse in school may be asked to cooperate with them by reporting her observations either directly or on paper, or possibly by setting up support groups for peer counselling. Parents will need to be kept in contact; their feelings of inadequacy, failure and possibly guilt will have been aroused. If these are expressed in aggressiveness or defensiveness their parenting of their other children may be affected. The focus of attention will be on the disturbed child, but it is the parents who may be both the source of pressure and the source of help, and it may be they who feel most neglected and misunderstood. The school nurse may be able to find openings for extending friendliness to them and confidence in their own insights. This in itself can sustain and strengthen their coping powers by reducing their feelings of guilt and failure. Such negative emotions cannot be judged as 'true' or not—their effect is destructive if it is not redirected.

When dealing with anxiety of any sort in either child or teacher, it is wise to develop interpersonal techniques that avoid confrontation. 'If' and 'perhaps' and 'may' and 'could' are easier versions of 'it is' or 'it does' or 'you must' or 'you didn't'. Simple ways around a possible offence such as 'I think it might have been'—rather than 'I know it was'—will often leave the way open for a change of direction.

Similarly, although it might come into the teacher's remit to discipline a child with disturbed behaviour, it is not the role of the school nurse to treat a child as 'naughty'. She has the advantage of being lateral and non-authoritarian, and can afford to be non-judgemental and accepting, on the other hand, that the teacher in charge of a large class has to keep it under control. There are various recognised methods of treating school phobia, for instance, but it may only be *because* an anxious child can find a safe haven for a few minutes when his difficulties are too much for him that he is able to come to school at all. Prescribed treatment must always be upheld, but feelings on the part of the child that he is disapproved of should not be confirmed by the nurse. Useful phrases for the listener which immediately convey an open-ended acceptance by her of what the child is trying to express, and also lead him to verbalise it further, are those which reflect his own words without introducing different ideas. Examples are 'I think you said you feel angry . . ?' '. . . is that how it is?' '. . . so your Dad said . . .' 'how did you feel? . . .'

Alleviation of Stress

Tension is useful, but when it builds up and threatens to overbalance spirited behaviour into antisocial behaviour, it needs to be depressurised. Cooling down the pressure cooker before it explodes is a useful analogy:

1. Turn off the source of heat. Identify and cut off the original tension, or reduce or deflect it.
2. Cool the vessel. Let off steam safely: allow the child to do the same. Take the heat out of the situation by running cool water over it: for example, introduce measured deep breathing, relaxation techniques, yoga; build skills in arts and crafts; exercise such as swimming or bicycling. When and where possible, we need to learn to laugh at ourselves.
3. Open it up and look at the contents. What are the ingredients that were 'cooking'? Which are cooked, nutritious and worth using? Which are harmed, burnt out and should be put away?

Connections and bonds that have become stuck or too tight should be relaxed and loosened. Allegiances and priorities can be reassessed and reasserted. Relationships which have broken down can be reformed and renewed. And the school nurse can be the upholder—it is too much to ask her to be the mould!—but not the stirrer.

Conclusion

It is not coincidental that the last few pages have in fact covered all the major themes of this present book. Stress is common to all of us; it can be used to add zest to our living and add thrust to our special efforts. But it is also one of the many 'good' ingredients of life that can be overused and misdirected. At the present time, minds, bodies, spirits and feelings are becoming overbalanced and some are in danger of becoming overstimulated, oversensitised, oversexed and overindulged.

It is a prime function of the nurse who works in school to take her part in keeping a balance. Balancing her own roles, balancing the needs of the child, and making sure that the balance between caring and schooling is kept in sight, is basic to the nurture of health. The nurse is in a position where the interlocking interests of the child can meet and be brought together to move smoothly as a whole. What a position to be in, and what a privilege to be able to make use of it!

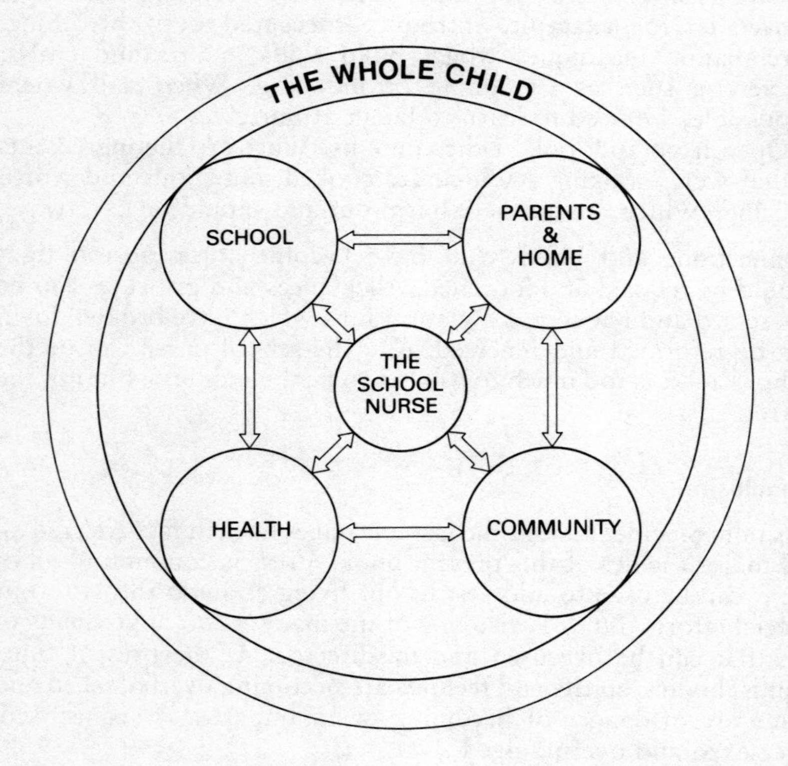
THE WHOLE CHILD
SCHOOL
PARENTS & HOME
THE SCHOOL NURSE
HEALTH
COMMUNITY

Appendix 1

DEVELOPMENT OF BASIC EDUCATIONAL PROVISION

1698 Society for Promotion of Christian Knowledge (SPCK).
1780 British and Foreign Schools Society.
National Society for Promoting the Education of the Poor (now the Society for Promoting Religious Education).
1800–1833 Monitorial system of teaching using older pupils as teachers.
1833–1893 Government grants given to above societies.
Education Committee of the Privy Council. Secretary Sir James Kay-Shuttleworth. Establishment of Teacher Training College at Battersea (now Polytechnic of the South Bank). Abolition of monitorial system.
Establishment of Schools Inspectorate.
1870 Foster Education Act. Establishment of School Boards to provide Elementary Education. School attendance not compulsory.
1890 Scotland—Education of Blind and Deaf Children Acts.
1893 England and Wales—required Authorities to provide elementary education from 5–16 years for blind children, and 7–16 years for deaf children.
1899 Establishment of National Board of Education.

1902–1944

1902 Balfour Education Act. Creation of Local Education Authorities (LEAs).
Statutory elementary education up to 14 years.
Permissive powers only for education other than elementary.
Grants could be given to religious and endowed schools in return for school scholarship places.
1918 Fisher Education Act—compulsory leaving age raised to 14 years.
Provisions for medical treatment and inspection.
1921 Education Act—consolidated provisions for Special Education, 4 categories.
1924 Haddow Committee. Enquiry into curriculum up to age of 15

years for schools other than Grammar Schools. Recommendations: primary school education up to 11 years, followed by either Senior or Modern School up to 15 years.

1939 Spens Committee—recommended secondary education to develop along three lines: Grammar, Modern and Technical.

1944 Butler Education Act—the establishment of Primary, Secondary and Further Education. Discretionary provision of Nursery Education for children from 2 years. Duty to make appropriate provision for all children over 5 years and to ascertain their needs.

1953 Education Act (Miscellaneous Provisions)—ascertainment of special educational needs to include all types of disability. Certification of defective children abolished. Compulsory school attendance for all between 5 and 16 years, and the right to remain beyond 16 years established. Use of Independent schools approved where appropriate, but subject to the Minister of State's veto.

1964–1965 Isle of Wight Study into education, health and behaviour.

1964 Education Act—powers granted to vary age limits within schools.

1970 Transfer of responsibility for education of all mentally handicapped children of school age from health to education authorities.

1974 Warnock Committee of Enquiry into Special Educational needs.

1976 Education Act—Secretary of State given power to compel reorganisation of Secondary Schools on Comprehensive lines. Section 10 of the act required LEAs to arrange for special education of all handicapped pupils to be given in county or voluntary schools, except where this was impractical, incompatible with efficient instruction, or unreasonably expensive; but this was not implemented, as the Secretary of State decided to await the findings of the Warnock Committee.

1978 Warnock Committee Report on Special Educational Needs.

1981 Education Act.

DEVELOPMENT OF CHILD HEALTH PROVISION

1769–1781 Infant Dispensary and Home Visiting Scheme. London. George Armstrong.

1816–1867 Early sporadic home visiting schemes offering care and health advice.

1833 Guys Hospital established a separate children's ward. Factory Act. Inspectorate set up to judge fitness of children for employment

1852 Hospital for Sick Children, Great Ormond Street, established by Charles West.

1867 All children under 16 years of age to be examined before employment. Manchester and Salford Ladies Sanitary Reform Association established home visiting service.

1884 Medical Officers of Schools Association founded; first Dental Surgeon appointed to Poor Law School.

1890 First fulltime School Medical Officer appointed.

1891 First certificated course of Health Visitors, North Buckinghamshire Technical Committee.

892 Metropolitan and National Nursing Association, founder William Rathbone, supplied a School Nurse to a London school in Chancery Lane.
899 St Helens Infant Milk Depot.
901 Huddersfield Infant Visiting Service.

902–1944

902 Continued proliferation of Maternity and Infant Welfare Clinics until 1916.
904 Interdepartmental Committee on Physical Deterioration.
905 London County Council School Medical Service established.
906 School Meals Act.
907 Education (Administrative Provisions) Act—School Medical Service established under Sir George Newman.
First School Dental Clinic, Cambridge.
Notification of Births Act—permissive powers to require registration of births within 36 hours. 1915 Extension Act gave compulsory powers.
908 Health Visitor/School Nurse Certificate established by Royal Sanitary Institute.
First School Clinic, Bradford.
909 First wholetime School Dentist appointed.
911 National Health Insurance Act. Provided General Practitioner services to some compulsorily insured workers, but not to their dependants.
1918 Maternity and Child Welfare Act—Local Authorities given powers to set up antenatal and postnatal clinics, with medical and health visitor staffing.
Fisher Education Act—established medical treatment and inspection in all elementary schools, and medical inspection in secondary schools.
1919 Health Visitor Training Regulations established by the Board of Education and the Ministry of Health.
Ministry of Health assumed overall control of the School Medical Service.
Sir George Newman appointed Chief Medical Officer of Health at the Board of Education. School Nurse provision varied. Many Local Authorities used Health Visitors by arrangement with Medical Officers of Health. London maintained a special scheme of training and employment for School Nurses. Register of Sick Children's Nurses established.
1925 Health Visiting established as Ministry of Health responsibility.
1928 All newly appointed health visitors required to hold HV Certificate.
British Paediatric Association formed.
Association of Sick Children's Hospital Nurses formed.
1929 Poor Law Authorities abolished.
Local Government Act empowered County and County Borough Councils to develop Municipal Hospitals alongside existing Voluntary Hospitals.
1934 Free milk in schools scheme.

1939–1945 Second World War

1940 National Milk Scheme for children and expectant mothers.
1942 Welfare Foods Scheme—orange juice, cod liver oil, milk.
Voluntary and Municipal Hospitals brought together as nationally organised hospital service with a regional administra-tion.
Beveridge Report—recommended system of social security for al
1944 Butler Education Act—School Medical Service renamed Schoo Health Service.
Provision of school meals and free milk became a Local Authorit responsibility for children between the ages of 2–15.
Free provision of medical services for minor ailments, chil guidance, orthopaedics, audiometry, speech therapy, orthoptic remedial exercises, chiropody, ENT clinics, services for asthma enuresis, and rheumatism; free dental services and treatment.
1945 School Health Services Regulations—nurses appointed as schoo nurses required to hold HV Certificate.
Eleven categories of Special Educational provision specified.

Post-war

1946 National Health Act—establishment of comprehensive healt service.
Tripartite service: 1. General Practitioner Service; 2. Hospital an Specialist Service; 3. Local Health Authority Services, includin specific provision for a health visiting service. Each service wa separately administered.
1956 Jameson Enquiry into Health Visiting.
1962 Health Visiting and Social Work (Training) Act—Council fo Training and Education of Health Visitors assumed responsibility
1967 Advisory Committee on Child Welfare Centres. Sir Wilfre Sheldon.
1973 National Health Service Reorganisation Act.
Integration of Local Authority Health Services with Hospita Services, including transfer of responsibility for the School Healt Service to Area Health Authorities, accountable to the Minister o State for Health and Social Services.
1970–1984 Setting up of Health Centres, development of Primary Health Care teamwork, Health Visitors attached to GP practice with consequent increase of nurses employed in schools an accountable to health visitors. First School Nurse Training Courses established by CETHV for State Registered Nurses o Registered Sick Children's Nurses.
1976 Court Committee Report on Child Health Services.
1979 Nurses, Midwives and Health Visitors Act. Established a Central Council, with National Boards responsible for training, further training, and professional discipline, and maintenance of a single professional register.
1982–1983 Reorganisation of NHS—abolished Area Health Author-ities, leaving Districts and Regions.

DEVELOPMENT OF SPECIAL EDUCATIONAL PROVISION

Deaf Children

1760–1783 Asylum for the Support and Education of the Deaf, established by Thomas Braidwood at Edinburgh.
1783 Transferred to London under Thomas Braidwood's nephew.
1809 Asylum for the support of Deaf and Dumb Children of the Poor, established at Margate.
1812 Braidwood School for the Deaf, Birmingham.
1820 Schools for the Deaf at Liverpool, Manchester, Exeter, Doncaster. In all these schools education was extremely limited and subordinated to training with a view to teaching pupils to earn a living.
1847 First School for the Deaf in Wales at Aberystwyth. Donaldson's Hospital (now school) Edinburgh.
1874–1888 First classes for the deaf at elementary schools.
1886 Royal Commission on the Blind and the Deaf, reported in 1889.
1890 Scotland Act—Education of Blind and Deaf Children, and 1983 England and Wales Education (Deaf Children) Act. These acts required Education Authorities to provide suitable elementary education in their own or other schools; for blind children from 5–15 years, and for deaf children from 7–15 years. It provided rights of inspection and made training recommendations.
1902 Education Act—School Board functions relating to Special Education transferred to Local Education Authorities for Elementary Education, and to County and County Borough Councils for Secondary Education.
1906 London County Council Provision for Partially Deaf Children. Bristol Special School for Partially Deaf Children.
1907 Establishment of Joint Examining Board for Teachers of the Deaf.
1909 Training diploma recognised. Teachers to obtain this qualification within two years of appointment.
1921 Education Act—statutory framework of Special Education set out. Four categories of handicap were recognised. The Act gave discretionary powers to provide secondary education after 16 years.
1934 Committee of Enquiry into Problems related to Children with Defective Hearing.
1937 Education (Deaf Children) Act—made education compulsory from 5 years.
1944 Education Act—imposed a duty upon LEAs to ascertain needs and make educational provision for all children from 5 years.
1945 Handicapped pupils and School Health Services Regulations specified 11 categories of Special Educational Provision, including deaf and partially hearing children.
1946 Mary Hare Grammar School for the Deaf was established for boys and girls.
1953 Education (Miscellaneous Provisions) Act—allowed LEAs to use independent schools where appropriate, but gave the Minister of State for Education the power of veto. (For further provisions see Basic Educational Provision.)
1955–1980 Increasing provision for partially hearing children and expansion of peripatetic teaching, especially between 2–5 years.

1978 Warnock Committee Report on Special Educational Needs.
1981 Education Act.

Blind Children

1791 School of Instruction for the Indigent Blind, established by Henr Dannett at Liverpool.
1793 Asylum for the Industrious Blind, Edinburgh and Bristol.
1800 School for the Indigent Blind, London.
1805 School for the Indigent Blind, Norwich.
In all these schools education was extremely limited, an subordinated to training with a view to teaching pupils to earn living.
1835 Yorkshire School for the Blind. First school which set out t educate; taught reading, writing, arithmetic and vocationa training.
1838 Formation of London Society for teaching the blind to read.
1847 Henshaw's Blind Asylum, Manchester, and General Institute fo the Blind, Birmingham. Offered educational subjects and voca tional training.
1866 Worcester College for Blind Sons of Gentlemen. Offered secon dary education.
1875 London School Board established a class for the blind in a elementary school; this was followed by 23 others. The childre were taught by blind teachers.
1886 Royal Commission on the Blind and the Deaf. Reported 1889.
1890 Education Act (Scotland).
1893 Education Act (England and Wales).
These Acts required Education Authorities to provide suitabl elementary education in their own or other schools—for blind children from 5–15 years, and for deaf children from 7–15 years. It also provided rights of inspection and made training recommendations. It also made per capita grants.
1902 Education Act—School Board functions relating to special education transferred to Local Education Authorities (LEAs) for elementary education, and secondary education powers transferred to County and County Borough Councils. Note—up to this time there was no nursery education provision; or provision for partially sighted children; nor was there any secondary education available for girls.
1907 London County Council made the first provision for partially sighted children who were taught reading and writing from large type instead of braille in the Authority's blind schools.
1908 London County Council set up a special higher class for myopic children, and by 1913 there were 13 classes, combining some teaching in ordinary classes.
1918 Nursery education for blind children was initiated by the Royal National Institute for the Blind, who opened residential Sunshine Homes.
1921 Chorley Wood College Secondary School for Girls was founded by the Royal National Institute.
1921 Education Act—statutory framework of Special Education set

out. Four categories of handicap were recognised. The Act gave discretionary powers to provide secondary education after 16 years.

1934 Committee of enquiry into problems relating to children with partial sight. Recommended education in ordinary schools as far as possible.

1944 Education Act—imposed a duty upon LEAs to ascertain special educational needs and to make educational provision for all children from 5 years.

1945 Handicapped Pupils and School Health Service Regulations specified 11 categories of Special Educational Provision, Blind and Partially Sighted being two of them.

1953 Education Act (Miscellaneous Provisions)—included the use of independent schools subject to the Minister's power of veto.

1978 Warnock Committee Report on Special Educational Needs.

1981 Education Act.

Physically Handicapped Children

1851 Cripples Home and Industrial School for Girls, Marylebone.

1865 Crippled Boys Home, Kensington.
Both mainly Industrial Training with rudimentary education.

1870 Education Act (Forster)—established School Boards to provide elementary education, but did not specifically include disabled children.

1892 London School Board opened a school for physically and mentally defective children. Mainly occupational activity. By 1896 there were 24 special schools in London.

1900 Six other boards established schools.

1902 Education Act—School Board functions relating to Special Education transferred to Local Education Authorities for elementary education and secondary education powers to County and County Borough Councils.

1903 Chailey Heritage Craft Schools and Hospital founded.

1905 Swinton House School of Recovery founded in Manchester.

1907 London Council Open Air School, Plumstead.

1908 Lord Mayor Treloar Cripples School, Alton.

1910 Manchester LEA opened a residential school for epileptics.

1918 Education (Physically Defective and Epileptic) Act—permissive powers to provide education now became a duty to provide.

1921 Education Act—set out framework of Special Educational Provision, recognising four categories of handicap and giving discretionary powers to provide secondary education after 16 years.

1941 Education After the War (Green Paper)—suggested that provision for many delicate and physically defective children should be in ordinary schools and the discussions which followed led to the agreement that there should be a single framework of provision in which special education would have a distinctive place.

1944 Education Act—imposed a duty on LEAs to ascertain special educational needs and make educational provision for all children from 5 years.

1945 Handicapped Pupils and School Health Service Regulations specified 11 categories of Special Educational Provision.

College of Speech Therapists was formed and a single training recognised. This led to an expansion of provision for all speech defective children.

1946 National Health Service Act empowered regional hospital boards and teaching hospitals to arrange for the education of children in hospital in collaboration with local education authorities.

1947 First State Grammar School for Speech Defectives.

1974 Warnock Committee of Enquiry into Special Educational Needs reported 1978.

1976 Court Committee Report on Child Health Services.

1981 Education Act.

Mentally Handicapped Children

1847 Asylum for Idiots, Highgate.

1870 Asylums at Caterham, Leavesden and Hampstead.

1852–1863 Institutions for the education of imbeciles established at Dundee and Edinburgh.

1862 Lunacy Act (Scotland)—authorised training and care licences for charitable institutions.

1889 Royal Commission distinguished between Feebleminded, Imbeciles and Idiots. Idiots were not considered to be educable.

1892 Leicester School Board established a special class for feebleminded pupils.

London School Board established schools for the Physically and Mentally Handicapped, and by 1986 there were 24 such special schools.

1896 National Association for Promoting the Welfare of the Feebleminded. Research Report. Dr Francis Warner. Recommended special provision for feebleminded children.

1896 Education Department Committee on Defective and Epileptic Children envisaged that an appointed school medical officer would decide whether a child should receive education either in ordinary or special school, or should be certified as ineducable and therefore admitted to an asylum.

1899 Education Act—gave discretionary powers to provide education for Defective and Epileptic Children and increased the grants available.

1902 Education Act—School Board functions relating to Special Education transferred to Local Education Authorities for elementary education, and secondary education powers transferred to County and County Borough Councils.

1914 Education Act (Mentally Defective and Epileptic)—discretionary powers to provide education for these categories now became a duty to provide.

1913 Mental Deficiency Act—required LEAs to ascertain and provide for educable children aged 7–16 years. Ascertainment in the hands of School Medical Officers. Those deemed ineducable became the responsibility of local mental deficiency committees. A similar act was passed for Scotland.

1921 Education Act—established the framework of Special Educational Provision, recognising four categories of handicap and giving discretionary powers to provide secondary education after 16 years.

924 Wood Committee of Enquiry into Mental Deficiency Provisions. Recommended abolition of certification system and development of special education according to needs; special schools to be considered as a helpful variation of normal school, not separate from mainstream education. Reported 1929.

941 Education After the War (Green Paper)—recommended that Maladjustment should be recognised as an additional category of handicap and that special schools should be established for this group. LEAs should cooperate in the joint use of special schools in the interests of effective and efficient provision.

944 Education Act—imposed a duty on LEAs to ascertain special educational needs and make educational provision for all children from 5 years. Certification of defective children was abolished, and children not considered capable of being educated in school were reported to the local authority for the purposes of the Mental Deficiency Act 1913. For these children local authorities began to set up Junior Training Centres for those who were not sent to institutions.

1945 School Health Services Regulations specified 11 categories of handicap, Educationally Subnormal being one of these categories.

1946 National Health Service Act empowered regional hospital boards and teaching hospitals to arrange for the teaching of children in hospital in collaboration with LEAs.

1953 Education Act (Miscellaneous Provisions)—included the use of independent schools subject to the Minister's power of veto.

1959 Mental Health Act—parents allowed extra time in which to appeal against school placement, and were given the right to call for a review after one year. Parents to be given more information regarding their child's future education; cooperation between LEAs and health authorities enforced by statute. Despite these measures exclusion of children from entitlement to education continued to give rise to increasing criticism.

1970 Education (Handicapped Children) Act—transferred responsibility for the education of all mentally handicapped children of school age from health authorities to the education service, together with the staff and buildings of junior training centres. The act also applied to children in hospitals, private homes and institutions. For the purposes of education, they were regarded as severely mentally subnormal, and special educational provision was made for them as of right.

1973 Guidance given to authorities on the training requirements of teachers for mentally handicapped pupils.

1976 Court Report on Child Health Services.

1977 Recognition of independent schools was discontinued.

1978 Warnock Committee Report on Special Educational Needs.

1981 Education Act—Special Educational Provision.

The Maladjusted

1893 University College, London—a psychological laboratory began to study the problems of difficult children.
British Child Study Association founded.

1913 London County Council appointed a school psychologist (Cyril

Burt) to examine individual cases. The concept of Child Guidance began to emerge on multiprofessional lines; this was mainly due to work done in America.

1927 Child Guidance Council was formed; this later merged into the National Association for Mental Health. Clinics were started by hospitals and voluntary bodies.

1928–1939 Child Guidance Clinics were developed as part of the School Medical Services. By 1939 there were 22 clinics wholly or party maintained by authorities.

1932 First school for Nervous and Difficult Children opened in Leicester.

1937 First fulltime Child Guidance Clinic established by Glasgow LEA.

1941 Education After the War (Green Paper)—recommended that Maladjustment should be recognised as an additional category of handicap, and that special schools should be established for this group. LEAs should cooperate in the joint use of special schools in the interests of effective and efficient provision.

1944 Education Act—acceptance of single framework for ordinary and special education. LEAs' duty to ascertain needs and make educational provision for all children from 5 years.

1945 Education (Scotland) Act—empowered Authorities to establish Child Guidance Clinics and services. Recognised the educational importance of early discovery and treatment of any disability.

1953 Education Act (Miscellaneous Provisions)—included the use of independent schools subject to the Minister's power of veto.

1945 Handicapped Pupils and School Health Service Regulations specified Maladjustment as one of the 11 categories of handicap.

1946 Government guidelines on treatment. The needs of maladjusted children should be assessed by an educational psychologist or a child guidance team; educational needs could be met by specialist teaching, attendance at another school or transfer to a boarding special school.

1945–1955 Expansion of services followed. Training courses for teachers and housestaff were commenced.

1950 Underwood Committee of Enquiry. Reported 1955. Recommended a comprehensive child guidance service available to every LEA, involving a school psychological service, school health service, and child guidance clinics working in close cooperation. Regional hospital boards and authorities should plan their provision in close cooperation. In the main authorities would provide premises, employ psychologists and psychiatric social workers, and hospitals would provide psychiatrists. There was a shortage of trained professional staff, and this continued for many years.

1964–1965 Isle of Wight Study on Education, Health and Behaviour.

1968 Summerfield Working Party recommended doubling the number of psychologists and expanded arrangements for training.

1974 Health Service Reorganisation recommended child guidance based on a multiprofessional team.

1976 Court Committee on Child Health Services reported.

1977 Recognition of independent schools discontinued.

1978 Warnock Committee Report on Special Education Needs.

Appendix 2

Court Report comparison with *Warnock Report*

Court Report outline of recommendations relating to Education and Health.

Parents

(a) The service to parents should provide professional advice and support that is readily available. The objectives of teachers, health visitors and doctors must be to increase both parents' understanding of their child's needs and their skills.

(b) Parents should have the right of access to the District Handicap Team and others concerned with the treatment of their child.

(c) The view of parents and pupils should at all times be taken into consideration by health care staff working in schools

Under 5s

(a) A basic programme of health surveillance should be offered to all children. Health surveillance to be shared between the doctor and the health visitor. A minimum programme would consist of health interviews at birth, 6 weeks, 7–8 months, 18 months, $2\frac{1}{2}$–3 years, $4\frac{1}{2}$–5 years immediately prior to school entry. Arrangements should be made for additional surveillance for vulnerable or disadvantaged children.

(b) The point at which the education service should make a contribution to assessment and management of the child cannot be related solely to chronological age. The legal limitation upon the power of the LEAs to make this contribution before the age of 2 years should be removed.

Coordination

(a) Joint Consultative Committees were established at the time of the NHS Reorganisation Act. They provide a forum for consultation planning and collaboration between health, education and social services. Joint Consultative Committees should consider how best to ensure that particular needs of children receive due attention, and in this context they may wish to appoint a subcommittee of members of health and local authorities to advise on the development of services for children.

(b) A District Handicap Team should be established in each district and should be regarded as a common service to which health, education and social service authorities contribute professional staff through whom they have direct access to the team.

Training

(a) Doctors and nurses providing health services in school should be required to have undertaken appropriate training.

(b) The CETHV (Council for the Training and Education of Health Visitors) or any educational body who may carry this responsibility in future should be asked to design a course leading to a Higher Certificate in Educational Nursing.

Warnock outline of recommendations relating to Health Provision

Parents

(a) One person should be designated as Named Person to provide a point of contact for the parents of every child who has been discovered to have a disability, or who is showing signs of having special needs. In most cases the health visitor should be the Named Person in the early years.

(b) The Named Person for the parents of a child recorded as requiring special educational provision shall be someone designated by the multiprofessional team which assessed the child's needs.

(c) A variety of forms of short-term relief should be available for parents of children with severe disabilities who are living at home.

Under 5s

(a) A basic programme of health surveillance should be provided for all children as recommended in the Court Report.

(b) The education of children with disabilities or significant difficulties must start as early as possible without any minimum age limit.

Coordination

(a) Joint Consultative Committees should be asked to advise health, education and social services authorities as soon as possible on the health and social services which will be needed by and can be provided for ordinary schools to meet the needs of children with disabilities or significant difficulties, and what priority their provision should be accorded.

(b) The Specialist in Community Medicine (Child Health) or a designated medical colleague should be responsible for coordinating contributions to Form SE2 by members of the health service.

(c) Where a District Handicap Team exists, it should be augmented as necessary so that it can carry out among its functions the assessment of children with special educational needs.

Training

(a) The practice of giving health visitors additional training to enable them to add an understanding of young children with special needs to their existing knowledge of child development and make the best possible use of developmental information acquired during the course of their visits should be extended.

(b) More opportunities for post-qualification training on an inter-professional basis should be made available to members of the health service concerned with children with disabilities or significant difficulties.

Information

(a) Health records should be maintained for every pupil, and relevant information made available to the education services.

(b) Consideration should be given to devising a standard health record for all children aged 0–15 years, in relation to both preventive and therapeutic health care, and the possibility and advantages of such a standardised health record being computer managed should be studied.

Practice and Provision

(a) Every school should have a doctor and nurse nominated as their school doctor and school nurse who are suitably qualified and knowledgeable about educational medicine and nursing, and have sufficient time to get to know their schools and meet the teachers regularly.

(b) The medical examination in relation to entry to school should be made statutory, and subsequent examinations of individual children should be carried out only when required.

(c) The school doctor should hold regular clinics in secondary schools for adolescent pupils to attend, if they choose, independently and in confidence.

(d) Every pupil should have an annual health care interview with the school nurse, and all 13 year old children should have an interview with the school doctor.

(e) Primary schools should have as a rule not less than 6 hours of nurse time per week, and secondary schools not less than 15 hours and preferably 30 hours (fulltime).

(f) Every special school should have a nominated school doctor who should be a consultant community paediatrician.

(g) A sufficient number of nurses should be appointed to each special school to meet its individual requirements, taking account both of the actual nursing involved and the need for nurses to participate in assessment and counselling.

(h) Regional Handicap Teams should be established in paediatric departments of university teaching hospitals under the direction of a consultant paediatrician with special experience of handicapped children.

Information

(a) Form 10(B)M or its equivalent (which provides an adequate summary by school doctors and nurses of health findings for educational use) should be used properly and consistently for all school children.

(b) The results of professional consultations and sensitive information given about a child's background or family relationships should be recorded in a separate confidential folder. The folder should be kept in the school and access to it should be controlled by the head teacher.

Practice and Provision

(a) There should be a named school doctor and a named school nurse for every school.

(b) Health authorities should make adequate resources available to promote effective child health services in ordinary and special schools.

(c) Local education and health authorities should provide the necessary space, equipment, nursing and secretarial help to enable medical specialists to hold their clinics in special schools.

(d) Health authorities should ensure that continuity of treatment and, where necessary, nursing support is provided for children during the school holidays.

(e) Arrangements should be made for all children to receive education as soon as possible after their admission to hospital.

(f) Wherever possible educational premises should be specially provided in hospital for children unable to leave hospital to attend school.

(g) Regional multiprofessional centres for children with relatively rare and particularly complex difficulties should be established in university hospitals, and the education services should be fully represented in these centres.

(h) Local education authorities in consultation with health authorities should satisfy themselves that adequate health care is available before placing children in non-maintained special schools or independent schools catering wholly or mainly for handicapped pupils.

(i) Health services comparable to those provided in special schools should be made available to establishments of further and higher education which cater for students with more severe disabilities or disorders.

(j) The Specialist in Community Medicine (Child Health) should ensure that arrangements are made for the transfer of responsibility for the medical surveillance of a young person with special needs to an appropriate branch of the health service when that young person leaves school or goes on to further education.

General Bibliography

Anderson C.A. *et al.* (1979). *Who Knows Best in Health Education?* Nottingham: Leverhulme Health Education Project.
Anderson D. C., ed. (1979). *Health Education in Practice*. London: Croom Helm.
Argyle M. (1969). *Social Interaction*. London: Tavistock Publications.
Baly M. E. (1983). *Professional Responsibility*. Edinburgh: Churchill Livingstone.
Berne E. (1964). *The Games People Play*. Harmondsworth: Penguin Books
Black D. (1979). 'The Paradox of Medical Care'; *Journal of the Royal College of Physicians*; 13:57–65.
Blaxter M. (1981). *The Health of the Children. A Review of Research on the Place of Health in Cycles of Disadvantage*. London: Heinemann Educational Books.
Brechin A., Liddiard P. (1981). *Look at it This Way: New Perspectives in Rehabilitation*. Sevenoaks: O.U. Press, Hodder and Stoughton.
Brierley J. (1976). *The Growing Brain*. Slough: NFER.
Burnett M. (1983). *Children Today, a factfile about children in GB and N. Ireland*. London: National Children's Home.
Button L. (1974). *Developmental Group Worth with Adolescents*. London: University of London Press.
Carr J. (1981). *Helping your Handicapped Child*. Harmondsworth: Penguin Books.
Croydon DHA (1979–80). *School Nurse Pilot Health Surveillance Project*. Croydon: DHA.
Dalzell-Ward A. (1974). *A Textbook of Health Education*. London: Tavistock Publications.
Davis A., Horobin G. (1977). *Medical Encounters: The Experience of Illness and Treatment*. London: Croom Helm.
Davies B. M. (1977). *Community Health and Social Services*. London: Hodder and Stoughton.
Davies J. (1979). 'Death of a Child'; *World Medicine*; Nov. 17:23–7.
Department of Education and Science (1978). *Social Educational Needs: the Warnock Report*. London: HMSO.

de Young M. (1982). *The Sexual Victimization of Children*. London: McFarland.
Dingwall R., McIntosh J., eds. (1978). *Readings in the Sociology of Nursing*. Edinburgh: Churchill Livingstone.
Dion K. K., Berscheid E. (1974). 'Physical Attractiveness and Peer Perception among Children'; *Sociometry*; **37**:1–12.
Dollery C. (1978). *The End of an Age of Optimism*. London: Nuffield Provincial Hospitals Trust.
Dorner S. (1975). 'The Relationship of Physical Handicap to Stress in Families with an Adolescent with Spina Bifida'; *Developmental Medicine and Child Neurology*; **17**:765–76.
Dorner S. (1976). 'Adolescents with Spina Bifida—how they see their situation'; *Archives of Diseases in Childhood*; **51**:439–44.
Dorner S. (1977). 'Sexual Interest and Activity in Adolescents with Spina Bifida'; *Journal of Child Psychology and Psychiatry*; **18**:229–37.
Draper P. *et al.* (1980). 'Three Types of Health Education'; *British Medical Journal*; 16 Aug.:493–5.
Durning (1951). 'An Enquiry into Over-dependence in Children'; *British Journal of Educational Psychology*; **21**:67–70.
Eisenberg N. (1980). 'What makes Persons "Patients" and Patients "Well"?'; *American Journal of Medicine*; **69**:277–86.
Erikson E. (1977). *Childhood and Society*. St Albans: Triad/Paladin.
Fieldhouse P. (1980). 'Health Interests of Children'; *Health Visitor*; **53**:313–5.
Finnie N. R. (1974). *Handling the Young Cerebral Palsied Child At Home*. London: William Heinemann Medical Books.
Flynn P. A. R. (1980). *Holistic Health*. New York: Brady.
Foott S., ed. (1976). *The Disabled School Child and Kitchen Sense*. London: William Heinemann Medical Books.
Freeman H. E., Levine S., Reeder L. G. (1972). *Handbook of Medical Sociology*. Englewood Cliffs NJ: Prentice-Hall.
Freire P. (1976). *Education: The Practice of Freedom*. London: Writers and Readers Publishing Cooperative.
Gagne R. M. (1977). *The Conditions of Learning*. New York: Holt, Rinehart, Winston.
George S., Hart B. (1983). *Physical Education for Handicapped Children*. London: Souvenir Press (Educational and Academic).
Gillis L. (1980). *Human Behaviour in Illness*. London: Faber.
Goffman E. (1957). *The Presentation of Self in Everyday Life*. Harmondsworth: Penguin.
Goffman E. (1967). *Interaction Ritual*. Harmondsworth: Penguin Books.
Goffman E. (1970). *Strategic Interaction*. Harmondsworth: Penguin Books.
Gordon J. S. (1981). 'Holistic Medicine: Toward a New Medical Model'; *Journal of Clinical Psychiatry*; **42**:3, 114–20.
Gordon N., McKinley I., eds. (1980). *Helping Clumsy Children*. Edinburgh: Churchill Livingstone.
Greengross W. (1976). *Entitled to Love*. London: National Marriage Guidance Council.
Gyulay J. E. (1978). *The Dying Child*. Maidenhead: McGraw-Hill.
Hadley B. J. (1974). 'Current Concepts of Wellness and Illness: their Relevance for Nursing'; *Image*; **6**:21.

Harris T. A. (1973). *I'm OK, You're OK*. London: Pan Books.
Hegarty S., Pocklington K., Lucas D. (1981). *Educating Pupils with Special Needs in the Ordinary School*. Windsor: NFER–Nelson.
Henderson V. (1978). *Principles and Practices of Nursing*, 6th edn. London: Macmillan.
Herzlich C., trans. Graham D. (1973). *Health and Illness, A Social Psychological Analysis*. London: Academic Press.
Holt J. (1964). *How Children Fail*. New York: Pitman.
Holt J. (1967). *How Children Learn*. London: Pitman.
Hopson B. H., Scally M. (1981). *Lifeskills Teaching*. Maidenhead: McGraw-Hill.
Illich I. (1975). *Medical Nemesis*. London: Calder and Boyars.
Igoe J., ed. (1980). *The School Nurse Achievement Program*. Denver: University of Colorado Health Sciences Center.
Jay P. (1979). *Help Yourselves*. London: Ian Henry.
Jones A., Owen F. (1984). *Handle with Care*. Henley-on-Thames: Gresham.
Kleinman A., ed. (1981). *The Relevance of Social Science for Medicine*. Holland: D. Reidel Publishing.
Levin S. L. (1977). *Self-Care*. London: Croom Helm.
Lipowski Z. P. (1969). 'Psychosocial Aspects of Disease'; *Annals of Internal Medicine*; **71**:1197–206.
Lonsdale G. (1978). 'Family Life with a Handicapped Child'; *Child: Care Health and Development*; **4**:99–120.
McConkey R., McCormack B. (1983). *Breaking Barriers, Educating People about Disability*. London: Souvenir Press.
MacFarlane J. (1982). 'Nursing Values and Nursing Action'; *Nursing Times Occasional Paper*; **78**(28):109–12.
McFarlane J., Casteldine G. (1982). *The Practice of Nursing Using the Nursing Process*. St Louis: C. V. Mosby.
Menzies I. E. P. (1970). *The Functioning of Social Systems as a Defence against Anxiety*. London: Tavistock Institute of Human Relations.
Nash W. E. (1984). 'The Perceptions of 14–15 Year-olds Concerning Stress'; In *Health Education and Youth* (Campbell G., ed) pp. 123–40. London: The Falmer Press.
Office of Health Economics (1975). *Am I Kranken Doctor? The Health Care Dilemma*. London: HMSO.
O'Moore M. (1980). 'Social Acceptance of the Physically Handicapped Child in the Ordinary School'; *Child: Care, Health and Development*; **6**:317–37.
Painter F. (1984). *Living with a Gifted Child*. London: Souvenir Press.
Parker G. (1983). Helping incontinent disabled children. *University of York Social Policy Research Unit, Working Paper* DHSS 136 3/83 GP.
Parker G. (1984). 'Incontinence Services for the Disabled Child'; *Health Visitor*; **57**,**2**:44–5; **3**:86–88.
Philip M., Duckworth D. (1982). *Children with Disabilities and Their Families, A Review of Research*. London: NFER-Nelson.
Pugh G., Russell P. (1979). *Shared Care; support services for families with handicapped children*. London: National Childrens Bureau.
Reid R. (1977). *My Children, My Children*. London: British Broadcasting Corporation.
Riehl J. P., Roy C. (1980). *Conceptual Models for Nursing Practice*. Englewood Cliffs NJ: Prentice-Hall.

Report of a Research Group, Inequalities in Health. (1980) (The Black Report). London: DHSS.
Report of the Committee on Child Health Services (1976). *Court Report: Fit for the Future*. London: HMSO.
Robinson D. (1971). *The Process of Becoming Ill*. London: Routledge and Kegan Paul.
Robinson D. (1977). *Self Help and Health: Mutual Aid for Modern Problems*. London: Martin Robertson.
Robinson D. (1980). 'Self Help in Health Care'; *Journal of Medical Ethics*; **6**:4–6.
Rogers C. R. (1969). *Freedom to Learn*. Ohio: Charles E. Merrill.
Russell P. (1984). *The Wheel-chair Child*. London: Souvenir Press.
Schurr M. C., Turner J. (1982). *Nursing—Image or Reality?* London: Hodder and Stoughton.
Shakespeare R. (1975). *The Psychology of Handicap*. London: Methuen.
Shearer A. (1981). *Disability: Whose Handicap?* Oxford: Basil Blackwell.
Slack A. P. (1978). *School Nursing*. London: Baillière Tindall.
Snowdon Working Party (1976). *Integrating the Disabled (Snowdon Report)*. Horsham: National Fund for Research into Crippling Diseases.
Society of Area Nurses (Child Health). (1981). *Review of the School Nursing Service*. London.
Stark G. D. (1977). *Spina Bifida, Problems and Management*. Oxford: Blackwell Scientific Publications.
Stein L. (1978). 'The Doctor–Nurse Game'; *Readings in the Sociology of Nursing*. (Dingwall R., McIntosh J., eds.) Edinburgh: Churchill Livingstone.
Sutherland I., ed. (1979). *Health Education Perspectives and Choices*. London: George Allen and Unwin.
Taylor D. C. (1982). 'Counselling the Parents of Handicapped Children'; *British Medical Journal*; **284**:1027–8.
Thomas D. (1978). *The Social Psychology of Childhood Disability*. London: Methuen.
Thurmott P. (1981). *Health in the School*. London: Society of Area Nurses (Child Health).
Tillich P. (1961). 'The Meaning of Health'; *Perspectives in Biology and Medicine*; **5**:92.
Townsend P. (1982). 'A Positive Approach to Health'; *Health Visitor*; **55**:97–101.
Tschudin V. (1982). *Counselling Skills for Nurses*. London: Baillière Tindall.
Thruston M. (1980). 'Court, Warnock, Jay—Words or Action for Children with Handicaps?'; *Royal Society of Health Journal*; **100(1)**:26–9.
Thruston M. (1982). 'The Seven Ages of Disability: the School Boy'; *Nursing Times*; Special Supplement. Aug. 4.
Tuckett D. (1976). 'Becoming a Patient'; *Introduction to Medical Sociology* (Tuckett D., ed.). London: Tavistock Publications.
Twaddle A. (1974). 'The Concept of Health Status'; *Social Science and Medicine*; **8**:29–38.
Twaddle A. (1979). *Sickness Behaviour and the Sickness Role*. Boston: Schenkman-Hall.

Varma V. P., ed. (1976). *Stresses in Children*. London: Hodder and Stoughton.

Vickery D. M., *et al.* (1979). *Take Care of Yourself*. London: George Allen and Unwin.

Walker K. (1954). *The Story of Medicine*. London: Hutchinson.

Warnock Report. Special Educational Needs. (1978). London: HMSO.

Whelan E., Speake B. (1979). *Learning to Cope*. London: Souvenir Press.

White J. (1979). *Parents in Pain*. Leicester: Inter-Varsity Press.

Whitehead T. (1979). *Fears and Phobias: what they are and how to overcome them*. London: Sheldon Press.

Whitmore K. (1982). 'Health Services in Primary Schools: the Nurse's Role'; *Nursing Times Occasional Papers*; 78(25):97–100 and 103–4.

Willis M., McLachlan M. E. (1977). *Medical Care in Schools*. London: Edward Arnold.

Wilson M. (1975). *Health is for People*. London: Darton, Longman and Todd.

Wold S. J. (1981). *School Nursing*. St Louis: C. V. Mosby.

Wolff S. (1981). *Children under Stress*, 2nd edn. Harmondsworth: Penguin Books.

Wood M. (1984). *Living with a Hyperactive Child*. London: Souvenir Press.

Wright B. (1959). 'A New Look at Over-protection and Dependency'; *Exceptional Children*; November: 115–22.

Index